THE HUMAN BRAIN CIRCULATION

Vascular Biomedicine

THE HUMAN BRAIN CIRCULATION

Functional Changes in Disease

A publication of the
University of Vermont
Center for Vascular Research

Edited by

Rosemary D. Bevan and John A. Bevan

Totman Laboratory for Human Cerebrovascular Research,
Department of Pharmacology, University of Vermont,
Burlington, Vermont

HUMANA PRESS • TOTOWA, NEW JERSEY

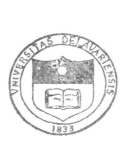

© 1994 Humana Press Inc.
999 Riverview Drive, Suite 208
Totowa, New Jersey 07512

Library of Congress Cataloging-in-Publication Data

The human brain circulation: functional changes in disease/edited by Rosemary D. Bevan and John A. Bevan
    p. cm.—(Vascular biomedicine)
    "A publication of the University of Vermont Center for Vascular Research."
    Includes index
    ISBN 0-89603-271-X
    1. Cerebral circulation.   2. Brain—Blood-vessels   3. Cerebrovascular disease.   I. Bevan, Rosemary D.   II. Bevan, John D., 1930– .
III. University of Vermont. Center for Vascular Research.   IV. Series.
    [DNLM: 1. Brain—blood supply.   2. Cerebrovascular Circulation—physiology.
3. Blood Vessels—physiopathology. WL 302 H918 1994]
QP108.5.C4H86   1994
612.8'24—dc20
DNLM/DLC   94-15788
for Library of Congress   CIP

Contents

Preface

Much of our knowledge of the cerebral circulation has been derived from studies of species other than human. There is increasing recognition of species differences and concern that studies in animals may be misleading if unquestioningly applied to the human. A dramatic example of this occurred in the early history of the study of the circulation of the brain.

Galen of Pergamo (131–201 AD) described a *rete mirabile* or "marvelous network" of blood vessels at the base of the human skull that he must have derived from observations of certain animals. This vascular structure was supplied by the carotid arteries which, after penetrating the cranium,"are divided into a large number of very small and thin branches in the region between the cranium and the dura matter. Then...intersecting one another they give the impression of having forgotten their way in the brain. But this is not the case. In fact, these numerous arteries rejoin and unite like the roots of a tree trunk...."

The authority of Galen's writings dominated scientific thought for about 1500 years. His description of a rete was unquestioned by Leonardo de Vinci, who included it in his anatomical sketches. William Harvey's remarkable observations led to his definitive account of the circulation of blood. Only a short time later, Thomas Willis, a medical practitioner as well as Professor of Natural Philosophy at Oxford and a founding fellow of the Royal Society, published an account of a vascular structure at the base of the brain very different from Galen's description and a hypothesis of its functional role. This arterial circle, later named after him, was illustrated by Sir Christopher Wren from direct observation of the human brain.

Such a dramatic instance is unlikely to occur today. However, there are many examples of functional differences of comparable cerebral arteries of different species and in many instances we do not know about the human. In *The Human Brain Circulation*, for this reason, we have complemented studies of the human with those of animals in order to emphasize where our knowledge of the former is deficient. It scarcely needs to be said that there is still much to discover concerning the processes involved in the dynamics of brain circulation.

The chapters in this book were contributed by the participants of a conference entitled "The Human Brain Circulation: Functional Changes in Disease" held at Basin Harbor, Vermont, October 4–7, 1992. Its purpose was to assemble current information on the brain circulation obtained by direct study and to define future directions for research into the nature of human cerebrovascular disease. Included also is a synopsis of the potentialities of the newer imaging techniques. When information on the human circulation was not available, the results of studies of other mammalian species were included. The meeting was convened under the auspices of the Totman Laboratory for Human Cerebrovascular Research in the Department of Pharmacology at the University of Vermont. Mr. Totman, who died April 2, 1988, was a resident of Malone, in upstate New York. He requested that a Trust be set up to support medical research in his name and that of his wife.

We gratefully acknowledge the support of the Trustees of the Ray and Ildah Totman Medical Research Fund in this International Conference.

Our thanks go to Roberta Anderson for the excellent general arrangements and organization of the Conference. In this she was ably assisted by Tammy Provencher, who handled the clerical responsibilities of the meeting and the preparation of this publication. Her perseverance and patience are truly appreciated.

Rosemary D. Bevan
John A. Bevan

Contributors

Gunvor Ahlborg · *Department of Clinical Physiology, Huddinge Hospital, Stockholm, Sweden*

Pierre Aubineau · *Laboratoire de Physiologie Cellulaire et Pharmacologie Moleculaire, Université de Bordeaux II, Bordeaux Cédex, France*

Gary L. Baumbach · *Department of Pathology, University of Iowa College of Medicine, Iowa City, IA*

Rosemary D. Bevan · *Department of Pharmacology, University of Vermont College of Medicine, Burlington, VT*

John A. Bevan · *Department of Pharmacology, University of Vermont College of Medicine, Burlington, VT*

Joseph E. Brayden · *Department of Pharmacology, Medical Research Facility, University of Vermont, Colchester, VT*

David W. Busija · *Department of Physiology and Pharmacology, Cardiovascular Program, Bowman Gray School of Medicine, Wake Forest University, Winston-Salem, NC*

Peter Coyle · *Department of Anatomy and Cellular Biology, University of Michigan, Ann Arbor, MI*

François Dauphin · *Laboratory of Cerebrovascular Research, Montreal Neurological Institute, Montreal, Quebec, Canada*

James R. Docherty · *Department of Physiology, Royal College of Surgeons in Ireland, Dublin, Ireland*

John T. Dodge · *Department of Pharmacology, University of Vermont College of Medicine, Burlington, VT*

Lars Edvinsson · *Department of Internal Medicine, University Hospital of Lund, Lund, Sweden*

Robert F. Furchgott · *Department of Pharmacology, State University of New York Health Science Center, Brooklyn, NY*

Sergio Gulbenkian · *Department of Internal Medicine, University Hospital of Lund, Lund, Sweden*

Edith Hamel · *Montreal Neurological Institute, Laboratory of Cerebrovascular Research, Montreal, Quebec, Canada*

xi

Daniel F. Hanley · *Departments of Anesthesiology and Critical Care Medicine, The Johns Hopkins University, Baltimore, MD*

Jan Erik Hardebo · *Department of Histology, University of Lund, Lund, Sweden*

Mark A. Helfaer · Departments of *Anesthesiology and Critical Care Medicine, The Johns Hopkins Medical Institutions, Baltimore, MD*

Annette Hémsen · *Department of Pharmacology, Karolinska Institute, Stockholm, Sweden*

Zhihong Huang · *Stroke Research Laboratory, Neurosurgery and Neurology Service, Massachusetts General Hospital, Harvard Medical School, Boston, MA*

Inger Jansen · *Department of Internal Medicine, University Hospital of Lund, Lund, Sweden*

Hiroshi Jino · *Pharmacology Division, Radioisotope Research Center, Kyoto University, Kyoto, Japan*

Jeffrey R. Kirsch · *Departments of Anesthesiology and Critical Care Medicine, The Johns Hopkins Medical Institutions, Baltimore, MD*

Alynn Klaasen · *Department of Pharmacology, University of Vermont College of Medicine, Burlington, VT*

Kazuyoshi Kurahashi · *Pharmacology Division, Radioisotope Research Center, Kyoto University, Kyoto, Japan*

Wolfgang Kuschinsky · *Physiologisches Institut der Universität, Heidelberg, Germany*

Ismail Laher · *Department of Pharmacology, University of Vermont College of Medicine, Burlington VT*

Tony J.-F. Lee · *Department of Pharmacology, Southern Illinois University School of Medicine, Springfield, IL*

Donald Linville · *Laboratory of Cerebrovascular Research, Montreal Neurological Institute, Montreal, Quebec, Canada*

Jan M. Lundberg · *Department of Pharmacology, Karolinska Institute, Stockholm, Sweden*

Pierrette Mathiau · *Laboratoire de Physiopathologie et Pharmacologie Vasculaire, Université Bordeaux II, Bordeaux, France*

Eiharu Morikawa · *Department of Neurology and Neurosurgery, Massachusetts General Hospital, Harvard Medical School, Boston, MA*

Michael A. Moskowitz · *Stroke Research Laboratory, Neurosurgery and Neurology Service, Massachusetts General Hospital, Harvard Medical School, Boston, MA*

Else Müller-Schweinitzer · *Pharmaceutical Division, Biological and Medical Research, SANDOZ Ltd., Basel, Switzerland*

Mark T. Nelson · *Department of Pharmacology, Medical Research Facility, University of Vermont, Colchester, VT*

Christer Nilsson · *Wallenberg Laboratory, Division of Molecular Neurobiology, University of Lund, Lund, Sweden*

Christopher S. Ogilvy · *Neurosurgical Service, Massachusetts General Hospital, Boston, MA*

George Osol · *Department of Obstetrics and Gynecology, University of Vermont College of Medicine, Burlington, VT*

Christer Owman · *Wallenberg Laboratory, Division of Molecular Neurobiology, University of Lund, Lund, Sweden*

William J. Pearce · *Department of Physiology, Loma Linda University School of Medicine, Loma Linda, CA*

Paul Penar · *Department of Surgery, University of Vermont, Burlington, VT*

Tina Poseno · *Department of Pharmacology, University of Vermont College of Medicine, Burlington, VT*

William J. Powers · *Department of Neurology, Jewish Hospital of St. Louis, St. Louis, MO*

John M. Quayle · *Department of Pharmacology, Medical Research Facility, University of Vermont, Colchester, VT*

Sami Rosenblatt · *Stroke Research Laboratory, Neurosurgery and Neurology Service, Massachusetts General Hospital, Harvard Medical School, Boston, MA*

William I. Rosenblum · *Department of Neuropathology, Medical College of Virginia, Richmond, VA*

Anders Rudehill · *Department of Anesthesiology, Karolinska Hospital, Stockholm, Sweden*

Hiroaki Shirahase · *Pharmacology Division, Radioisotope Research Center, Kyoto University, Kyoto, Japan*

Norihiro Suzuki · *Departments of Medical Cell Research and Neurology, University of Lund, Lund, Sweden*

Vincent Ting · *Laboratory of Cerebrovascular Research, Montreal Neurological Institute, Montreal, Quebec, Canada*

Noboru Toda · *Department of Pharmacology, Shiga University of Medical Science, Seta, Ohtsu, Japan*

Richard J. Traystman · *Department of Anesthesiology and Critical Care Medicine, The Johns Hopkins Medical Institutions, Baltimore, MD*

Rolf Uddman · *Department of Internal Medicine, University Hospital of Lund, Lund, Sweden*

Mauro Ursino · *Dipartimento di Elettronica ed Automatica via Brecce Bianche, Ancona, Italy*

Hachiro Usui · *Pharmacology Division, Radioisotope Research Center, Kyoto University, Kyoto, Japan*

Dee A. Van Riper · *Department of Internal Medicine, University of Virginia Health Sciences Center, Division of Cardiology, Charlottesville, VA*

Peter Vorkapic · *Nordstadt Hospital, Hannover, Germany*

Carrie L. Walters · *Neurological Surgeons P. C., Phoenix, AZ*

Eddie Weitzberg · *Department of Pharmacology, Karolinska Institute; and Department of Anesthesiology, Karolinska Hospital, Stockholm, Sweden*

Theresa Wellman · *Department of Pharmacology, University of Vermont College of Medicine, Burlington, VT*

David A. Wilson · *Departments of Neurology and Anesthesia and Critical Care Medicine, The Johns Hopkins Medical Institutions, Baltimore, MD*

Kenneth K. Wu · *University of Texas Medical School, Division of Hematology, Houston, TX*

Tazuka Yoshida · *Stroke Research Laboratory, Neurosurgery and Neurology Service, Massachusetts General Hospital, Harvard Medical School, Boston, MA*

Nadim Zamar · *Laboratory of Cerebrovascular Research, Montreal Neurological Institute, Montreal, Quebec, Canada*

Chapter 1

Positron Emission Tomography of the Brain

In Vivo Techniques
for Studying Cerebrovascular Pathophysiology

William J. Powers

Positron Emission Tomography

Radiotracers have been utilized extensively for many years to investigate physiology and pathology in vivo. These radioactive molecules or particles are administered to the organism in such small quantities that they do not affect the physiologic process under study, and yet the radioactivity is sufficient that it can be measured by an appropriate detection system. Utilization of radiotracer technology for physiologic investigation requires three components—a radiotracer, a radiation detection system, and a mathematical model that relates the physiologic process under study to the radiation detected. Of the three, it has been the radiation detection system that historically has been the major barrier to the application of radiotracer methods to quantitative in vivo investigation of human cerebrovascular pathophysiology. For experimental animal studies, radiotracers in the brain are most often measured *ex vivo* after sacrificing the animal. This is done either by counting the radioactivity in individual samples or by autoradiography of tissue slices. Autoradiography requires exposure of the slice to special film, which produces a photographic image with

From *The Human Brain Circulation*, R. D. Bevan and J. A. Bevan, eds.
©1994 Humana Press

intensity proportional to the radioactivity in each region. Both of these *ex vivo* methods provide accurate quantitative regional measurements of brain radioactivity. However, they only provide one measurement per animal and require sacrifice of the animal. Obviously, some method to measure accurately regional brain radioactivity in vivo, preferably at multiple different time-points in the same subject, is necessary for application to human studies. This is not easy. Radionuclides that decay by electron emission, such as ^{3}H and ^{14}C, cannot be detected externally because the electrons are all absorbed by a few millimeters of surrounding tissue. Radionuclides that decay by photon (γ) emission can be detected externally, but present several problems. A variable fraction of the photons is absorbed by the surrounding tissue depending on the photon energy, tissue composition, and path length. Furthermore, with conventional planar detection systems, the radioactivity from overlapping superficial and deep structures is superimposed and cannot be distinguished. Nevertheless, such detection systems have been used extensively for radiotracer investigation of cerebral blood flow (CBF) and other physiologic variables.[1–5]

In the early 1970s, X-ray computed tomography (CT) was developed by Godfrey Hounsfield.[6] The ability of X-ray CT to provide accurate, three-dimensional images led to a great deal of interest in developing similar techniques for application to the external detection of internally administered radiotracers. Application of CT technology to this end is not straightforward. Computed tomography is based on the reconstruction of a sectional image from a series of two-dimensional projections taken at different angles around an object.[7] In X-ray CT, the profiles used in the image reconstruction represent the attenuation of X-rays by the object being studied. For external detection of the radiation emitted by internal radiotracers (or emission CT), the desired information in the reconstructed image is the quantitative spatial distribution of the radioactivity. Unfortunately, the profiles externally recorded will represent the desired information on spatial distribution of radioactivity altered by the variable absorption (attenuation) of this radiation by the surrounding tissue. Furthermore, the reconstruction process in CT assumes that the spatial resolution of the radiation detectors does not vary with the distance from the detector.

Although this is very close to true for X-ray CT, it is simply not the case for conventional single-photon (γ) detectors. The resolution of these detectors decreases as the distance from the detector increases.[7,8] Nevertheless, a variety of single-photon emission computed tomography (SPECT) systems have been built incorporating empiric or other corrections for attenuation and mathematical adjustments for distance-dependent resolution.

A major advance in the quantitative accuracy of emission CT came with the development of positron emission tomography (PET). Certain radionuclides decay by emission of a positron, a small particle with the same mass as an electron, but the opposite charge. After traveling a few millimeters through tissue, the positron interacts with an electron, resulting in the destruction of both. This annihilation creates two photons that travel away from the annihilation site in opposite directions. A pair of external radiation detectors positioned on either side of a positron emitting source will register these photons at almost the same time. (The difference in time is equivalent to the difference in the distance the two photons travel divided by the speed of light.) If this detector pair is connected by an electronic circuit that records a signal only when two photons arrive within this short time interval, then only photons arising from positron annihilations occurring between the detector pair will be recorded. Annihilation coincidence detection presents the solution to the problems encountered with single-photon emission computed tomography. The spatial resolution of a pair of annihilation coincidence detectors is nearly uniform for most of the region located between the two detectors.[7,9,10] The fraction of radioactivity lost because of absorption by surrounding tissue can be measured accurately and then corrected for. For an individual photon, this attention fraction depends on the tissue composition and the distance the photon travels through the tissue. For a pair of annihilation photons, the tissue composition and total distance traveled by both γ photons will be the same regardless of where between the detector pair the annihilation occurs. The attenuation fraction for a given path through an object will, therefore, be the same whether the annihilation occurs internally or externally to the object. The attenuation fraction for any pair of coincidence detectors relative to a specific object can be measured accurately prior to the internal administration of any radiotracers. First, a positron emitting source is placed between the detector pair, and the total number of coincidences per unit time is recorded. The head (or other part of the body to be studied) is then also placed between the detector pair, and the number of coincidences per unit time is again measured. The fractional reduction in the initial radioactivity represents the annihilation photons absorbed by the head for the tissue path between the detector pair. When a radiotracer is administered, this individually measured attenuation fraction is used to correct the number of coincidence events recorded by the detector pair to yield the actual number of positron annihilations that took place with its field of view.

A positron emission tomograph consists of a large number of detector pairs connected by coincidence circuits. After corrections for attenuation, the information obtained from each of these detector pairs is used to construct a series of projections, each representing the distribution of regional radioactivity as viewed from a different angle. These projections are then combined to produce a two-dimensional reconstruction of the regional radioactivity within the combined field of view of all the detectors. Tomographs with multiple rings of detectors can generate multiple reconstructed slices simultaneously, each depicting a different level of the brain and together providing a true three-dimensional image.

The accuracy of the reconstructed PET image as a quantitative measure of regional radioactivity depends on a variety of technical factors beyond the scope of this chapter.[10,11] There is one technical concept, however, that is crucial for the proper interpretation of any PET measurement. This is the effect of image resolution on the accuracy of the measurement of regional radioactivity. In the PET image, radioactivity from a given region in the object is redistributed or smeared over a larger area. For a point source of radioactivity, this redistribution approximates the form of a Gaussian (bell-shaped) curve with the maximum value occurring at the original point. The resolution of the reconstructed image is described in terms of this point-spread function. It is usually given as the width of the point-spread function at one-half its maximum amplitude (full width, half maximum, abbreviated FWHM). The FWHM is a description of the degree of smearing or redistribution of radioactivity in the reconstructed image, not a description of the smallest size structure that can be delineated or measured accurately. The latter will depend not only on the image resolution, but also on the amount and distribution of radioactivity in the region of interest and surrounding areas. As a consequence of this redistribution of radioactivity, a given region in the reconstructed image, regardless of its size, contains only a portion of the radioactivity actually within that region in the original structure. The remainder has been redistributed into surrounding regions of the image. Similarly, some radioactivity originally in these surrounding regions has been redistributed into the region of interest. Thus, the regional radioactivity measurement made with PET represents some portion of the radioactivity actually within that region plus a contribution from radioactivity in surrounding regions.[8,12,13] This is known as the partial volume effect. Thus, PET will always demonstrate a gradual transition of values between two structures even when there is an abrupt change, such as at the edge of a cerebral infarct or hemorrhage.

As a result of the partial volume effect, it is therefore difficult to obtain values that truly represent either pure gray matter or pure white matter. This is especially true for cortical regions, which will always contain a heterogeneous mixture of cortical gray matter and contiguous subcortical white matter. Furthermore, in areas of brain adjacent to cerebrospinal fluid (CSF), there will be a reduction in the radioactivity measured in the brain owing to the usually low or absent radiotracer accumulation in CSF. This is particularly a problem in patients with cerebral atrophy or hydrocephalus.[14,15] The influence of the partial volume effect on regional quantitation depends on both the pattern of distribution of radioactivity and the image resolution. Truly accurate PET measurements of regional radioactivity can be made only when the contribution from surrounding areas is absent. This will occur in the center of a homogeneous region with a diameter of twice the FWHM, providing that the surrounding radioactivity is zero.[12] If the surrounding radioactivity is greater than zero, a homogeneous region of interest must be even larger to achieve accurate quantitation at its center. Because of this contribution from surrounding regions, areas of low activity surrounded by areas of high activity are particularly difficult to measure accurately and, if small enough, may not be detected at all.

The second requirement for PET measurements of physiology is a radiotracer containing a positron emitting radionuclide. For biologic radiotracer applications, positron emitting radionuclides can be divided into two groups—radioisotopes of elements that are normal constituents of biological molecules (^{11}C, ^{13}N, ^{15}O) or radioisotopes of nonbiologic elements that can be attached to biologic molecules as radiolabels (^{18}F, ^{68}Ga, ^{75}Br). Most positron emitting radionuclides have half-lives of minutes to a few hours. This allows relatively large amounts of radioactivity to be administered while keeping the radiation dose to the subject at a safe level. Since the radioactivity often decays rapidly, sequential studies may be easily performed. The disadvantage to these short-lived radionuclides is obvious. In most cases, they must be prepared on site or shipped only short distances. Since production of the more commonly used positron emitters (^{11}C, ^{15}O, and ^{18}F) requires a cyclotron or linear accelerator, their availability depends on proximity to one of these facilities. Synthesis of molecules incorporating short-lived radionuclides is a specialized field requiring great expertise. The synthesis must be performed rapidly and, at the same time, yield substances that are of sufficient purity to be safe for administration to human subjects.

The third requirement for PET measurements of physiology is a mathematical model that quantitatively relates tissue concentration of the positron emitting radiotracer (as measured by PET) to the physiologic variable under study. This model must take into account a variety of factors, including delivery of the tracer to the tissue, distribution and metabolism of the tracer within the tissue, egress of tracer and metabolites from the tissue, recirculation of metabolized and unmetabolized tracer, and the amount of tracer and metabolites remaining in the blood. Furthermore, the model must be practically applicable given the constraints imposed by PET designs and the amount of radioactivity that can be safely administered to human subjects. Finally, the validity of the underlying assumptions and possible sources of error for each model when applied to the study of both normal physiology and disease states must be clearly understood. Ideally, each PET technique should be validated by pair-wise comparison to a "gold standard" under the conditions for which it will be used.

The following sections will deal with some of the more common PET methods used to study cerebrovascular physiology and pathophysiology directly by measuring cerebral blood flow (CBF) and cerebral blood volume (CBV), to investigate the metabolic regulation of cerebral blood vessels by measuring the cerebral metabolic rate of oxygen ($CMRO_2$) and glucose (CMRGlu), and to investigate the blood–brain barrier by measuring the flux of different radiotracers from the blood into the brain.

PET Measurements of CBF and CBV

Cerebral Blood Flow

The most widely used method for measuring regional cerebral blood flow (rCBF) with PET involves the continuous inhalation of ^{15}O-labeled carbon dioxide.[16-18] In the pulmonary vessels, ^{15}O-CO_2 is rapidly converted to water by carbonic anhydrase in red blood cells. The resultant ^{15}O-H_2O circulates throughout the body. After 5–10 min, a steady state is reached in the brain such that the amount of radioactivity entering as ^{15}O-H_2O is equal to the amount lost via radioactive decay and venous outflow.

During this equilibrium, the relationship between rCBF and regional radioactivity can be expressed by a simple, nonlinear equation. Calculation of quantitative values for rCBF requires, in addition to the regional radioactivity data obtained by PET, measurement of the arterial concentration of ^{15}O-H_2O and knowledge of the specific volume of distribution of water (often called the partition coefficient and symbolized as λ). The latter is derived from previous experimental data. This method has many practical advantages. First, its use is not limited by machine design. Scanning can be performed with radioactivity levels low enough to be within the range of any tomograph and at the same time can be carried out long enough (typically 5 min) to provide enough counts for statistical accuracy. Second, only a single arterial blood sample needs to be collected during steady-state conditions, although in practice, several are usually obtained and averaged since the method is sensitive to errors in measurement of the arterial concentration of $^{15}O\text{-}H_2O$. The major disadvantages of the steady-state $^{15}O\text{-}CO_2$ method stem from the nonlinear relationship between regional radioactivity and rCBF. This has two consequences. First, inaccuracies in measurement of regional brain radioactivity and blood radioactivity cause errors in rCBF that become progressively larger as the blood flow increases. Use of an inaccurate value for λ (which may change in pathologic conditions) causes similar errors.[19–22] Second, in any region containing a mixture of cerebral tissues with different blood flows, the measured rCBF will deviate by up to 30% from the true mean value for rCBF in that region. This deviation will also increase at higher rates of rCBF.[23] As noted previously, the resolution of PET tomographs is such that virtually any region will contain a heterogeneous mixture of gray and white matter. A further problem with this technique, unrelated to nonlinearity, arises because the blood–brain barrier is incompletely permeable to water.[23] As a result, $^{15}O\text{-}H_2O$ is incompletely extracted at high rates of flow causing underestimation of rCBF.[19]

An alternative method for measuring rCBF with $^{15}O\text{-}H_2O$ that we have extensively employed at Washington University is based on the classic tissue autoradiographic technique of Kety and coworkers.[24,25] This method utilizes a bolus iv injection of $^{15}O\text{-}H_2O$ followed by a 40-s PET scan.[26,27] During this period, sequential samples of arterial blood are collected to determine the time–activity curve for $^{15}O\text{-}H_2O$. In order to achieve adequate statistical counting accuracy with such a short scan time, a large amount of $^{15}O\text{-}H_2O$ (typically 50–75 mCi) must be injected. Implementation of this technique is therefore restricted to tomographs that remain accurate when counting such high levels of radioactivity. Because of the almost linear relationship between regional radioactivity and rCBF with this model, there is little error resulting from tissue heterogeneity; the measured regional rCBF closely approximates the weighted mean for tissues within the region. Errors in the estimation of λ also have very little effect. As with the steady-state technique, this method is limited by the incomplete extraction of water at high CBF. When blood flow is in excess of 65 mL 100 g^{-1} min,$^{-1}$ rCBF is progressively underestimated. This problem can be obviated by the use of ^{15}O-butanol, a completely extracted inert radiotracer.[28] The major disadvantage of the modified, autoradiographic technique is its dependence on the arterial time–activity curve. This curve, obtained by sampling from a peripheral artery, is assumed to be the same as that for the cerebral circulation. Any difference between the peripheral curve and the cerebral curve will lead to errors in calculated rCBF, the worst errors occurring when the radiotracer bolus arrives in the brain at a different time than it arrives in the peripheral artery. This problem can largely be overcome by timing the arrival of the radiotracer bolus in the brain by the sudden increase in PET counts and shifting the peripheral curve to match. Several other PET methods for measuring rCBF involving multiple scans obtained in sequence and more complex mathematical formulations have also been described.[29]

Cerebral Blood Volume

Measurement of rCBV is performed following inhalation of air containing trace amounts of carbon monoxide labeled with either ^{11}C or [15]O. The labeled carbon monoxide binds to hemoglobin in red blood cells and circulates throughout the body. When equilibrium between arterial and venous circulations is reached, the regional radioactivity in the brain will be equal to the amount of labeled carboxyhemoglobin and therefore proportional to the regional red cell mass. By measuring the amount of radioactivity in a peripheral blood sample and correcting for the difference between the peripheral vessel hematocrit and the mean hematocrit of cerebral vessels, the blood volume of intraparenchymal cerebral vessels can be determined.[30–32] The principal source of error in this measurement stems from the use of a single standard value as the correction factor for the difference between peripheral (or large vessel) and the tissue (or small vessel) hematocrit. Recent evidence indicates that there are not only regional differences in cerebral hematocrit, but that the regional cerebral hematocrit may change from one physiologic state to another.[33,34]

Regional CBV measurements provide an index of local vasodilation. When intraparenchymal blood vessels dilate, CBV increases. When intraparenchymal vessels constrict, CBV decreases. The relative distribution of intraparenchymal CBV has been estimated as 16% arterial, 1% capillary, and 83% venous.[35] In addition, rCBV can be incorporated into mathematical models to correct other

PET measurements for the amount of radiotracer remaining within the intravascular space.

CBF and CBV Measurements in Health and Disease

PET measurements of CBF and CBV have been used to investigate basic mechanisms of cerebrovascular control in both human subjects and animals. These studies have confirmed known mechanisms, and also provided some new insights into both normal physiology and pathophysiologic states.

Standard autoregulatory curves to changes in systemic arterial pressure can be obtained easily by repeat PET measurements of CBF. We have carried these studies out in nonhuman primates, and plan to perform further studies of the regional autoregulatory limits in human subjects with normal aging, Alzheimer's disease, Binswanger's disease, and following treatment with various antihypertensive drugs. Rhodes et al. have produced the expected relationship between $PACO_2$ and CBF in six anesthetized dogs.[36] At Washington University, similar studies were carried out in baboons in concert with CBV measurements.[35] These data show a decline in CBV as CBF declines, indicating intraparenchymal vasoconstriction. The importance of arterial oxygen content in regulating CBF was demonstrated in a study of six patients with sickle cell anemia. Both CBF and CBV were increased as compared to nonanemic controls indicating intraparenchymal vasodilation. There was no correlation between CBF and blood viscosity.[37] We have recently studied the response of CBF to stepped arterial hypoglycemia in nine normal subjects and have found no change with values as low as 2.3 mM. Because of its accuracy for detecting regional changes, PET has been very useful for detecting the changes in rCBF that accompany normal brain activity. This has led to widespread use in investigating human cortical organization.[38,39] We have recently demonstrated that the increase in rCBF that accompanies somatosensory stimulation is not changed by moderate decreases in arterial glucose concentration.[40]

The effect of different pharmacologic agents on regional cerebrovascular beds can also be studied, as has been done with adenosine.[41] Such pharmacologic studies must be interpreted with some caution, however. The observed CBF effects may be the result of direct pharmacological stimulation of blood vessels, but alternatively, may reflect a local change in metabolism with secondary changes in blood flow. Thus, changes in regional CBF following administration of L-dopa to patients with hemiparkinsonism are likely not the result of direct vascular effects of the drug, but of alterations in metabolism caused by receptor stimulation.[42]

In the investigation of human disease, PET measurements of CBF and CBV have most extensively been used to investigate cerebrovascular disease. Once cerebral infarction has occurred, any conclusions regarding mechanisms of cerebrovascular control become difficult. However, a study of patients with occlusive carotid artery disease without evidence of tissue damage has demonstrated consistent evidence of autoregulatory dilation of intraparenchymal vessels (increased CBV) under conditions of reduced CBF or poor collateral circulation.[43] Investigations of similar patients with following aneurysmal subarachnoid hemorrhage who have angiographic evidence of large vessel vasospasm have demonstrated that CBV declines as CBF decreases.[44] This is a response similar to that seen with hypocapnia and suggests that vasospasm also occurs in small, angiographically invisible, interparenchymal vessels.

PET Measurements of Cerebral Metabolism

Cerebral Oxygen Metabolism

Regional cerebral oxygen consumption ($rCMRO_2$) is most commonly measured by an extension of the steady-state ^{15}O-CO_2 inhalation CBF method.[16] Following the ^{15}O-CO_2 scan, a second continuous inhalation of ^{15}O-O_2 is performed. ^{15}O-O_2 binds to hemoglobin and circulates throughout the body. A fraction of the ^{15}O-O_2 in the blood is extracted by the brain and locally metabolized to water. This ^{15}O-H_2O exits the brain, and a portion then recirculates back to the brain where it is distributed in proportion to rCBF. By using rCBF data from the ^{15}O-CO_2 image to correct for recirculating ^{15}O-H_2O, the fraction of ^{15}O-O_2 extracted from the blood (rOEF) can be calculated and is, in fact, proportional to the ratio of the regional radioactivities measured by the two scans, $(^{15}O$-$O_2)/(^{15}O$-$CO_2)$. Regional $CMRO_2$ can then be calculated by multiplying rOEF × rCBF × the arterial oxygen content measured from a peripheral arterial sample. This method of measuring cerebral oxygen metabolism has the same technical advantages as the steady-state ^{15}O-CO_2 method. It is suitable for most PET instruments and requires only a single arterial blood sample during each scan. As originally described and implemented, this method failed to correct for radioactivity from intravascular ^{15}O-O_2 still bound to hemoglobin. As a result, rOEF and rCMRO$_2$ were overestimated. This overestimation of rOEF depends on the local intravascular volume, and is greatest at low values of rOEF and rCBF. The error varies from 5 to 20% in normal subjects, but may be as high as 50% in patients with acute cerebral infarction.[19,45–47] Correction for the effect of intravascular ^{15}O-O_2 hemoglobin using data from a separately performed rCBV measurement has been described.[45–47] This correction is being used increasingly with concomitant increase in the accuracy of reported measurements.

At Washington University, we have used a different method for measuring rOEF and rCMRO$_2$ employing a brief inhalation of air containing ^{15}O-O_2.[35] Following inhalation, a 40-s PET scan is performed, and arterial blood samples are collected. As with the modified autoradiographic method for measuring rCBF, this method also requires a tomograph capable of performing accurately at high counting rates. Data from separately performed ^{15}O-H_2O CBF and ^{15}O-CO CBV studies are also required. A two-compartment model describing the production and egress of water of metabolism in cerebral tissue, recirculating water of metabolism in the brain, and the arterial, venous, and capillary contents of ^{15}O-hemoglobin is used to calculate rOEF. Other methods for measuring CMRO$_2$ using dynamic multiple-scan sequences and more complex mathematical models have also been described.[29,48]

Cerebral Glucose Metabolism

Methods for measuring regional cerebral glucose metabolism (rCMRGlu) with PET have relied heavily on modifications of the ^{14}C-deoxyglucose (^{14}C-DG) autoradiographic method as originally described by Sokoloff and colleagues.[49] This method is based on the fact that deoxyglucose is transported into the brain and phosphorylated in a manner similar to glucose, but is then not further metabolized and remains trapped in the tissue. The metabolic rate for glucose was calculated by Sokoloff et al. from three rate constants (RCs) describing the influx, efflux, and phosphorylation of deoxyglucose plus a lumped constant (LC) that corrected for the difference between the kinetics of glucose and deoxyglucose.

The ^{14}C-DG method has been adapted to PET using ^{18}F-fluoro-deoxyglucose (^{18}F-DG) as the radiotracer.[50-52] RCs for ^{18}F-DG (including a fourth rate constant describing the dephosphorylation of ^{18}F-DG-6-phosphate) for normal human subjects have been determined by sequential scanning. By using the average value for each RC determined from these experiments, the value of LC necessary to make the calculated global CMRGlu equal to a mean literature value of 5.38 mg 100^{-1} min^{-1} was determined.[51,52] Subsequent direct measurement of LC in humans has given a slightly different value.[53] These previously determined normal values for RC and LC, together with a single PET scan performed 45 min after injection of ^{18}F-DG and a blood time–activity curve, have been used with the operational equation of Sokoloff et al. (or minor modifications thereof) to determine rCMRGlu in humans under a variety of conditions. Huang et al. have shown that the accuracy of this method depends on how close the average values for RC and LC used in the operational equation are to the true values in the brain region under study. Small deviations in RC produce little change in rCMRGlu.[52] However, measurements of the regional RC by sequential scanning in patients with cerebral infarction have produced values that differ markedly from normal values and that also vary from patient to patient. Substantial differences in the estimation of rCMRGlu occur when normal RC or averaged "ischemia" RC are used in place of the individually measured regional RC for each patient.[54] Therefore, in order to ensure maximum accuracy in the measurement of rCMRGlu with ^{18}F-DG in patients with disease, RC must be measured individually by sequential scanning.

Since CMRGlu is inversely proportional to the LC, accurate measurement of the LC is also essential for accurate measurement of CMRGlu. Under normal conditions, the LC at rest differs little among species.[55] However, in pathophysiological conditions, the LC has been shown to vary significantly. Theoretically, the LC can be expected to increase when glucose supply approaches glucose demand. Thus, in experimental conditions of ischemia and hypoglycemia, the LC increases by 50% or more.[56–58] Application of the [18]FDG method to measure CMRGlu in these situations using the resting (and thus incorrect) LC value will produce proportionate overestimation of CMRGlu. Thus, the PET-FDG method is not suitable to measure CMRGlu in ischemia and hypoglycemia.

These problems can, of course, be avoided by the use of glucose itself as the radiotracer. ^{11}C-glucose has been produced in sufficient quantities by the photosynthetic method[59,60] for PET studies in adult human subjects. This synthetic method results in the ^{11}C label being distributed among all six carbons. Attempts to use this photosynthetically labeled glucose to measure CMRGlu have been unsuccessful because of the early efflux of labeled metabolites from the brain.[61–64]

The use of ^{11}C-glucose labeled specifically at the 1-carbon position (1-^{11}C-glucose) obviates this problem. The loss of radioactive label is <2% in the first 10 min, since the 1 and 6 carbons are the last to be metabolized to CO_2.[65] This offers a distinct advantage over the use of photosynthetically labeled glucose. Blomqvist et al. have recently published results of PET studies of seven normal volunteers employing 1-^{11}C-glucose and a three-rate-constant model in which correction for the loss of labeled metabolites is carried out by subtracting the quantity measured in blood samples simultaneously obtained from the jugular bulb.[66] The requirement for jugular venous sampling and the inability to deal with regional differences in loss of labeled metabolites make this approach less than ideal. These authors also demonstrated that the rate of loss of [11]CO_2 is a constant function of the quantity of labeled compound in the metabolic compartment. Thus, a fourth, time-invariant rate constant can be used to describe [11]CO_2 egress from the brain. The rate of loss of ^{11}C acid metabolites (presumably lactate) varied with time, but remained of small magnitude.[66]

We have undertaken a series of experiments in macaques comparing direct measurements of arterio-jugular venous glucose differences to PET measurements using 1-^{11}C-glucose and a modification of the model of Mintun et al. employing a fourth rate constant to describe the egress of all labeled metabolites from the brain.[62] Preliminary data indicate that our method is accurate.

CMRO$_2$ and CMRGlu in Health and Disease

By combining PET measurements of CMRO$_2$ and CMRGlu with CBF, it has been possible to investigate further the "metabolic" control of cerebral blood vessels in both normal and pathophysiologic conditions. In the normal human brain at rest, there is a close regional correlation among CBF, CMRGlu, and CMRO$_2$. Approximately one-third of the oxygen and one-tenth of the glucose delivered to the brain (CBF × arterial content) is utilized.[43] With task-related increased regional brain activity, CBF and CMRGlu increase to approximately the same degree, but CMRO$_2$ increases little if at all. Thus, local tissue hypoxia cannot be the sign for local vasodilation during increased neuronal activity.[67]

Reductions in CBF owing to hypocapnia produced concomitant increases in OEF such that CMRO$_2$ is maintained.[35] Similarly, with reduction in arterial oxygen content because of anemia, CBF increases to maintain rOEF and CMRO$_2$ constant.[37] The measurement of regional metabolic rate in the resting brain permits differentiation between changes in CBF that are the result of primary vascular effects from those that are the result of primary metabolic effects. Thus, in patients with carotid artery disease and no tissue damage, CBF decreases more than CMRO$_2$ and OEF increases.[43] The same is true for similar patients with vasospasm following aneurysmal subarachnoid hemorrhage.[44] On the other hand, in areas of the brain with reduced metabolic activity owing to destruction of afferent or efferent pathways, both CBF and CMRO$_2$ are reduced to the same degree, and OEF is normal.[68]

PET Investigations of the Blood–Brain Barrier

PET studies of radiotracer movement from blood into brain are ideally suited to evaluate the blood–brain barrier (BBB) and its alterations in disease. A variety of specific substances, both passively and actively transported, have been evaluated. Herscovitch et al. have described a method for determining the blood–brain permeability to water (PS$_W$) using the ratio of the cerebral uptakes of ^{15}O-water and ^{11}C-butanol.[69] Using a modification of this technique, Jakobsen et al. demonstrated increased PS$_W$ during visual stimulation of occipital cortex in diabetic as compared to normal subjects.[70]

Lammertsma and colleagues have used the potassium analog [82]Rb to investigate the BBB to small cations. They found an
increase of Rb uptake in brain tumors that showed enhancement
with iodinated contrast by X-ray CT, but not in nonenhancing
tumors or in other conditions.[71,72] Kessler et al. demonstrated
reversible opening of the BBB to the radiolabeled macromolecule
^{68}Ga-EDTA in rhesus monkeys given intracarotid infusions of
hypertonic mannitol.[73]

Lockwood and colleagues have evaluated the BBB to ammo-
nia using ^{13}N-ammonia and found increased permeability in
patients with liver disease.[74,75] Koeppe et al. have described the use
of ^{11}C-aminocyclohexanecarboxylate, a nonmetabolized amino acid
analog, to study the transport of large neutral amino acids across
the BBB. They were able to show competitive inhibition by high
phenylalanine levels in a patient with phenylketonuria.[76] ^{18}F-fluoro-
dopa has similarly been used to investigate BBB amino acid transport in patients with Parkinson's disease.[77]

Several PET investigations of glucose transport across the
BBB in human subjects have been carried out using somewhat
different methodologies. PET methods for measuring CMRGlu
with [18]FDG or ^{11}C-glucose allow calculation of a rate constant
that describes the fractional transport of radiotracer from the
blood to the brain per unit time. For [18]FDG, this rate constant
provides a nonquantitative, relative index of the BBB transport
of glucose. For ^{11}C-glucose, the rate constant can be used to
calculate blood-to-brain-glucose flux directly in mmol 100 g^{-1}
min.$^{-1}$ An alternative approach uses ^{11}C-3-O-methylglucose, a
glucose analog that is transported back and forth across the BBB
by the hexose transporter, but not metabolized at all.[78–81] This
analog, like FDG, provides a relative, nonquantitative measure
of glucose transport.

To date, studies in patients with hypoglycemia or diabetes have
suffered from methodologic inadequacies and have produced data
that are difficult to interpret.[64,82–84] The effect of chronic hyperglycemia or diabetes itself on glucose transport across the BBB in
humans remains to be determined. FDG has been used to study
the effect of insulin on BBB glucose transport in normal subjects[85]

and to demonstrate an increase in transport during visual stimulation of occipital cortex.[86]

In Alzheimer's disease and in myotonic dystrophy, FDG studies have shown reduced transport as well as reduced CMRGlu.[87-89] It is believed that the reduced transport is a consequence (downregulation), not the cause, of reduced CMRGlu.

Conclusions

PET provides an accurate quantitative method for measuring regional brain radioactivity in vivo in human subjects. When combined with an approximate radiotracer and a valid mathematical model, PET provides a means to carry the practice of tissue autoradiography into living human subjects. Although technically complex to implement, PET, with its ability to obtain regional values from both deep and superficial structures for a variety of important physiology variables and to make sequential measurements in the same subject in vivo provides an unparalleled opportunity to further our understanding of cerebrovascular physiology and the pathophysiology of human disease.

Acknowledgments

This research was supported by USPHS grants (NS06833, NS28947, NS28700) and The Jewish Hospital of St. Louis.

References

1 Hoedt-Rasmussen, K., Sveinsdottir, E., and Lassen, N. A. (1966) *Circ. Res.* **18**, 237–247.

2 Obrist, W. D., Thompson, H. K., Wang, H. S., and Wilkinson, W. E. (1975) *Stroke* **6**, 245–256.

3 Eichling, J. O., Raichle, M. E., Grubb, R. L., Jr., and Ter-Pogossian, M. (1974) *Circ. Res.* **35**, 358–364.

4 Eichling, J. O., Raichle, M. E., Grubb, R. L., Jr., Larson, K. B., and Ter-Pogossian, M. M. (1975) *Circ. Res.* **37**, 707–714.

5 Raichle, M. E., Grubb, R. L., Jr., Eichling, J. O., and Ter-Pogossian, M. M. (1976) *J. Appl. Physiol.* **40**, 638–640.

6 Hounsfield, G. N. (1973) *Br. J. Radiol.* **46**, 1016–1022.

7 Ter-Pogossian, M. M. (1977) *Semin. Nucl. Med.* **7**, 109–127.

8 Budinger, T. F., Derenzo, S. E., Gullberg, G. T., Greenberg, W. L., and Huesman, R. H. (1977) *J. Comput. Assist. Tomogr.* **1**, 131–145.

9 Ter-Pogossian, M. M. (1985) *Positron Emission Tomography* (Reivich, M. and Alavi, A., eds.), Liss, New York, pp. 43–61.

10 Hoffman, E. J. and Phelps, M. E. (1986) *Positron Emission Tomography and Autoradiography: Principles and Applications for the Brain and Heart* (Phelps, M., Mazziotta, J., and Schelbert, H., eds.), Raven, New York, pp. 237–286.

11 Lammertsma, A. A. and Frackowiak, R. S. J. (1985) *CRC Crit. Rev. Biomed. Eng.* **13**, 125–169.

12 Hoffman, E. J., Huang, S. C., and Phelps, M. E. (1979) *J. Comput. Assist. Tomogr.* **3**, 299–308.

13 Mazziotta, J. C., Phelps, M. E., Plummer, D., and Kuhl, D. E. (1981) *J. Comput. Assist. Tomogr.* **5**, 734–743.

14 Herscovitch, P., Auchus, A. P., Gado, M., Qin, D., and Raichle, M. E. (1986) *J. Cereb. Blood Flow Metabol.* **6**, 12–124.

15 Brooks, W., Beaney, R. P., Powell, M., Leenders, K. L., Crockard, H. A., Thomas, G. T., Marshall, J., and Jones, T. (1986) *Brain* **109**, 613–628.

16 Frackowiak, R. S. J., Lenzi, G. L., Jones, T., and Heather, J. D. (1980) *J. Comput. Assist. Tomogr.* **4**, 727–736.

17 Jones, T., Chesler, D. A., and Ter-Pogossian, M. M. (1976) *Br. J. Radiol.* **49**, 339–343.

18 Subramanyam, R., Alpert, N. M., Hoop, B., Brownell, G. L., and Taveras, J. M. (1978) *J. Nucl. Med.* **19**, 48–53.

19 Lammertsma, A. A., Jones, T., Frackowiak, R. S. J., and Lenzi, G. L. (1981) *J. Comput. Assist. Tomogr.* **5**, 544–550.

20 Huang, S. C., Phelps, M. E., Hoffman, E. J., and Kuhl, D. E. (1979) *Phys. Med. Biol.* **24**, 1151–1161.

21 Jones, S. C., Greenberg, J. H., and Reivich, M. (1982) *J. Comput. Assist. Tomogr.* **6**, 116–124.

22 Lammertsma, A. A., Heather, J. D., Jones, T., Frackowiak, R. S. J., and Lenzi, G. L. (1982) *J. Comput. Assist. Tomogr.* **6**, 566–573.

23 Herscovitch, P. and Raichle, M. E. (1983) *J. Cereb. Blood Flow Metab.* **3**, 407–415.

24 Landau, W. M., Freygang, W. H., Jr., Rowland, L. P., Sokoloff, L., and Kety, S. S. (1955) *Trans. Am. Neurol. Assoc.* **80**, 125–129.

25 Kety, S. S. (1960) *Methods Med. Res.* **8**, 228–236.

26 Herscovitch, P., Markham, J., and Raichle, M. E. (1983) *J. Nucl. Med.* **24**, 782–789.

27 Raichle, M. E., Martin, W. R. W., Herscovitch, P., Mintun, M. A., and Markham, J. (1983) *J. Nucl. Med.* **24**, 790–798.

[28] Berridge, M. S., Adler, B. L., Nelson, A. D., Cassidy, E. H., Muzic, R. F., Bednarczyk, E. M., and Miraldi, F. (1991) *J. Cereb. Blood Flow Metabol.* **11,** 707–715.

[29] Baron, J., Frackowiak, R. S. J., Herholz, K., Jones, T., Lammertsma, A. A., Mazoyer, B., and Wienhard, K. (1989) *J. Cereb. Blood Flow Metabol.* **9,** 723–742.

[30] Grubb, R. L., Raichle, M. E., Higgins, C. S., and Eichling, J. O. (1978) *Ann. Neurol.* **4,** 322–328.

[31] Phelps, M. E., Huang, S. C., Hoffman, E. J., and Kuhl, D.E. (1979) *J. Nucl. Med.* **20,** 328–334.

[32] Martin, W. R. W., Powers, W. J., and Raichle, M. E. (1987) *J. Cereb. Blood Flow Metabol.* **7,** 421–426.

[33] Sakai, F., Nakazawa, K., Tazaki, Y., Ishii, K., Hino, H., Igarashi, H., and Kanda, T. (1985) *J. Cereb. Blood Flow Metabol.* **5,** 207–213.

[34] Lammertsma, A. A., Brooks, D. J., Beaney, R. P., Turton, D. R., Kensett, M. J., Heather, J. D., Marshall, J., and Jones, T. (1984) *J. Cereb. Blood Flow Metabol.* **4,** 317–322.

[35] Mintun, M. A., Raichle, M. E., Martin, W. R. W., and Herscovitch, P. (1984) *J. Nucl. Med.* **25,** 177–187.

[36] Rhodes, C. G., Lenzi, G. L., Frackowiak, R. S. J., Jones, T., and Pozzilli, C. (1981) *J. Neuro. Sci.* **50,** 381–389.

[37] Herold, S., Brozovic, M., Path, F. R. C., Gibbs, J., Lammertsma, A. A., Leenders, K., Carr, D., Fleming, J. S., and Jones, T. (1986) *Stroke* **17,** 692–698.

[38] Mintun, M. A., Fox, P. T., and Raichle, M. E. (1989) *J. Cereb. Blood Flow Metabol.* **9,** 96–103.

[39] Raichle, M. E. (1990) *Semin. Neurosci.* **2,** 307–315.

[40] Powers, W. J., Hirsch, I. B., and Cryer, P. E. (1991) *J. Cereb. Blood Flow Metabol.* **11,** S362.

[41] Sollevi, A., Ericson, K., Eirksson, L., Lindqvist, C., Lagerkranser, M., and Stone-Elander, S. (1987) *J. Cereb. Blood Flow Metabol.* **7,** 673–678.

[42] Perlmutter, J. S. and Raichle, M. E. (1985) *Neurology* **35,** 1127–1134.

[43] Powers, W. J. (1991) *Ann. Neurol.* 29, 231–240.

[44] Carpenter, D. A., Grubb, R. L., Jr., Tempel, L. W., and Powers, W. J. (1991) *J. Cereb. Blood Flow Metabol.* **11,** 837–844.

[45] Lammertsma, A. A. and Jones, T. (1983) *J. Cereb. Blood Flow Metabol.* **13,** 416–424.

[46] Lammertsma, A. A., Wise, R. J. S., Heather, J. D., Gibbs, J. M., Leenders, K. L., Frackowiak, R. S. J., Rhodes, C. G., and Jones, T. (1983) *J. Cereb. Blood Flow Metabol.* **3,** 425–431.

[47] Pantano, P., Baron, J.-C., Crouzel, C., Collard, P., Sirou, P., and Samson, Y. (1985) *Eur. J. Nucl. Med.* **10,** 387–391.

48 Ohta, S., Meyer, E., Thompson, C. J., and Gjedde, A. (1992) *J. Cereb. Blood Flow Metabol.* **12,** 179–192.

49 Sokoloff, L., Reivich, M., Kennedy, C., Des Rosiers, M. H., Patlak, C. S., Pettigrew, K. D., Sakurada, O., and Shinohara, M. (1977) *J. Neurochem.* **28,** 897–916.

50 Reivich, M., Kuhl, D., Wolf, A., Greenberg, J., Phelps, M., Ido, T., Casella, V., Fowler, J., Hoffman, E., Alavi, A., Som, P., and Sokoloff, L. (1979) *Circ. Res.* **44,** 127–137.

51 Phelps, M. E., Huang, S. C., Hoffman, E. J., Seline, C., Sokoloff, L., and Kuhl, D. E. (1979) *Ann. Neurol.* **6,** 371–388.

52 Huang, S. C., Phelps, M. E., Hoffman, E. J., Sideris, K., Selin, C. J., and Kuhl, D. E. (1980) *Am. J. Physiol.* **238,** E69–E82.

53 Reivich, M., Alavi, A., Wolf, A., Fowler, J., Arnett, C., MacGregor, R. R., Shiue, C. Y., Atkins, H., Anand, A., Dann, R., and Greenberg, J. H. (1985) *J. Cereb. Blood Flow Metabol.* **5,** 179–192.

54 Hawkins, R., Phelps, M. E., Huang, S. C., and Kuhl, D. E. (1981) *J. Cereb. Blood Flow Metabol.* **1,** 37–52.

55 Gjedde, A. (1987) *Biochem. Pharmacol.* **12,** 1853–1861.

56 Gjedde, A., Wiehard, K., Heiss, W.-D., Kloster, G., Diemer, N. H., Herholz, K., and Pawlik, G. (1985) *J. Cereb. Blood Flow Metabol.* **5,** 163–178.

57 Suda, S., Shinohara, M., Miyaoka, M., Lucignani, G., Kennedy, C., and Sokoloff, L. (1990) *J. Cereb. Blood Flow Metabol.* **10,** 499–509.

58 Greenberg, J. H., Hamar, J., Welsh, F. A., Harris, V., and Reivich, M. (1992) *J. Cereb. Blood Flow Metabol.* **12,** 70–77.

59 Lifton, J. F. and Welch, M. J. (1971) *Radiat. Res.* **45,** 35–40.

60 Ehrin, E., Stone-Elander, S., Nilsson, J. L. G., Bergstrom, M., Blomqvist, G., Brismar, T., Eriksson, L., Greitz, T., Jansson, P. E., Litton, J. E., Malmborg, P., af Ugglas, M., and Widen, L. (1983) *J. Nucl. Med.* **24,** 326–331.

61 Raichle, M. E., Welch, M. J., Grub, R. L., Jr., Higgins, C. S., Ter-Pogossian, M. M., and Larson, K. B. (1978) *Science* **199,** 986–987.

62 Mintun, M. A., Raichle, M. E., Welch, M. J., and Kibourn, M. R. (1985) *J. Cereb. Blood Flow Metabol.* **5,** S623–S624.

63 Blomqvist, G., Bergstrom, K., Bergstrom, M., Ehrin, E., Eriksson, L., Garmelius, B., Lindberg, B., Lilja, A., Litton, J. E., Lundmark, L., Lundqvist, H., Malmborg, P., Mostrom, U., Nilsson, L., Stone-Elander, S., and Widen, L. (1985) *The Metabolism of the Human Brain Studied with Positron Emission Tomography* (Greitz, T., Ingvar, D. H., and Widen, L., eds.), Raven, New York, pp. 185–194.

64 Gutniak, M., Blomqvist, G., Widen, L., Stone-Elander, S., Hamberger, B., and Grill, V. (1990) *Am. J. Physiol.* **258,** E805–E812.

65 Hawkins, R., Mans, A., Davis, D., Vina, J., and Hibbard, L. (1985) *Am. J. Physiol.* **248**, C170–C176.

66 Blomqvist, G., Stone-Elander, S., Halldin, C., Roland, P. E., Widen, L., Lindqvist, M., Swahn, C. G., Langstrom, B., and Wiesel, F. A. (1990) *J. Cereb. Blood Flow Metabol.* **10**, 467–483.

67 Fox, P. T., Raichle, M. E., Mintun, M. A., and Dence, C. (1988) *Science* **241**, 462–464.

68 Powers, W. J. and Raichle, M. E. (1985) *Stroke* **16**, 361–376.

69 Herscovitch, P., Raichle, M. E., Kilbourn, M. R., and Welch, M. J. (1987) *J. Cereb. Blood Flow Metabol.* **7**, 527–542.

70 Jakobsen, J., Hirsch, I., Snyder, A., Cryer, P., and Raichle, M. E. (1991) *J. Cereb. Blood Flow Metabol.* **11**, S492.

71 Lammertsma, A. A., Brooks, D. J., Frackowiak, R. S. J., Heather, J. D., and Jones, T. (1984) *J. Cereb. Blood Flow Metabol.* **4**, 523–534.

72 Brooks, D. J., Beaney, R. P., Lammertsma, A. A., Leenders, K. L., Horlock, P. L., Kensett, M. J., Marshall, J., Thomas, D. G., and Jones, T. (1984) *J. Cereb. Blood Flow Metabol.* **4**, 535–545.

73 Kessler, R. M., Goble, J. C., Bird, J. H., Girton, M. E., Doppman, J. L., Rapoport, S. I., and Barranger, J. A. (1984) *J. Cereb. Blood Flow Metabol.* **4**, 323–328.

74 Lockwood, A. H., Bolomey, L., and Napoleon, F. (1984) *J. Cereb. Blood Flow Metabol.* **4**, 516–522.

75 Lockwood, A. H., Yap, E. W. H., and Wong, W. H. (1991) *J. Cereb. Blood Flow Metabol.* **11**, 337–341.

76 Koeppe, R. A., Mangner, T., Betz, A. L., Shulkin, B. L., Allen, R., Kollros, P., Kuhl, D. E., and Agranoff, B. W. (1990) *J. Cereb. Blood Flow Metabol.* **10**, 727–739.

77 Leenders, K. L., Poewe, W. H., Palmer, A. J., Brenton, D. P., and Frackowiak, R. S. J. (1986) *Ann. Neurol.* **20**, 258–262.

78 Brooks, D. J., Beaney, R. P., Lammertsma, A. A., Herold, S., Turton, D. R., Luthra, S. K., Frackowiak, R. S. J., Thomas, D. G. T., Marshall, J., and Jones, T. (1986) *J. Cereb. Blood Flow Metabol.* **6**, 230–239.

79 Vyska, K., Magloire, J. R., Freundlieb, C., Hock, A., Becker, V., Schmid, A., Feinendegen, L. E., Kloster, G., Stocklin, G., Schuier, F. J., and Thal, H. U. (1985) *Eur. J. Nucl. Med.* **11**, 97–106.

80 Feinendegen, L. E., Herzog, H., Wieler, H., Patton, D. D., and Schmid, A. (1986) *J. Nucl. Med.* **27**, 1867–1877.

81 Herholz, K., Wienhard, K., Pietrzyk, U., Pawlik, G., and Heiss, W. D. (1989) *J. Cereb. Blood Flow Metabol.* **9**, 104–110.

82 Blomqvist, G., Gjedde, A., Gutniak, M., Grill, V., Widen, L., Stone-Elander, S., and Hellstrand, E. (1991) *Eur. J. Nucl. Med.* **18**, 834–837.

[83] Shapiro, E. T., Cooper, M., Chen, C. T., Given, B. D., and Polonsky, K. S. (1990) *Diabetes* **39,** 175–180.

[84] Brooks, K. J., Gibbs, J. S., Sharp, P., Herold, S., Turton, D. R., Luthra, S. K., Kohner, E. M., Bloom, S. R., and Jones, T. (1986) *J. Cereb. Blood Flow Metabol.* **6,** 240–244.

[85] Hasselbalch, S., Knudsen, G. M., Jakobsen, J., Holm, S., Hogh, P., and Paulson, O. (1991) *J. Cereb. Blood Flow Metabol.* **11,** S465.

[86] Horii, H., Imahori, Y., Miukawa, N., Ueda, S., Oki, F., Inaba, T., and Nakahashi, H. (1991) *J. Cereb. Blood Flow Metabol.* **11,** S381.

[87] Fukuyama, H., Kameyama, M., Harada, K., Nishizawa, S., Senda, M., Mukai, T., Yonekura, Y., and Torizuka, K. (1989) *Acta. Neurol. Scand.* **80,** 307–313.

[88] Jagust, W. J., Seab, J. P., Huesman, R. H., Valk, P. E., Mathis, C. A., Reed, B. R., Coxson, P. G., and Budinger, T. F. (1991) *J. Cereb. Blood Flow Metabol.* **11,** 323–330.

[89] Fiorelli, M., Duboc, D., Mazoyer, B. M., Blin, J., Eymard, B., Fardeau, M., and Samson, Y. (1992) *Neurology* **42,** 91–94.

Chapter 2

Some Features
of the Functional Anatomy
# of Human Cerebral Blood Vessels

William I. Rosenblum

Introduction: Special Problems in Defining Form
and Function in Human Cerebral Vessels

The study of human blood vessels presents some problems that are not usually encountered in animal studies. For example, the human life-span is many times longer than that of laboratory animals. Blood vessels of humans undergo many age-related changes. These changes may not reflect the preprogrammed result of aging *per se*, but may represent diseases that require the passage of time for their induction or expression. Such considerations are especially important now that endothelium-dependent dilation and endothelium-dependent constriction have been demonstrated in cerebral blood vessels.[1-3] We have shown that endothelium-dependent responses may be impaired by lesions that cannot be appreciated by or that are barely discernible by conventional electron microscopy.[2-4] Consequently, whenever a disease is present that may injure the endothelium, one must worry that the disease produced abnormal responses to a variety of vasoactive stimuli. Atherosclerosis and/or hypercholesterolemia represent common human diseases that may produce endothelial injury and consequently aberrant vasomotor responses.[5] Hypertension is also common and may produce abnormal responses to a given agonist,

From *The Human Brain Circulation*, R. D. Bevan and J. A. Bevan, eds.
©1994 Humana Press

perhaps by inducing prostaglandin formation, whose vasomotor consequences overcome the effects of endothelium-derived relaxing factor released by the same agonist.[6]

Factors like those just enumerated may limit the determination of normal function in human vessels. A description of the functional morphology of human cerebral vessels is also limited because ultrastructural artifacts result from delay in fixation, which occurs when tissue is immersed in, rather than perfused by, fixative. In order to be effective, perfusion fixation must be begun in living tissue. Hence, it cannot be carried out in humans. Therefore, human cerebral vessels must be immerse fixed, and hence, some aspects of their ultrastructure may be artifactually altered. Because of this problem, electronmicroscopists have generally been reluctant to examine human cerebral tissue—including vessels—except for purposes of making medical diagnoses. Consequently, there is relatively little published, detailed information about the functional microscopic anatomy of human cerebral vessels. This handicaps a reviewer attempting to report relevant data.

Normal Morphologic Features and Their Possible Functional Significance

Size of Vessels

When discussing human brain blood vessels, it is important to note that they fall for the most part within the "microcirculation." That is, they are <300 μm and indeed are usually <100 μm in internal diameter.[7] This is true for the smallest surface branches (the smallest "pial vessels") and for virtually all of the vessels once they have entered the parenchyma. In fact, the intraparenchymal vessels of the human brain and the rodent brain fall essentially within the same size class (<100 μm diameter) as do the parenchymal vessels of most mammals.[7] A relationship of size of brain to diameter of vessel is only present in the Circle of Willis and the larger pial vessels. Thus the pial vessels of small mammals, for example, mice, will be <100 μm in diameter and will resemble in size the parenchymal vessels rather than representative, pial vessels of humans.

Innervation

Size, however, is not the sole parameter of interest when comparing vessels between species. The larger vessels of the Circle of Willis and the small pial arteries and arterioles are covered by networks of nerves carrying diverse mediators, sometimes with several mediators in a single nerve. This is true irrespective of species, so in the mouse, for example, an adrenergic nerve net accompanies the pial arterioles even though they are usually <60 μm in internal diameter. However, in mammals generally and presumably including humans,[8] vessels of similar size, if they have penetrated the brain (i.e., parenchymal vessels), lose their adrenergic innervation, at least in many brain regions. Therefore, when one utilizes pial vessels of small mammals, one is studying vessels that resemble the pial vessels of humans with respect to innervation, but that resemble the parenchymal vessels of humans with respect to size.

Anastomoses

Once vessels enter the brain, they are interconnected by so many connections that the vascular bed is a meshwork resembling a mass of "Brillo" or steel wool (Fig. 1A). The level of the anastomoses has been a subject of controversy.[9] The vast majority of connections occur at the capillary level. Numerous connections occur between precapillary vessels, but these are still generally <15 μm in size. Larger interarterial anastomoses are rare, as are arteriovenous shunts. The numerous capillary and precapillary anastomoses mean that in theory a red blood cell can travel from one end of the brain to the other. In humans and most other mammals, occlusion of a single penetrating arteriole by an embolus should not result in necrosis (infarction) of surrounding brain if adjacent penetrating arterioles and the precapillary anastomoses are patent.[10] Moreover, the irregular, complex pathway of the vessels in the "mesh" and the frequent close passage between these vessels render invalid, in the author's opinion, any attempt to "model" oxygen delivery using the conventional Krogh assumptions, which assume a microvessel with the proximal end having higher oxygen levels than the distal end. In the human brain, and that of most mammals, there are simply too many opportunities for oxygen to be shunted between close neighboring vessels.

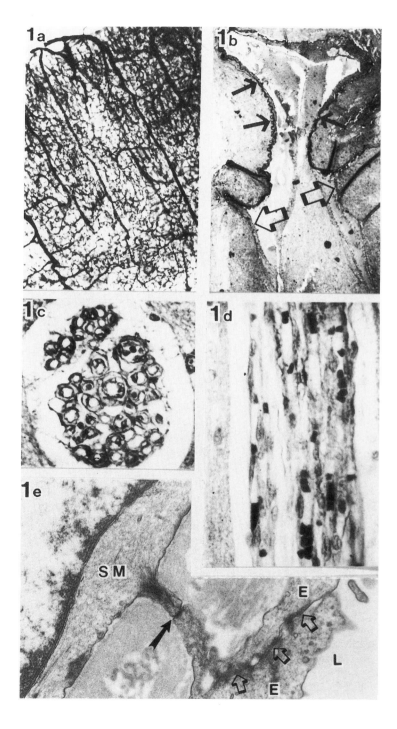

Elastica

Brain arteries and arterioles, unlike other arteries and arterioles, have only a single (internal) elastic lamella. This may provide the explanation for the location of so-called berry aneurysms[11] only in the cerebral circulation (Fig. 1B). These saccular aneurysms occur at branch points at vessels in or near the Circle of Willis. Their rupture can be devastating. The absence of a media at branch points is a characteristic of many vascular beds and cannot account for the development of these aneurysms only in brain. However, the absence of an outer elastica in brain vessels, coupled with the absence of media at branch points, might make these branch points more susceptible to the hemodynamic forces that produce aneurysms.

The Blood–Brain Barriers

The endothelium of cerebral vessels is specially adapted to maintain certain barrier functions.[12] Supposedly the term blood–brain barrier" was coined to denote a barrier to large molecules, e.g., proteins. However, the barrier is more extensive than this and is really a set of barriers—probably diverse mechanisms—that regulate passage of materials between plasma and brain parenchyma. In spite of a large number of studies using contemporary techniques, the location and nature of the barrier to large molecules is still a matter of controversy in animals, so no definitive statement can be made concerning humans.

It is generally believed that tight junctions between endothelial cells account for the barrier to large molecules. These zonulae

---

Fig. 1. (A) *(previous page)* Human cerebral cortex with vessels filled by India ink. Shows dense mesh of anastamosing capillary and precapillary vessels filling space between penetrating arterioles and exiting draining venules. (B) Human artery from base of brain. Single elastic lamella (black arrows) ends abruptly (open arrows) along with media where berry aneurysm begins. (C and D) Two vascular wickworks: one in cross-section, and the other in longitudinal section. These consist of bundles of intertwined capillaries. (E) Electron microphotograph of human arteriole 40 µ in diameter. A myoendothelial junction (dark arrow) is present between smooth muscle (SM) and endothelial cell (E). Two endothelial cells are seen with tight junctions (open arrows) between them. L = Lumen of vessel.

occludens have a pentalaminar ultrastructure. However, to be truly tight, such junctions must form a circumferential band totally separating adjoining endothelial cells. Since such junctions take a tortuous path as they circle the vessel, their demonstration requires serial sections of well fixed material. This has not been done to the best of the author's knowledge using human material. Nevertheless, junctions that appear tight in single sections can be found throughout the cerebrovascular endothelium. Often gaps appear along these junctions, but we must keep in mind that because the junctional "belt" is tortuous, an apparent gap in any one section may not represent a passage, but merely a space trapped within a tortuous "belt." Such a space would not communicate with both the lumen and the extravascular tissue. If tight junctions are the barrier to large molecules, then these junctions must open if such molecules are to pass. It remains an open question as to whether pathologic breakdown of the barrier depends on opening of these junctions and which segments of the brain's vasculature-arteriole—capillary or venule—are involved. Moreover, different pathologic states might alter barrier functions and/or affect different segments of the vasculature.

The reason for doubting that the barrier to large molecules resides solely at tight junctions has to do with the question of the importance of vesicular[12,13] or canalicular transport of large molecules by endothelial cells. Normal cerebrovascular endothelium is characterized by a paucity of such vesicles or canaliculi in contrast to endothelium from many other organs. This paucity is seen in humans as well as other mammals. If, as many believe, vesicular transport is important, then the barrier in the cerebral vessels is characterized not only by what the vessels have—i.e., tight junctions—but by what they do not have—i.e., vesicles in the endothelium. However, in diseased states, at least in animals, the number of vesicles may increase and a role for them in transport—although abnormal transport—becomes a consideration. Thus, it is possible, but not proven, that a breakdown in the barrier to large molecules consists of enhanced vesicular transport.

The barriers to small molecules depend on diverse transport systems, usually based on the presence of carrier molecules, or on the presence of enzyme systems in endothelium that destroy compounds as they pass through the endothelium. Glucose and many amino acids have specialized carrier systems in animals, and presumably in humans. Biogenic amines are among those compounds thought to be catabolyzed by enzymes within the endothelium.[14]

In animals, astrocytes have been shown to induce enzyme activity in endothelium of adjacent capillaries.[15-17] The close apposition of astrocytic foot processes to cerebral microvessels may reflect the structural arrangement necessary to maintain a normal level of several barrier regulating carriers or enzymes within the nearby endothelium. One such inducible enzyme, γ glutamyl transpeptidase (GGTP), has a variety of functions. One of these may be to convert leukotrienes that disrupt the blood–brain barrier into other inactive leukotrienes.[18] Recently, an elegant animal study demonstrated histochemically that γ glutamyl transpeptidase activity was absent in microvessels proliferating at a site of brain injury, but the GGTP activity then appeared in these vessels once proliferating astrocytes contacted them.[19] Attempts should be made to perform analogous studies using human material.

At least some of the enzymatic barrier functions seem to be absent from pial vessels of animals, although present in parenchymal vessels.[14] We have studied (unpublished) GGTP activity in humans and animals, and found it missing from many pial vessels. This is expected if the enzyme is induced by astrocytes, since their processes do not contact many pial vessels. Perhaps this is the explanation for other differences between the content of barrier enzymes in pial vs parenchymal vessels. In any case, it is no longer believed that astrocyte foot processes are a physical barrier to transport from blood to brain.

Myoendothelial Junctions

The structure of cerebral vessels, like that of vessels elsewhere, is characterized by junctions between endothelial cells and vascular smooth muscle. Recently, when these myoendotholial junctions (MEJ) were reported in humans by the author's laboratory,[20] we were not aware of other reports concerning humans. Since then, older reports have been found from one other laboratory describing MEJ in humans' cerebral blood vessels.[21] The author had previously observed MEJ in the pial arterioles of mice and cats, and they had been described by Dahl in nonhuman primates.[22]

The author's interest in MEJ originated with in vivo observations of propagated constriction between two zones of endothelial injury in pial arterioles of mice.[23] The constriction appeared to be caused by substances released from platelets aggregating at the upstream site. The constriction never extended below the downstream injury. This was powerful evidence that the effect was initiated by agonists released by the platelets at the upstream site, but that these agonists were diluted in the flowing blood and were not themselves the cause of constriction downstream, close to the downstream site of injury. If agonists passed downstream in concentrations adequate to produce constriction, then constriction should not have ended abruptly at the downstream injury. Surely, there then should have been a number of instances in which the agonists, passing further downstream, would have produced constriction below the downstream injury. This was never seen. Thus, we concluded that the agonists released by the platelet aggregate upstream directly induced a constriction over a very small zone of vascular smooth muscle, and that this constriction was then propagated until it reached the downstream site of endothelial damage, which blocked the propagated response.

Propagated responses have recently been demonstrated in other microvascular beds.[24] Both propagated dilation and constriction have been observed.[24] Propagation occurs in both the upstream and downstream direction from the site of initiation.[25] In our case, there is endothelial damage beneath the platelet aggregate at the upstream site. Failure of constriction to occur upstream from the aggregate is consistent with our conclusion that endothelial damage blocks propagation.

If this scenario is correct, then a healthy endothelium is essential for the propagation of a contractile wave. The MEJ, already observed in mice, might represent a structure essential to the propagation. Perhaps electrical impulses do not simply pass longitudinally through the vascular smooth muscle, but rather pass from muscle to endothelium and back through MEJs along a longitudinal path. It is also possible that some chemical mediator passes from endothelial cell to muscle cell via MEJs in response to an electrical impulse and that this chemical is essential to the continuance of the electrical wave. Certainly, the evidence from other vascular beds suggests that propagated responses are electrotonic in nature.[24]

In any case, our observations of propagation and MEJs in mice, coupled with our finding that propagation was blocked by endothelial damage, led us to search for MEJs in human cerebral vessels. This search was confined to small arteries and arterioles, and was successful.[20]

As was the case with mice or cats, immersion fixation was perfectly adequate to preserve these junctions (Fig. 1E). In addition other structural features were well preserved, such as apparently tight interendothelial junctions (Fig. 1E) and Weibel-Palade bodies within the endothelial cytoplasm. However, fixation limitations and/or the lack of serial sections precludes our drawing conclusions about the fine structural detail of the junctions. Three types of MEJs were identified based on their broad structural characteristics. These were called types I, II, and III, and consisted either of a downward peg of endothelium, an upward peg of smooth muscle, or a meeting between pegs of each cell type at an intermediate point within the subendothelial basal lamina or elastica. Multiple MEJs were sometimes seen between a single pair of endothelial and smooth muscle cells.

MEJ were not looked for in venules or in arteries larger than about 1 mm. From here down to capillaries, MEJs were identified. When their number was related to the length of vascular segments that were examined, a much greater frequency of MEJ was found in the narrower segments than in the wider segments. Location in the pial or parenchymal portion of the bed was not as important as the size of vessel in determining the frequency of MEJ.

These data provide a morphologic basis for communication between endothelium and vascular smooth muscle. This communication may be essential for propagation of waves of muscle hyperpolarization or depolarization with consequent propagation of dilation or constriction. The endothelial cytoplasm on either side of the MEJ may play a role also in conducting impulses. In either event, endothelial injury by modifying either MEJ, endothelial cytoplasm, or both might then block propagated responses as we have reported in animals.[23]

Propagation may be clinically important for at least two reasons. It may amplify the increased cerebrovascular resistance caused by local accumulation of blood at the base of the brain in subarachnoid hemorrhage. This would amplify the adverse effects of "vasospasm" in some instances of subarachnoid hemorrhage. Second, propagated responses could account for deviations from the well-known coupling between metabolism and blood flow in the brain. Apparently, global responses to changes in metabolism may sometimes be exaggerated, and the explanation for such exaggerations is unknown.[26] It is possible that local alterations in vascular tone, produced by local changes in metabolism, may propagate into adjacent areas whose metabolism is unchanged. If this were to occur and the metabolic and flow measurements involved both areas of brain, the alteration in flow would be disproportionate to the alteration in metabolism.

Pathologic Findings

At the beginning of this chapter, conditions, such as atherosclerosis or hypertension, which change the structure of cerebral blood vessels and alter endothelial structure and/or function, were referred to. These conditions, common to humans, may alter the behavior of human blood vessels selected for study, and may even lead to confusing the common but abnormal with the less common but normal (i.e., unaltered) behavior of the vessels. In closing this chapter, two other morphologic changes that are common and that must alter the function of the cerebral vascular bed will be added.

Amyloidosis

The first of these is amyloidosis[27] caused by deposition of β amyloid in the vessel wall. This amyloid is a specific type of amyloid whose precursor protein is coded by a gene on chromosome 21. This amyloid is identical to that produced in Alzheimer's disease. Its appearance in cerebral vessels as well as brain tissue increases with age, particularly after age 60. It is invariably present, although in variable amounts, in patients with dementia caused by Alzheimer's disease. However, cerebrovascular involvement may be severe in the elderly without dementia. The process by which the precursor protein is converted to amyloid is not yet established. The brain and its vessels are selective sites for production and/or deposition of this amyloid, even though its gene is present in all cells. Persons with cerebrovascular deposition are often said to have amyloid angiopathy (or Congophilic angiopathy because the amyloid stains with Congo Red). However, the angiopathy differs greatly in severity from person to person and vessel to vessel. Some vessels show frank disarrangement of all layers of the vessel wall with fibrosis of the wall, whereas other vessels show only a mild deposition of amyloid whose location with respect to endothelium, media, or adventitia has been variously described. It is difficult to imagine that any vessel infiltrated by amyloid can have normal responses to vasoactive mediators, changes in pressure or flow, and so forth. Consequently, the author believes this change in addition to the atherosclerosis (affecting arteries) and the hypertensive arteriolosclerosis (affecting arterioles) may skew the results obtained when the vessels come from the elderly.

Vascular Wickworks

The last change that will be mentioned also occurs in the elderly. It has been called a vascular "wickworks" by analogy to the wrapping or braiding of fibers in a candle wick.[28,29] For unknown reasons, capillaries proliferate and wrap around each other or around the parent arteriole (Fig. 1C,D). Numerous intertwined vessels form a single wick, and numerous wicks can be present in a microscopic field. The consequences of all this must surely be an increase in cerebrovascular resistance. Since the components of the wick appear to be capillaries, it is not likely that they respond to humoral or neural mediators by changing tone. Nevertheless, their existence and effect on resistance should be considered when one examines the relationship between form and function in brain blood vessels.

Acknowledgments

This work was supported by grants HL 35935 and HL 45617 from the National Heart, Lung, and Blood Institute.

References

1 Rosenblum, W. I. (1986) *Stroke* **17**, 494–497.
2 Rosenblum, W. I., Nelson, G. H., and Povlishock, J. T. (1987) *Circ. Res.* **60**, 169–176.
3 Rosenblum, W. I. and Nelson, G. H. (1988) *Circ. Res.* **63**, 837–843.
4 Povlishock, J. T., Rosenblum, W. I., Sholley, M. M., and Wei, E. P. (1983) *Am. J. Path.* **110**, 148–160.
5 Forstermann, U., Mugge, A., Alheid, U., Haverick, A., and Frolich, J. C. (1988) *Circ. Res.* **62**, 185–190.
6 Faraci, F. M. and Heistad, D. D. (1991) *Hypertension* **17**, 917–922.
7 Alexander, L. and Putnam, T. J. (1938) *The Circulation of the Brain and Spinal Cord*, Proc. Assoc. Res. Nervous Mental Diseases, vol. 18, Williams & Willkins, Baltimore, pp. 471–543.
8 Peerless, S. J. and Kendall, M. J. (1976) *The Cerebral Vessel Wall* (Cervos-Navarro, J., Betz, E., Matakas, F., and Wullenweber, R., eds.), Raven, New York, pp. 175–181.
9 Raven, J. R. (1974) *Pathology of Cerebral Microcirculation* (Cervos-Navarro, J., ed.), de Gruyter, Berlin, pp. 26–38.
10 Kennedy, J. C. and Taplin, G. V. (1967) *Am. Surg.* **33**, 763–771.
11 Stebbens, W. E. (1972) *Pathology of the Cerebral Blood Vessels*, C. V. Mosby, St. Louis, MO.
12 Rapoport, S. I. (1976) *Blood–Brain Barrier in Physiology and Medicine*, Raven, New York.
13 Westergaard, E. (1980) *Advances in Neurology, vol. 28, Brain Edema* (Cervos-Navarro, J. and Ferszt, R., eds.), Raven, New York, pp. 55–74.
14 Edvinsson, L. and MacKenzie, E. T. (1977) *Pharm. Rev.* **28**, 275–348.
15 DeBault, L. E. and Cancilla, P. A. (1980) *Science* **207**, 653–655.
16 Beck, D. W., Vinters, V., Hart, M. N., and Cancilla, P. A. (1984) *J. Neuropath. Exp. Neurol.* **43**, 219–224.
17 Maxwell, K., Berliner, J. A., and Cancilla, P. A. (1989) *J. Neuropath. Exp. Neurol.* **48**, 69–80.
18 Baba, T., Black, K. L., Ikezaki, K., Chen, K., and Becker, D. S. (1991) *J. Cereb. Blood Flow Metab.* **11**, 638–643.

19 Cancilla, P. A., Berliner, J. A., and Bready, J. V. (1990) *Pathophysiology of the Blood Brain Barrier* (Johansson, B. B., Owman, C., and Widener, H., eds.), Elsevier, Amsterdam, pp. 31–40.

20 Aydin, F., Rosenblum, W. I., and Povlishock, J. T. (1991) *Stroke* **22,** 1592–1597.

21 Raggendorf, W., Cervos-Navarro, J., and Rozas, J. R. I. (1981) *Cerebral Microcirculation and Metabolism* (Cervos-Navarro, J. and Fritschka, E., eds.), Raven, New York, pp. 443–453.

22 Dahl, E. (1973) *Z. Zelforsch.* **145,** 577–586.

23 Rosenblum, W. I., Weinbrecht, P., and Nelson, G. H. (1990) *Microcirc. Endoth. Lymph.* **6,** 369–386.

24 Segal, S. S. and Duling, B. (1989) *Am. J. Physiol.* **256,** H838–H845.

25 Segal, S. S. and Duling, B. R. (1986) *Science* **234,** 868–870.

26 Low, C., Edvinsson, L., and MacKenzie, E. T. (1987) *Ann. Neurol.* **22,** 289–297.

27 Yamaguchi, H., Yamazaki, T., Lemere, C. A., Frosch, M. P., and Selkoe, D. J. (1992) *Am. J. Path.* **141,** 249–259.

28 Hassler, O. (1965) *Acta Neuropathol. (Berl.)* **5,** 40–53.

29 Saunders, R. L. de C. H. and Bell, M. A. (1971) *J. Neurosurg.* **35,** 128–140.

Chapter 3

Neural Pathways
to the Cerebral Circulation in Humans

Jan Erik Hardebo and Norihiro Suzuki

As elsewhere in the body, the blood vessels to the brain are innervated by autonomic and sensory fibers. The fibers participate in regulation of local vascular tone, in pain transmission, and in the natural growth of the vessel wall. The possible presence of central nerves innervating brain parenchymal vessels is not discussed here.

Sympathetic Nerves

It has long been known that the main supply of sympathetic fibers to the cerebral vessels originates in the superior cervical ganglion. This is also true in humans. The fibers—visualized by antero- and retrograde tracing technique and immunohistochemical staining of their transmitters norepinephrine and neuropeptide Y— run in the adventitia along the internal carotid artery (ICA) extracranially and in the carotid canal as a solid nerve, the internal carotid nerve.

As soon as the nerve enters intracranially, branches are issued that form a terminal network in the vessel wall.[1,2] The main nerve continues along the intracranial ICA and its arborizations to issue branches along these vessels that end as terminal networks. The fibers follow the pial arteries and arterioles, and also their penetrating cortical arterial and arteriolar branches[3] (Fig. 1). There is little spread over the midline via the Circle of Willis of fibers originating in the ganglion on one side.

From *The Human Brain Circulation*, R. D. Bevan and J. A. Bevan, eds.
©1994 Humana Press

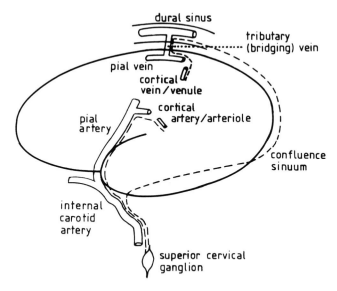

Fig. 1. Schematic illustration of the pathways for the sympathetic innervation of the arterial and venous vascular trees in the human brain.

All but vascular fibers to the orbit leave the ICA wall at the
cavernous level to follow the ophthalmic nerve—and not the ophthalmic artery—to the eye[4-6] and probably the oculomotor nerve to
the smooth muscle portion of the levator palpebrae muscle (Fig. 2).

The sympathetic pathways to the cerebral veins have been
revealed in some detail in recent years, as studied in laboratory
animals and monkey. When the internal carotid nerve courses with
ICA through the cavernous sinus, a branch is issued that follows
the trochlear nerve backwards in the frontolateral origins of the
tentorium cerebelli[6-8] (Fig. 2). After leaving the nerve, this branch
divides and runs as bundles together with trigeminal fibers (nervi
tentorii) toward the epiphysis and confluence sinuum.[6-8] From here,
they follow the sinuses and their connections to the brain surface
(the cerebri magna vein and tributary veins),[9] and distribute with
sensory fibers along the venous vessels on the brain surface and in
the brain parenchyma (Fig. 1).

Ultrastructural observations of the sympathetic cerebrovascular innervation have been performed also in human vessels.[10]

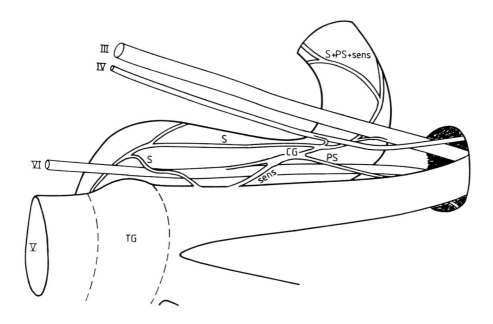

Fig. 2. Schematic representation of sympathetic (S), parasympathetic (PS), and sensory (sens) fiber branches in the human cavernous sinus walls, of relevance for the cerebral arterial and venous innervation, and sympathetic fibers to orbital structures. The three nerve types actually form a plexus in the cavernous walls before joining the different cranial nerves and the internal carotid artery, whereas nervi tentorii probably take a separate course through the cavernous sinus (not shown) to the trochlear nerve. TG = trigeminal ganglion.

Adrenergic nerve fibers and terminals, with granular electron dense neurotransmitter vesicles, are confined to the adventitial-medial transitional zone and the outer layer of the media.[10]

Perivascular adrenergic fibers are present in human internal carotid, pial, and cortical penetrating arteries, and arterioles already in fetuses from 12–28 wk of gestation.[11] At this age, fibers can be traced even in 50-μm diameter lenticulostriate vessels. It is possible that perivascular fibers in the brain are more numerous during growth than in the adult.

It has been demonstrated by histochemistry that serotonin is present in spread preparations of pial perivascular nerve fibers. This represents either a natural uptake of small quantities in the sympathetic fibers or inadvertent uptake into these nerves from ruptured platelets during the preparation, rather than the presence of specific serotonergic nerves.

Parasympathetic Nerves

Until recent years, little has been known about a parasympathetic innervation of cerebral vessels, in contrast to the sympathetic innervation. Recent histochemical and biochemical studies on cerebrovascular parasympathetic nerves have revealed their sources and pathways. Histochemical studies have demonstrated nerve fibers containing choline acetyltranferase (ChAT), a reliable marker for cholinergic nerves, and vasoactive intestinal polypeptide (VIP) in the cerebral vessels. By combining histochemistry with retrograde tracer technique and selective denervations, the cerebrovascular parasympathetic innervation has been mapped in the rat, cat, and monkey. By comparison with findings in monkey, a similar mapping can be made also in humans.

The histochemical demonstration of parasympathetic nerves in the cerebral blood vessels has been hindered for many years by the lack of suitable markers for the specific cholinergic nerves. Staining of acetylcholinesterase has been utilized for the demonstration of acetylcholine in the nerves presumed to be parasympathetic in nature. However, this enzyme is not solely confined to cholinergic nerves and may have functions other than those that are transmitter-related.[12]

Utilizing specific antibodies against ChAT, it has been shown that cholinergic nerves are localized in the adventitia of the cerebral vessels in the rat, cat, pig, dog, and monkey.[13-15] In the rat, ChAT-immunoreactive nerve fibers are observed in all branches of the Circle of Willis and in the vertebro-basilar artery, where they mostly run along the axis of vessels with few terminal varicosities. They are most abundant in the anterior part of the pial arteries.[15] Biochemical measurements in pial arteries and arterioles from several species, including humans, have demonstrated that ACh and VIP are present as transmitters in cerebrovascular nerves.[16,17] ChAT-immunoreactive fibers are observed close to or in the same nerve fibers as those containing immunoreactive VIP.[15] Perivascular fibers are present already in human fetuses from 12–28 wk of gestation, and run as far out in penetrating cerebral vessels as 50 μm in diameter.

Ultrastructural distribution of granular and agranular synaptic vesicles within perivascular nerve terminals in cerebral blood vessels has been shown in cat and rabbit.[18–20] The agranular vesicles, which have been assumed to be associated with cholinergic nerves and which remain after sympathectomy, have a diameter of approx 55 nm. Since the fixation used for electron microscopy is not specific for any particular neurotransmitter, it is not clear to which extent these agranular vesicles contain ACh. However, some of the vesicles have been shown to be associated with VIP.[21]

Retrograde axonal tracing studies have been utilized to elucidate the origins for ChAT- or VIP-containing nerves in the cerebral arteries of rat, cat, and monkey.[13,15,22–25] These studies have demonstrated several sources for cerebrovascular parasympathetic nerves, primarily the spheno(pterygo)palatine, otic, and internal carotid ganglia. In monkey, no clear evidence for an origin in the otic ganglion has been obtained. By combining histochemical demonstration of ChAT- and VIP-containing fibers with retrograde tracer techniques and denervation experiments, an extensive mapping of the cerebrovascular parasympathetic innervation has been made in rats and monkeys.[13,15,23]

Corresponding anatomical evidence has been obtained for the parasympathetic innervation in human cerebral arteries[26] (Fig. 3). They appear to have several origins:

1. The fibers from the sphenopalatine ganglion reach the cavernous segment of ICA as rami orbitales through the supraorbital fissure in humans. Along these rami, miniganglia may contribute with fibers to the innervation of large pial arteries; the most distant miniganglion along this pathway is named the cavernous ganglion (Figs. 2,3). The fibers join trigeminal sensory and sympathetic fibers in the cavernous sinus walls before reaching the ICA wall.
2. Fibers from the internal carotid ganglion along the greater superficial petrosal nerve reach the bypassing ICA through a short course in the (greater) deep petrosal nerve.

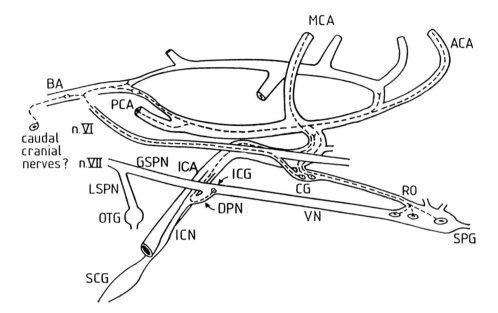

Fig. 3. Schematic representation of origins and pathways of cerebrovas-cular postganglionic parasympathetic nerves in humans. The fibers origi-nate in the sphenopalatine ganglion (SPG), to take a course in rami orbitales (R) through the supraorbital fissure to reach the internal carotid artery (ICA) and the basilar artery (BA) and their pial branches, via the cavernous gan-glion (CG), located in a plexus of sympathetic, parasympathetic, and sen-sory fibers in the cavernous sinus walls. In the internal carotid ganglion (ICG) along the greater superficial petrosal nerve (GSPN), to bridge via the (greater) deep petrosal nerve (DPN) to the adjacent ICA just above the carotid canal. Other possible origins are the otic ganglion (OTG)—to take a course along the lesser superficial petrosal nerve (LSPN), GSPN, and GDPN to the ICA—and caudal cranial nerves. ACA, anterior cerebral artery; ICN, inter-nal carotid nerve; MCA, middle cerebral artery; PCA, posterior cerebral artery; SCG, superior cervical ganglion; VN, Vidian nerve.

3. Possibly, fibers from the otic ganglion may reach ICA after a course in the lesser and greater superficial and deep petrosal nerves (Fig. 2).
4. Some autonomic fibers from the cavernous plexus, together with trigeminal sensory fibers from this plexus (*see* next section), join the abducent nerve to follow it backward to the brainstem to reach the basilar artery, as found in the monkey.[27] In this way, parasympathetic

postganglionic fibers from the sphenopalatine ganglion and the mini-ganglia along the rami orbitales (including the cavernous ganglion) may innervate the basilar artery and its branches (Fig. 3).

5. Possibly, the glossopharyngeal and vagal nerves may send parasympathetic fibers to innervate the proximal basilar artery.

It is likely that the scarce parasympathetic innervation of the cerebral veins derives from the cavernous plexus. The fibers may follow the sympathetic and sensory fibers along the trochlear nerve and tentorum cerebelli to the confluence sinuum,[8] and run along the sinuses[28] and the tributary veins to reach cerebral veins.

Sensory Nerves

It is well known that the intracranial ICA and its pial arterial branches, and some veins at the brain surface, are pain-sensitive for stimuli applied at single locations along their course.[29] The discovery of substance P, neurokinin A, and calcitonin gene related peptide (CGRP) being present as transmitters in pain fibers, together with the possibility to demonstrate immunohistochemically their presence in nerve fibers, has during the last decade made it possible to visualize and map out cerebrovascular pain fibers.

It has been found that the fiber density is markedly decreasing with smaller pial vessel diameters,[30] in line with a lower pain sensitivity. Whether sensory fibers progress down to intraparenchmal vessels is not known with certainty from histological studies, but physiological blood flow studies indicate that this is likely.[31] Also, biochemical measurements have demonstrated the presence of substance P and CGRP in pial arteries.[17,26]

Substance P-containing nerve endings in the adventitia of pial arteries have been demonstrated by electron microscopy.[30,32-34] There is ultrastructural evidence for the presence of trigeminal fibers also transferring other sensory modalities[30] in the pial vessels of the monkey.

1. Substance P- and CGRP-containing sensory fibers to the intracranial ICA and its branches in humans are mainly derived from the ophthalmic trigeminal division, leaving the ophthalmic trunk shortly distal to the ganglion and running a short course through the nerve plexus in the cavernous sinus walls.[26]

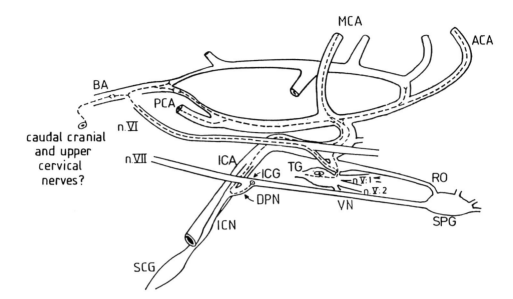

Fig. 4. Schematic overview of the origins and pathways in humans of sensory nerve fibers to the intracranial segment of the internal carotid artery, the basilar artery, and their pial arterial branches. TG, trigeminal ganglion. Other abbreviations are as in Fig. 3.

2. Some of these fibers join and follow the abducent nerve backwards to innervate the basilar artery and branches[26,27] (Figs. 2,4).
3. In monkey, a contribution from the maxillary division has been found, as well as aberrant trigeminal microganglia in the cavernous region.[27]
4. The internal carotid ganglion along the greater superficial petrosal nerve also contributes with sensory fibers to the ICA tree in humans and monkeys[13,26] (Fig. 4).
5. The proximal basilar artery may receive pain fibers from caudal cranial nerves and the upper cervical dorsal root ganglia (Fig. 4).

The cerebral veins appear to be innervated from the nervi tentorii (Arnold's nerve), which comprise a few branches issued from the ophthalmic nerve trunk into the connective tissue between the vessels of the cavernous sinus. In contrast to the situation in the monkey,[8] these nervi do not appear to join the cavernous nerve plexus in humans,[26] but run independently to the trochlear nerve to follow it backwards and then run in the tentorium cerebelli to the confluence sinuum.[8,35] Thereafter, the fibers run along and innervate the dural sinuses,[28,35] and it is likely that some fibers diverge to follow the tributary veins and cerebri magna vein, to distribute along the cerebral veins with terminal branches.

References

1 Handa, Y., Hayashi, M., Nojyo, Y., Tamamaki, N., and Caner, H. H. (1990) *Exp. Brain Res.* **82,** 493–498.

2 Yasargil, M. G. (1984) *Microneurosurgery,* vol. I, Georg Thieme Verlag, Stuttgart, p. 57.

3 Hardebo, J. E. (1989) *Neurotransmission and Cerebrovascular Function,* vol. II (Seylaz, J. and Sercombe, R., eds.), Elsevier, Amsterdam, pp. 193–210.

4 Parkinson, D. (1988) *Anat. Rec.* **220,** 108–109.

5 Marfurt, C. F., Zaleski, E. M., Adams, C. E., and Welther, C. L. (1986) *Brain Res.* **366,** 373–378.

6 Tamamaki, N. and Nojyo, Y. (1987) *Brain Res.* **437,** 387–392.

7 Kenny, G. C. T. (1985) *The Pineal Gland. Current State of Pineal Research* (Mess, B., Rúzsás, C., Tima, L., and Pévet, P., eds.), Elsevier, Amsterdam, pp. 341–345.

8 Ruskell, G. L. (1988) *J. Anat.* **157,** 67–77.

9 Keller, J. T., Marfurt, C. F., Dimlich, R. W., and Tierney, B. F. (1989) *J. Comp. Neurol.* **290,** 310–321.

10 Cuevas, P., Gutierrez-Diaz, J. A., Reimers, D., Dujovny, M., Diaz, F. G., and Ausman, J. I. (1987) *Surg. Neurol.* **27,** 113–116.

11 Kawamura, K., Sakata, N., and Takebayashi, S. (1991) *Angiology* **42,** 35–43.

12 Silver, A. (1974) *The Biology of Cholinesterase. Frontier of Biology,* vol. 36, North Holland Publ. Co., Amsterdam, pp. 355–388.

13 Hardebo, J. E., Arbab, M., Suzuki, N., and Svendgaard, N. A. (1991) *Stroke* **22,** 331–342.

14 Saito, A., Wu, J.-Y., and Lee, T. F. J. (1985) *J. Cereb. Blood Flow Metab.* **5,** 327–334.

15 Suzuki, N., Hardebo, J. E., and Owman, C. (1990) *J. Cereb. Blood Flow Metab.* **10,** 399–408.

16 Hamel, E. and Estrada, C. (1989) *Neurotransmission and Cerebrovascular Function, vol. II,* (Seylaz, J. and Sercombe, R., eds.), Elsevier, Amsterdam, pp. 151–173.

17 Edvinsson, L., Ekman, R., Jansen, I., Ottosson, A., and Uddman, R. (1987) *Ann. Neurol.* **21,** 431–437.

18 Lee, T. F.-J. (1981) *Circ. Res.* **49,** 971–979.

19 Nielsen, K. C., Owman, C., and Sporrong, B. (1971) *Brain Res.* **27,** 25–32.

20 Suzuki, N. (1983) *Jap. J. Stroke* **5,** 87–98.
21 Lee, T. F.-J., Saito, A., and Berezin, L. (1984) *Science* **224,** 898–901.
22 Edvinsson, L., Hara, H., and Uddman, R. (1989) *J. Cereb. Blood Flow Metab.* **9,** 212–218.
23 Suzuki, N., Hardebo, J. E., and Owman, C. (1988) *J. Cereb. Blood Flow Metab.* **8,** 697–712.
24 Suzuki, N. and Hardebo, J. E. (1991) *Auton. Nerv. Syst.* **36,** 39–46.
25 Walters, B. B., Gillespie, S. A., and Moskowitz, M. (1986) *Stroke* **17,** 488–494.
26 Suzuki, N. and Hardebo, J. E. (1991) *J. Neurol. Sci.* **104,** 19–31.
27 Ruskell, G. L. and Simons, T. (1987) *J. Anat.* **155,** 23–27.
28 Keller, J. T. and Marfurt, C. F. (1991) *J. Comp. Neurol.* **309,** 555–566.
29 Dalessio, D. J. (1980) *Wolff's Headache and Other Head Pain,* 4th ed., Oxford University Press, New York.
30 Simons, T. and Ruskell, G. L. (1988) *J. Anat.* **159,** 57–71.
31 Sakas, D. E., Moskowitz, M., Wei, E. P., Kontos, H. A., Kano, M., and Ogilvy, C. S. (1989) *Proc. Natl. Acad. Sci. USA* **86,** 1401–1405.
32 Itakura, T., Okuno, T., Nakakita, K., Kamei, I., Naka, Y., Nakai, K., Imai, H., Komai, N., Kimura, H., and Maeda, T. (1984) *J. Cereb. Blood Flow Metab.* **4,** 407–414.
33 Liu-Chen, L. Y., Liszczak, T. M., King, J. C., and Moskowitz, M. A. (1986) *Brain Res.* **369,** 12–20.
34 Matsuyama, T., Shiosaka, S., Wanaka, A., Yoneda, S., Kimura, K., Hayakawa, T., Emson, P. C., and Tohyama, M. (1985) *J. Comp. Neurol.* **235,** 268–276.
35 McNaughton, F. L. (1938) *Proc. Assoc. Res. Nerv. Ment. Dis.* **18,** 178–200.

Chapter 4

Neuropeptides in Human Cerebral Arteries

Occurrence, Characterization, and Receptors

Lars Edvinsson, Sergio Gulbenkian, Inger Jansen, and Rolf Uddman

Introduction

Four major mechanisms are considered the prime regulators of the cerebral circulation: metabolic, myogenic, chemical and neurogenic. In addition, recent studies have also suggested that the endothelium may have an important role in the regulation of cerebral blood flow.[1] For the past two decades, the neurogenic mechanisms that evoke vasomotor effects have been our main field of research. However, more recently, the putative influence of the endothelium has also attracted our attention.

Initial investigations have focused on the "classical" autonomic transmitters noradrenaline and acetycholine.[2] With the development of immunocytochemical techniques, attention has been directed toward new neurotransmitter candidates, such as amines and neuropeptides. There is now ample immunocytochemical evidence that peptides, such as neuropeptide Y (NPY), vasoactive intestinal peptide (VIP), substance P (SP), and calcitonin gene related peptide (CGRP), are present in nerve fibers supplying the cerebral vasculature of laboratory animals.[3] On the other hand, only a few studies have been carried out on human cranial ves-

From *The Human Brain Circulation*, R. D. Bevan and J. A. Bevan, eds.
©1994 Humana Press

sels.[4-8] In the present chapter, we will briefly describe the distribution of cerebrovascular nerve fibers, the characterization of the neuropeptides, and the effects of various neurotransmitters on human cerebral arteries.

Methods

Immunocytochemistry

Human cerebral (cortex pial) arteries were removed from macroscopically intact regions during neurosurgical tumor resections. Vessel segments were fixed in a mixture of 2% formaldehyde and 15% of a saturated aqueous picric acid solution in $0.1M$ phosphate buffer, rinsed in cold Tyrode buffer containing 10% sucrose for 48 h, frozen on dry ice, and sectioned in a cryostat (15 μm thick sections). For the demonstration of NPY, VIP, SP, or CGRP immunoreactivity, an indirect immunofluorescence method was used.[9] The antisera used have been characterized previously.[5,7] In control experiments, no immunostaining was observed when primary antisera were preabsorbed with their corresponding antigen (10–100 mg/mL diluted antiserum).

Radioimmunoassay

The material (mainly large cerebral arteries, removed during autopsy) was weighed and boiled in $0.5M$ acetic acid for 15 min. The specimens were homogenized (Polytron 1–2 min) and centrifuged at 2000g for 15 min. The supernatants were collected and lyophilized. For radioimmunoassay, the freeze-dried material was dissolved in 3 mL of $0.05M$ phosphate buffer, pH 7.5, containing 0.25% human serum albumin and centrifuged at 2000g for 15 min. Each tissue extract was assayed in serial dilutions in the respective neuropeptide assay. Immunoreactive NPY was quantitated using a rabbit antiserum at a final dilution of 1:40,000 (P. C. Emson, Cambridge, UK).[10] Immunoreactive VIP was quantitated using antiserum No 7852 (MILAB, Malmö, Sweden) at a final dilution of 1:72,000.[11] Immunoreactive SP was quantitated using a rabbit antiserum SP-2 at a final dilution of 1:50,000, and (Tyr8)-SP was used as a tracer (E. Brodin, Stockholm, Sweden).[12] Immunoreactive CGRP was quantitated using a rabbit antiserum (R-8429), raised against synthetic rat CGRP (MILAB, Malmö, Sweden), conjugated to bovine serum albumin, and used at a final dilution of 1:37,500. Iodinated CGRP was purified by high-performance liquid chromatography (HPLC).[13] Each tissue extract was assayed in serial dilutions in the respective neuropeptide assay.

Vasomotor Responses in Vitro

Segments of human cerebral arteries were examined using a sensitive in vitro system.[14] Arterial segments (2–3 mm) were suspended between two L-shaped metal prongs (0.1–0.2 mm) in small tissue baths containing a buffer solution aerated with 5% CO_2 in O_2, pH 7.4, and kept at 37°C. Mechanical activity was recorded by force displacement transducers (Grass FT03C) connected to a Grass polygraph. The vessels were given a passive load of 2 mN, and allowed to stabilize at this tension for 1.5 h before testing. The contractile capacity of the preparations was first tested by exposure to a buffer solution containing 60 mM potassium; this resulted in strong and reproducible contractions that were 8.1 ± 0.9 mN ($n = 56$). In experiments with NPY, the peptide was either applied alone in increasing concentrations, or given in a concentration of $10^{-8}M$ 5 min prior to NA administration. When VIP, SP, or human α-CGRP was tested, none were able to induce relaxation of vessels at the resting level of tension. Therefore, the vessels were precontracted with $3 \times 10^{-6}M$ prostaglandin $F_{2\alpha}$ ($PGF_{2\alpha}$), which induced strong and sustained contractions amounting to 6.4 ± 1.0 mN in cerebral arteries. The data are expressed below as mean EC_{50} or IC_{50} values (concentrations of agonist eliciting half-maximum contraction or relaxation, respectively) and as E_{max} or I_{max} (mean of the maximum responses) and given as mean values $\pm$ SEM of responses from a given number (n) of vessel segments (one or two from each patient).

The Sympathetic System

In humans, numerous NPY-immunoreactive varicose nerve fibers were observed in the adventitia and adventitial-medial border of cerebral arteries (Fig. 1). NPY-containing fibers were somewhat more numerous in temporal than in the cerebral and meningeal arteries.[5,7,8]

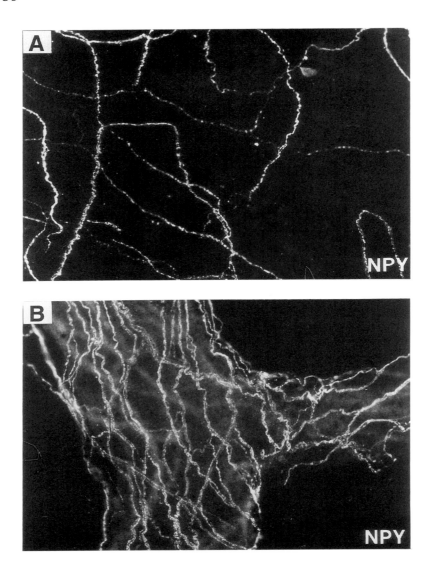

Fig 1. Whole mount preparations of human cortical veins **(A)** and arteries **(B)**, obtained during neurosurgical tumor resections, immuno-stained for NPY. A dense network is seen in arteries and a sparse supply is seen in veins.

Previous studies revealed that the cerebral arteries of laboratory animals were supplied by an extensive plexus of noradrenaline (NA)-containing fibers.[15] In contrast, veins were sparsely innervated. It was also observed that small arteries and arterioles were innervated by single fibers only.[15,16] Denervation experiments performed on animals showed that the majority of NA-containing fibers supplying forebrain vessels arise from the ipsilateral superior cervical ganglion.[17] Furthermore, double immunostaining for NPY and the catecholamine-synthesizing enzymes tyrosine hydroxylase and dopamine β hydroxylase (markers for adrenergic neurons) showed that NPY and NA coexisted in the same perivascular nerve fibers.[18]

Quantitative measurements of NPY in extracts of human cerebral arteries revealed higher concentrations of NPY in the temporal artery (13.5 ± 2.2 pmol/g) as compared to the cerebral (3.0 ± 2.4 pmol/g) and middle meningeal arteries (6.5 ± 1.6 pmol/g) ($p < 0.05$).[8] HPLC analysis revealed that NPY-LI eluted as one major component with the same elution volume as synthetic human NPY (Fig. 2A).

In cerebral arteries, the administration of NPY elicited concentration-dependent contractions (Fig. 3A). The NPY-induced contraction was somewhat stronger in magnitude when compared with that of NA. NPY was markedly more potent than NA. A low concentration of NPY ($10^{-8}M$) added 15 min before the NA concentration response curve did not modify the contraction induced by NA. A small additive effect was seen. The contractile responses to NA were antagonized by the α_1-adrenoceptor blocker prazosin ($10^{-7}M$). Neither this antagonist nor the 5-hydroxytryptamine blocker ketanserin ($10^{-7}M$) caused the blockade of contractions induced by NPY. However, PP56, a novel NPY blocker, showed antagonism of NPY-induced contractions (Fig. 3A).

The NPY-induced constriction of human cerebral and middle meningeal arteries[8] is more pronounced than that noted for NA and occurs at much lower concentrations. In human temporal arteries, NPY potentiated adrenergically mediated responses,[7,8] a feature that was not seen in experiments performed on human

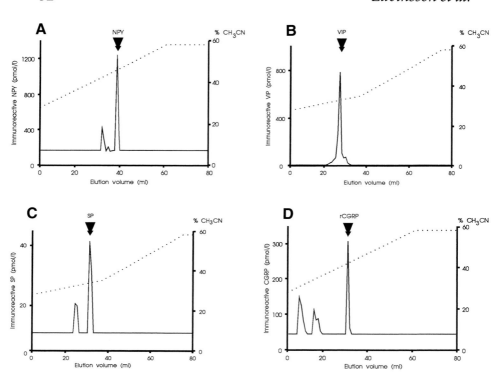

Fig 2. HPLC profiles of extracts of human cerebral arteries. The respective elution position of synthetic NPY **(A)**, VIP **(B)**, SP **(C)**, and CGRP **(D)** is indicated by an arrow, and the gradient is depicted by the broken line. Number of experiments $n = 4$ of each.

cerebral and middle meningeal arteries.[8] Thus, NPY and NA appear to act synergistically in human cerebral and middle meningeal arteries, since no potentiation of the NA-induced contraction was seen. Other studies have shown that NPY-induced contractions in feline cerebral arteries are markedly reduced by calcium antagonists or by calcium depletion, whereas adrenoceptor or 5-hydroxytryptamine antagonists are without effects.[19] In contrast, the potentiating effect of NPY on peripheral arteries is not directly dependent on extracellular calcium, but is attenuated by oubain and is absent in a sodium-free buffer solution.[20] The administra-

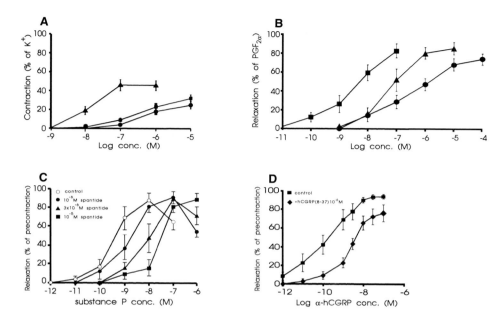

Fig 3. **(A)** Concentration-dependent contraction of human cerebral arteries to NA (●), NPY (▲), and NA in the presence of $10^{-8}M$ NPY (■). **(B)** Concentration-dependent relaxation of human cerebral arteries following the administration of VIP, PHM-27 (▲), and ACh (●) to vessels precontracted with $3 \times 10^{-6}M$ $PGF_{2\alpha}$. **(C)** Antagonistic effects of Spantide 10^{-6}–$10^{-5}M$ on SP-induced relaxation. **(D)** Antagonistic effects of human α-CGRP 8–37 $10^{-6}M$ on human α-CGRP-induced relaxation. Mean values ± SEM of five to eight experiments.

tion of NPY elicits strong concentration-dependent contractions of cerebral arteries. These NPY contractions can be blocked by D-myo-inositol-1.2.6-trisphosphate, a NPY blocker.[19,21] The present results revealed that there is a different mode of action of NPY on cerebral and middle meningeal as compared to temporal arteries. In the cerebrovascular bed, NPY may participate with NA in maintaining the upper limit of autoregulation during acute increases in arterial blood pressure. In temporal arteries, NPY may serve as a modulator of adrenergically mediated responses.

The Parasympathetic System

Nerve fibers containing immunoreactivity for vasoactive intestinal peptide (VIP) and peptide histidine isoleucine (PHI) were found to innervate cerebral arteries from several mammalian species.[22-26] It has also been shown that VIP immunoreactive nerve fibers are positive for the cholinergic markers choline acetyl transferase (ChAT) and acetylcholinesterase (AChE).[27,28] However, in a recent study, contradictory results were obtained showing that in the cerebral vasculature, VIP and ChAT immunoreactivities generally occurred in distinct nerve populations. ChAT and VIP immunoreactivity was found colocalized in <5% of the perivascular nerve fibers.[29]

Denervation experiments showed that the extirpation of the sphenopalatine ganglion causes a decrease in the density of AChE and ChAT-positive nerve fibers.[27-31] It should be noted, however, that some AChE positive nerve fibers arise from both the otic and internal carotid ganglia.[28,32-34] Perivascular nerve fibers containing VIP and PHI immunoreactivity were also found to originate from the sphenopalatine, otic, and internal carotid ganglia.[27,34,35] In humans, we found that cerebral, middle meningeal and temporal arteries were innervated by a sparse to moderate supply of VIP-immunoreactive nerve fibers,[5,6,8] which are typically located in the adventitia and at the adventitial-medial border.

Quantitative radioimmunoassay measurements revealed higher concentrations of VIP in the cerebral (2.3 ± 0.7 pmol/g) and middle meningeal arteries (1.2 ± 0.4 pmol/g) as compared to the temporal arteries (0.5 ± 0.2 pmol/g).[8] The extracted material coeluted with authentic VIP, and the HPLC peak was in the same position as the authentic peptide for all three cranial vessels (Fig. 2B).

ACh, VIP, and the human form of PHI, peptide histidine methionine (PHM-27), act as potent vasodilators in human cranial arteries. In the middle meningeal and cerebral arteries VIP was consistently more potent than PHM-27 and ACh. A different pattern of potency was found in the temporal artery where VIP, PHM-27, and ACh were equipotent. However, the two peptides resulted in the same maximum effect in the three regions. ACh, on the other hand, resulted in a lower maximum effect in the middle meningeal as compared to cerebral and temporal arteries. When VIP was given in increasing concentrations to $PGF_{2\alpha}$-contracted arteries, concentration-dependent relaxations occurred (Fig. 3B). The relaxation induced by VIP and PHM-27 was not affected by the β-adrenoceptor antagonist propranolol ($10^{-7}M$), the histamine H_2-blocker cimetidine ($10^{-6}M$), or the cholinergic antagonist atropine ($10^{-6}M$). The mechanism of action of VIP and PHI-27/PHM-27 involves an increase in the activity of adenylate cyclase[36,37] and is unrelated to the release of an endothelium-derived factor (through which ACh induces dilatation).[37,38] Previous studies in laboratory animals have shown that lower ACh concentrations cause endothelium-dependent relaxation by binding to endothelial muscarinic M3 receptors.[39] High concentrations of ACh induce nonendothelium dependent constriction by binding to muscarinic M2 receptors probably located on the vascular smooth muscle.

Exogenously applied VIP and PHI dilate cerebral arteries both in vitro and *in situ*.[23,24,40,41] VIP activates smooth muscle adenylate cyclase, and this effect correlates well with the potent vasodilator action of VIP.[36,37] In brain vessels, the relaxant response to VIP is unaffected by the removal of the endothelium,[37,42] thus suggesting that VIP acts directly on the smooth muscle. Specific PHI receptors have not been identified in cerebral arteries. The effect of PHI on cellular cAMP levels appears to be the result of the action of the peptide on cerebrovascular VIP receptors.[43] Using radioiodinated VIP, specific VIP binding sites have been observed in the medial layers of bovine cerebral arteries.[44]

The Sensory System

Cerebral arteries of laboratory animals are innervated with a moderate supply of SP-immunoreactive nerve fibers[45–47] and a moderate supply of CGRP-immunoreactive nerve fibers,[3,48,49] which are located in the adventitia and at the adventitial-medial border. Nerve fibers containing SP and CGRP immunoreactivity have also been found in human cerebral, middle meningeal, and temporal arteries[5,7,8] with a similar distribution to the one observed in laboratory animals. From the results of recent immunoelectron microscopical studies, it appears that sensory nerve fibers are mainly located in the distal part of the adventitia, whereas sympathetic and parasympathetic nerve fibers are generally found at the adventitial–medial border.

Although several origins for cerebrovascular nerves containing CGRP, SP, and neurokinin A (NKA) immunoreactivity have been described, it appears that sensory neurons of the trigeminal ganglion are the most important source, sending fibers to the Circle of Willis and its anterior and caudal branches. It has also been demonstrated that SP, NKA, and CGRP immunoreactivities are colocalized in the same neurons of the trigeminal ganglion of several mammalian species, including humans.[49,50]

The concentration of CGRP was in general higher than the concentration of SP.[8] It was noted that the level of SP was higher in the cerebral arteries (2.3 ± 0.8 pmol/g) as compared to middle meningeal (0.3 ± 0.06 pmol/g) and temporal arteries (0.5 ± 0.2 pmol/g). The level of CGRP was higher in the cerebral (3.9 ± 1.1 pmol/g) than in middle meningeal (1.7 ± 0.3 pmol/g) and temporal arteries (1.0 ± 0.3 pmol/g).

Substance P-LI eluted as two peaks, one major peak with the same retention as synthetic SP and a second peak with the same elution volume as oxidased SP (Fig. 2C). CGRP eluted in one major peak close to the elution position of rat and human synthetic α-CGRP (Fig. 2D).

Both SP and CGRP acted as potent relaxant agents on all arteries examined. NKA exerted a vasodilator action as strong as SP, but had lower potency (Fig. 3C,D). The middle meningeal artery showed a higher sensitivity to SP as compared to both the cerebral and temporal arteries. However, the reverse was seen for CGRP, for which cerebral arteries were more sensitive as compared to middle meningeal and temporal arteries. Three types of tachykinin receptors have been described: neurokinin 1 (NK-1), neurokinin 2 (NK-2), and neurokinin 3 (NK-3). These have been differentiated on the basis of the order of potency for a series of agonists. NK-1 receptors have the following rank order of potencies: SP > NKA > neurokinin B (NKB); NK-2 receptors have NKA > NKB > SP; and NK-3 receptors, NKB > NKA > SP. At the NK-1 receptor, SP is the most potent tachykinin, whereas NKA and NKB show high affinity for the NK-2 and NK-3 binding sites, respectively.[51,52] The order of agonist potency of SP and NKA in the human cranial vessels suggests that they are equipped with the NK-1 type of receptor. In a previous study performed on human cerebral arteries, we also included NKB and neuropeptide K (NPK) agonist responses; it was suggested that this tissue was supplied with a mixture of NK-1 and NK-2 receptors.[53] Furthermore, Spantide, an SP-antagonist that has been suggested to act via the NK-1 and NK-2 receptor subtypes, competitively blocked the response to SP in human cerebral arteries[53] (Fig. 3C).

The relaxation induced by human α-CGRP was blocked by the CGRP antagonist human α-CGRP$_{8-37}$ (Fig. 3D). However, the response to human β-CGRP was not blocked by this antagonist. These findings suggest that the human cerebral artery is equipped with two types of receptors for CGRP, one being sensitive to human α-CGRP$_{8-37}$ called the CGRP-1 receptor,[54,55] and the other not being sensitive to this antagonist. This has been shown in detail for cerebral arteries from guinea pig.[56] Tachykinins and CGRP exert their relaxant actions via different mechanisms. In laboratory animals, the vasomotor responses to α-CGRP, but not to SP, occur concomitantly with the activation of adenylate cyclase, whereas SP, but not CGRP, requires an intact endothelium for an adequate response.[37] These pharmacological observations are indicative of how the trigeminal system may modulate differently the responses in the intra- and extracranial circulations. As suggested by Markowitz and coworkers,[57] it is possible that SP may induce an inflammatory response in the meningeal circulation, although such a reaction is not seen in the cerebral circulation. In contrast, CGRP was found to be involved in a dynamic reflex aimed at protecting the brain against excessive vasoconstriction.[58] It was recently shown in humans, that during the headache phase of migraine with and without aura,[59] there is a marked and selective increase in craniovascular levels of the powerful vasodilator peptide CGRP, but not of NPY, VIP, and SP. Furthermore, the elevation of CGRP levels is reduced after sumatriptan administration in parallel with amelioration of the headache.[60] We have, furthermore, demonstrated that there is a selective release of CGRP that parallels the development of cerebral vasospasm in patients that have suffered a subarachnoid hemorrhage.[61,62] These findings give the first direct evidence of a peptidergic perivascular involvement clinically in cerebrovascular disorders.

Acknowledgments

This work was supported by grants from the Swedish Medical Research Council (no. 5958,6859), the Medical Faculty, Lund University, the Söderberg Foundation Sweden, and the Laerdal Foundation, Norway.

References

1   Edvinsson, L., MacKenzie, E. T., and McCulloch, J. (1993) *Cerebral Blood Flow and Metabolism,* Raven, New York.
2   Edvinsson, L., Owman, C., and Sjöberg, N.-O. (1976) *Brain Res.* **115,** 337–393.
3   Edvinsson, L. (1985) *Trends Neurosci.* **8,** 126–131.
4   Allen, J. M., Todd, N., Crockard, H. A., Schon, F., Yeats, J. C., and Bloom, S. R. (1984) *Lancet* **ii,** 550–552.
5   Edvinsson, L., Ekman, R., Jansen, L., Ottosson, A., and Uddman, R. (1987) *Ann. Neurol.* **21,** 431–437.
6   Edvinsson, L. and Ekman, R. (1984) *Peptides* **5,** 329–331.
7   Jansen, I., Uddman, R., Hocherman, M., Ekman, R., Jensen, K., Olesen, J., Stiernholm, P., and Edvinsson, L. (1986) *Ann. Neurol.* **20,** 496–501.
8   Jansen, I., Uddman, R., Ekman, R., Olesen, J., Ottosson, A., and Edvinsson, L. (1992) *Peptides* **13,** 527–536.
9   Coons, A. H., Leduc, E. H., and Connolly, J. M. (1955) *J. Exp. Med.* **102,** 49–60.
10 Widerlöv, E., Heilig, M., Ekman, R., and Wahlestedt, C. (1988) *Nord Psykiatr. Tidsskr.* **42,** 131–137.
11 Ekman, R. and Tornquist, K. (1985) *Invest. Ophtalmol. Visual. Sci.* **26,** 1405–1409.
12 Brodin, E., Lindefors, N. E., Dalsgaard, C.-J., Theodorsson-Norheim, E., and Rosell, S. (1986) *Regul. Pept.* **13,** 253–272.
13 Grunditz, T., Ekman, R., Håkanson, R., Rerup, C., Sundler, F., and Uddman, R. (1986) *Endocrinology* **119,** 2313–2323.
14 Högestätt, E. D., Andersson, K.-E., and Edvinsson, L. (1983) *Acta Physiol. Scand.* **117,** 49–61.
15 Nielsen, K. C. and Owman, C. (1967) *Brain Res.* **6,** 773–776.
16 Edvinsson, L. (1975) *Acta Physiol. Scand.* **(Suppl. 427),** 1–35.
17 Edvinsson, L., Owman, C., Rosengren, E., and West, K. A. (1972) *Acta Physiol. Scand.* **85,** 201–206.

[18] Ekblad, E., Edvinsson, L., Wahlestedt, C., Uddman, R., Håkanson, R., and Sundler, F. (1984) *Regul. Pept.* **8**, 225–235.

[19] Edvinsson, L., Emson, P., McCulloch, J., Tatemoto, K., and Uddman, R. (1983) *Neurosci. Lett.* **43**, 79–84.

[20] Wahlestedt, C., Edvinsson, L., Ekblad, E., and Håkanson, R. (1986) *J. Pharmacol. Exp. Ther.* **234**, 735–741.

[21] Edvinsson, L., Adamsson, M., and Jansen, I. (1990) *Neuropeptides* **17**, 99–105.

[22] Kobayashi, S., Kyoshima, K., Olshowka, J. A., and Jacobowitz, D. M. (1983) *Histochemistry* **79**, 377–381.

[23] Edvinsson, L. and McCulloch, J. (1985) *Regul. Pept.* **10**, 345–356.

[24] Edvinsson, L., Fahrenkrug, J., Hanko, J., Owman, C., Sundler, F., and Uddman, R. (1980) *Cell. Tissue Res.* **208**, 135–142.

[25] Larsson, L. I., Edvinsson, L., Fahrenkrug, J., Håkanson, R., Owman, C., Schaffalitsky de Muckadell, O. B., and Sundler, F. (1976) *Brain Res.* **113**, 400–404.

[26] Matsuyama, T., Shiosaka, S., Matsumoto, M., Yoneda, S., Kimura, K., Abe, H., Hayakawa, T., Inowe, H., and Tohyama, M. (1983) *Neuroscience* **10**, 89–96.

[27] Hara, H., Hamill G. S., and Jacobowitz, D. (1985) *Brain Res.* **14**, 179–188.

[28] Suzuki, N., Hardebo, J. E., and Owman, C. (1990) *J. Cereb. Blood Flow Metab.* **10**, 399–408.

[29] Miao, F. J.-P. and Lee, T. J.-P. (1990) *J. Cereb. Blood Flow Metab.* **10**, 32–37.

[30] Hara, H. and Weir, B. (1986) *J. Comp. Neurol.* **250**, 245–252.

[31] Saito, A., Wu, J.-Y., and Lee, T. J.-F. (1985) *J. Cereb. Blood Flow Metab.* **5**, 327–334.

[32] Keller, J. T., Boduk A., and Saunders, M. C. (1985) *Neurosci. Lett.* **58**, 263–268.

[33] Walters, B. B., Gillespie, S. A., and Moskowitz, M. A. (1986) *Stroke* **17**, 488–494.

[34] Edvinsson, L., Hara, H., and Uddman, R. (1989) *J. Cereb. Blood Flow Metab.* **9**, 212–218.

[35] Suzuki, N., Hardebo, J. E., and Owman, C. (1988) *J. Cereb. Blood Flow Metab.* **8**, 697–712.

[36] Huang, M. and Rorstad, O. P. (1984) *J. Neurochem.* **43**, 849–856.

[37] Edvinsson, L., Fredholm, B. B., Hamel, E., Jansen, I., and Verrecchia, C. (1985) *Neurosci. Lett.* **58**, 213–217.

[38] Furchgott, R. F. and Zawadzki, J. V. (1980) *Nature* **288**, 373–376.

[39] Hamel, E. and Estrada, C. (1989) *Neurotransmission and Cerebrovascular Function II* (Seylaz, J. and Sercombe, R., eds.), Elsevier, Amsterdam, pp. 151–173.

[40] Heistad, D. D., Marcus, M. L., Said, S. I., and Gross, P. (1980) *Am J. Physiol.* **239**, 73–80.

[41] McCulloch, J. and Edvinsson, L. (1980) *Am. J. Physiol.* **238**, H449–H456.

[42] Lee, T. J.-F., Saito, A., and Berezin, I. (1984) *Science* **224**, 898–901.
[43] Fahrenkrug, J. (1987) *Scand. J. Clin. Lab. Invest.* **47 (Suppl. 186)**, 43–50.
[44] Poulin, P., Suzuki, Y., Lederis, K., and Rorstad, O. P. (1986) *Brain Res.* **381**, 382–384.
[45] Edvinsson, L., McCulloch, J., and Uddman, R. (1981) *J. Physiol.* **318**, 251–258.
[46] Uddman, R., Edvinsson, L., Owman, C., and Sundler, F. (1981) *J. Cereb. Blood Flow Metab.* **1**, 227–232.
[47] Gibbins, I. L., Furness, J. B., Costa, M., MacIntyre, I., Hillyard, C. J., and Girgis, S. (1985) *Neurosci. Lett.* **57**, 125–130.
[48] Hanko, J., Hardebo, J. E., Kåhrström, J., Owman, C., and Sundler, F. (1985) *Neurosci. Lett.* **57**, 91–95.
[49] Uddman, R., Edvinsson, L., Ekman, R., McCulloch, J., and Kingman, T. A. (1985) *P. Neurosci. Lett.* **62**, 131–136.
[50] Lee, T., Kawai, Y., Shiosaka, S., Takami, K., Kiyama, H., Hillyard, C. J., Girgis, S., MacIntyre, I., Emson, P. C., and Tohyama, M. (1985) *Brain Res.* **330**, 194–196.
[51] Lee, C.-M., Campbell, N. J., Williams, B. J., and Iversen, L. L. (1986) *Eur. J. Phamacol.* **130**, 209–217.
[52] Regoli, D., Drapeau, G., Dion, S., and D'Orleans-Juste, P. (1987) *Life Sci.* **40**, 109–117.
[53] Jansen, I., Alafaci, C., McCulloch, J., Uddman, R., and Edvinsson, L. (1991) *J. Cereb. Blood Flow Metab.* **11**, 567–575.
[54] Donoso, V. M., Fournier, A., St. Pierre, S., and Huidobro-Toro, J. P. (1990) *Peptides* **11**, 885–889.
[55] Dennis, T., Fournier, A., Cadieux, A., Pomerleau, F. B., Jolicoeur, F. B., St. Pierre, S., and Quirion, R. (1990) *J. Pharmacol. Exp. Ther.* **254**, 123–128.
[56] Jansen, I. (1992) *Neuropeptides* **21**, 73–79.
[57] Markowitz, S., Saito, K., and Moskowitz, M. A. (1987) *J. Neurosci.* 4129–4136.
[58] McCulloch, J., Uddman, R., Kingman, T. A., and Edvinsson, L. (1986) *Proc. Natl. Acad. Sci. USA* **83**, 5741–5745.
[59] Goadsby, P. J., Edvinsson, L., and Ekman, R. (1990) *Ann. Neurol.* **28**, 183–187.
[60] Goadsby, P. J. and Edvinsson, L. (1991) *Cephalalgia* **11 (Suppl. 11)**, 3–4.
[61] Juul, R., Edvinsson, L., Gisvold, S. E., Ekman, R., Brubakk, A. O., and Fredriksen, T. A. (1990) *Br. J. Neurosurg.* **4**, 171–180.
[62] Juul, R., Gisvold, S. E., Brubakk, A. O., Fredriksen, T., Waldemar, G., Schmidt, J. F., Ekman, R., and Edvinsson, L. (1993) *Regul. Pept.* (submitted).

Chapter 5

Norepinephrine and Neuropeptide Y as Neurotransmitters to Cerebral Arteries

Dee A. Van Riper

The role of adrenergic nerves in controlling cerebral blood flow has for years been somewhat of an enigma. The discovery that peptide transmitters are coreleased with classical neurotransmitters in the cerebral circulation has served to both clarify and confound our understanding of cerebrovascular neuroeffector mechanisms. In this chapter, I will focus on neuropeptide Y (NPY) and norepinephrine (NE) in cerebral vessels—examining innervation, tissue responses, and the interaction of these transmitters in controlling smooth muscle tone.

By most estimates, the density of noradrenergic innervation of major cerebral arteries is comparable to, and in some cases greater than, peripheral arteries. In addition, innervation density varies between different regions of the brain: In the rat, for example, rostral vessels receive greater innervation than caudal arteries.[1] Innervation is greatest in the vicinity of the Circle of Willis, and extends along major cerebral arteries for several branches and into the parenchyma. Innervation density diminishes with increasing distance from the Circle of Willis.[2,3] However, since innervation density parallels smooth muscle mass in these arteries, the nerve/muscle ratio of small distal vessels may be comparable to that of larger, more proximal arteries. The development of adrenergic innervation of cerebral arteries is similar to peripheral systems.

From *The Human Brain Circulation*, R. D. Bevan and J. A. Bevan, eds.
©1994 Humana Press

Tsai et al.[1] compared the adrenergic innervation of cerebral arteries, iris, heart, and vas deferens of the rat, and found that innervation density of all tissues went from moderate in the fetus and neonate, to dense at 7–8 d postnatal, to very dense in the 15 d old to adult.

The in vitro responses of isolated cerebral arteries to exogenous NE are variable to a remarkable degree.[4] Variations exist both inter- and intraspecies: Arteries from humans, cats, dogs, and rabbits will contract, those from pigs relax, and both responses can be produced in bovine, rat, and monkey arteries. Furthermore, in the bovine brain, arteries from rostral regions contract to norepinephrine, whereas more caudal arteries relax. Variations in responsiveness to NE (assessed as either sensitivity or maximal response) also occur within the cerebral circulation. In sheep, for example, maximal responses to NE fall in the order: pial arteries, common carotid > middle cerebral > basilar.[5,6] With successive branches of rabbit middle cerebral artery, responses to NE diminish to the point that no response is seen in the smaller branches.[2] In terms of development, the responses of cerebral arteries to NE show a general decrement with increasing age. In comparisons of cerebral arteries from fetal, newborn, and adult sheep, two studies have shown that NE response decreases with each stage.[6,7] Similarly, as monkeys develop from premature to adult, both maximal response and sensitivity to NE diminish.[8] These findings are especially intriguing, since innervation density increases over these same stages.

The responses to NE (both contraction and relaxation) of cerebral arteries from adult animals consistently display low sensitivity and only modest maximal response (Fig. 1).[9] Although the sensitivity to norepinephrine (as estimated by pD_2) is within the range of peripheral arteries, it is among the lowest. The differences in response in terms of contraction or relaxation are clearly based on the presence of α or β receptor populations, respectively. Contractile responses are mediated by α_1 and α_2 receptors—some species having exclusively one subtype, e.g., rabbit (α_1), dog (α_2), or a mixture, as in the cat.[10] Since the varied receptor populations display comparable sensitivities (Fig. 1), the generally low respon-

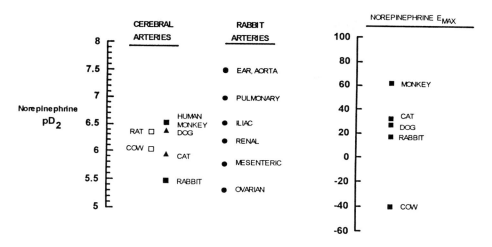

Fig. 1. Left panel: Inter- and intraspecies differences in NE sensitivity of isolated cerebral arteries. ■, α_1- and α_2-mediated contractile responses, respectively; □ β-mediated relaxation; ● contractile responses of rabbit arteries. Right panel: Species differences of maximum NE-mediated responses. Values for cerebral arteries are means derived from a non-exhaustive survey of published values; values of rabbit arteries from ref. 9.

siveness of cerebral vessels to NE is probably not the result of differences in receptor subtype populations.

The lack of responsiveness to NE may arise from several factors: active amine uptake systems, release of vascular endothelial substances, receptor characteristics, i.e., affinity and density, and receptor coupling. Although cerebral vessels are richly innervated, the response to NE is for the most part unaffected by uptake blockers. The effects of endothelium removal are inconclusive. In dog arteries, contractile responses may be endothelium-mediated[11] or endothelium-independent.[12] In perfused rabbit vessels, endothelium removal caused enhanced responses.[13] However, in ring preparations, no effects were observed.[2]

The sensitivities (pD_2) of adrenergic postjunctional receptors in cerebral arteries span at least an order of magnitude, but are within the range of peripheral arteries (Fig. 1) The affinity of rabbit basilar α adrenoceptors for NE as measured by dissociation constant (K_A) is comparable to that of peripheral arteries.[9] Adrenoceptor characterization using antagonists to yield pA_2 and K_B estimates have also produced parameters that agree well with those of peripheral arteries.[9,14] Taken together, these findings indicate that the adrenoceptors mediating norepinephrine responses in cerebral vessels are probably the same as those found in peripheral arteries.

The contribution of receptor density has been addressed in two ways. Receptor occlusion techniques in the rabbit basilar have shown that the limit of maximum response to NE is determined by the number of receptors on the artery.[15] Receptor binding experiments have been limited in scope. However, estimates of receptor density are within the range of peripheral arteries and are consistent with in vitro mechanical responses.[16,17] With regard to receptor coupling, there are few studies specifically addressing postreceptor events in cerebral arteries. This area is of potential significance in explaining weak responses, since receptor populations may exist on cerebral arteries that are poorly coupled or not coupled at all to a mechanical response.

Neuropeptide Y

The 36 amino acid peptide neurotransmitter Neuropeptide Y (NPY) is widely distributed in adrenergic neurons and is present in the cerebral vessels of all species examined so far. NPY innervation of the cerebrovasculature is in many ways similar to that of norepinephrine. The perivascular innervation is located in the adventitia and adventitial/medial border. NPY innervation is abundant and may exceed that of peripheral vessels. Innervation density parallels arterial diameter. The innervation of rostral arteries is greater than those more caudal.[3,18] Neuropeptide Y is codistributed with dopamine-β-hydroxylase (DβH) in the cerebral vasculature, and the destruction of sympathetic adrenergic innervation by ganglionectomy, reserpine, or 6-OHDA diminishes or eliminates NPY innervation. In peripheral as well as cerebral vessels, NPY and DβH are costored in the same subcellular location—large, dense vesicles (LDV). In spite of these similarities, NPY and NE appear to have different storage and release mechanisms. Lundberg et al.[19] examined various innervated tissues following treatment with reserpine and 6-OHDA, and found that although the levels of norepinephrine decreased universally, NPY levels showed no change in spleen and vas deferens, decreased in heart, and increased in the stellate ganglion. In addition, in perfused organ preparations, the ratio of NPY/NE released with nerve stimulation increases with increasing stimulus frequency.[20]

The response of isolated arteries to NPY is varied—most peripheral vessels contract weakly, if at all. However, cerebral arteries consistently contract to exogenous NPY. EC_{50} values are in the 10 nM range for most species, and maximum responses are modest—being in the range of 20–50% of tissue maximum. The response is typically a slowly developing contraction, and repeated exposure yields tachyphylaxis. *In situ* responses of cerebral arteries to NPY are consistent with in vitro results: Microapplication via pial window in cats results in long-lasting, concentration dependent contractions with maximum reductions in diameter of $\approx 35\%$.[21]

A notable quality of NPY is its potential for augmenting the vascular responses of other agonists. Edvinsson et al.,[22] using various rabbit arteries, showed that NPY by itself caused no or small responses, but potentiated NE responses in some but not all arteries. Investigations of cerebral arteries have generally shown that NPY does not enhance NE-mediated contraction.[18]

It is not clear if NPY is involved in pathological states. Edvinsson and Goadsby[23] looked for an association between migraine headache and NPY levels in jugular blood, and found that although changes were observed in other peptide neurotransmitters, there was no change in NPY levels. Experimentally induced subarachnoid hemorrhage (SAH) caused a generalized sharp decline in nerve density, and after sufficient recovery periods (>9 wk), the levels of VIP- and SP-containing nerves, but not NPY nerves, returned to baseline values.[24] In a subgroup of post-SAH patients, there was a close correlation between changes in blood flow velocity and jugular NPY levels.[25] Although these findings are suggestive, any definitive role for NPY in cerebrovascular pathology awaits further investigation.

The functional participation of NPY in the adrenergic neuro-effector mechanism has been carefully investigated in systems such as kidney and gracillus muscle. Sympathetic nerves release both NE and NPY, and prejunctional receptors for each agent mediate negative feedback control of the release of both transmitters. Blockade of pre- and postjunctional adrenergic receptors leads to enhanced neural NPY release and an NPY-mediated tissue response.[26,27] There have been few investigations of this nature of cerebral arteries. However, it has been shown that fractional release of ^{3}H-NE in response to nerve stimulation was reduced 80% by administration of NPY.[26]

We explored the possibility that such a neuroeffector system may be active in the cerebral circulation by subjecting isolated segments of rabbit middle cerebral artery to electrical field stimulation (EFS).[28] Previous studies of cerebral arteries using EFS have shown that in spite of obvious adrenergic innervation and participation, contractile responses are refractory to blockade by adrenergic antagonists. We confirmed these findings in rabbit MCA by treatment with phenoxybenzamine (PBZ) (Fig. 2) and also demonstrated that PBZ had no effect on NPY-mediated contraction. NPY desensitization (achieved by repeated exposure to high NPY concentrations) affected neither the EFS-mediated contraction nor the response to NE. When these treatments were combined, the EFS-mediated contraction was eliminated (Fig. 3). The same results were obtained with the specific α_1-antagonist prazosin. These findings demonstrate a functional NE/NPY neuroeffector mechanism in cerebral arteries that is consistent with that described for peripheral adrenergic systems. They also demonstrate that the EFS-mediated contraction of cerebral vessels observed in the presence of adrenergic blockade was most likely mediated by neurally released NPY.

Given that NPY is present in perivascular adrenergic nerves, what role does neurally released NPY play in modulating cerebrovascular tone? The responses of cerebral arteries to nerve stimulation are only modest in spite of their considerable innervation. This conclusion has followed from studies using either isolated tissues or intact animals, each of which can yield only limited or

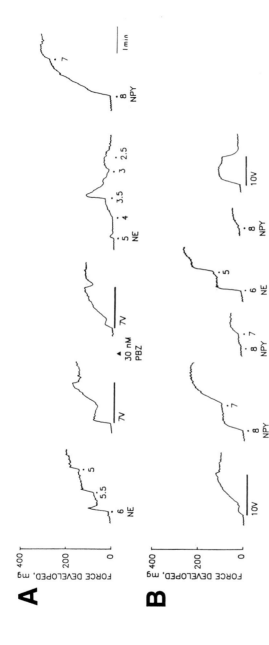

Fig. 2. Experimental tracings showing effects of phenoxybenzamine (PBZ) and NPY on electric field stimulation contraction of rabbit middle cerebral artery. Electrical field stimulation of two arterial segments (A and B) was done at the designated voltages; duration indicated by horizontal bars. NE and NPY concentrations given as -log [agonist]. (A) Treatment with PBZ (30 nM) for 20 min, and 15 min washout resulted in elimination of NE response, but no effect on NPY contraction. (B) NPY response is desensitization by repeated exposure with no effect on NE response. Data from ref. 28.

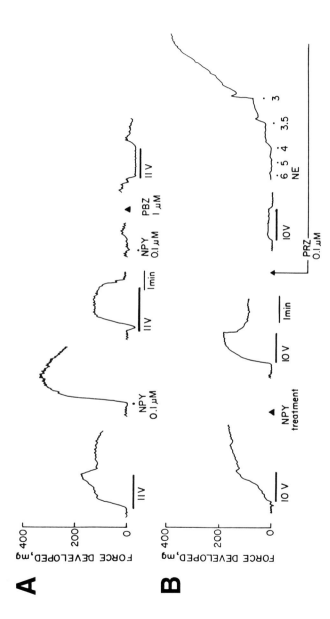

Fig. 3. Experimental records of combined NPY desensitization and adrenoceptor blockade in two segments of rabbit middle cerebral artery. Stimulation and agonist doses as in Fig. 2. **(A)** Following NPY desensitization, treatment with PBZ eliminates the electrical field stimulation response. **(B)** Vessel treated as in A, but prazosin (PR, 0.1 μM) blocked NE contractions at concentrations ≤10^{-4} M. Data from ref. 28.

suggestive data. When an isolated artery is subjected to field stimulation, all nerves are stimulated, and any number of amine, peptide, cholinergic, and as yet unknown transmitters are released—all of which sum, both pre- and postjunctionally, to produce a response. Until such time as each of these transmitters can be accounted for, field stimulation studies will be descriptive, but not definitive. There are several potential mechanisms underlying the weak responses to nerve stimulation, and the participation of NPY is consistent with these mechanisms. The neuroeffector mechanism, as considered here, consists of the prejunctional neural elements, the junction space itself, and the postjunctional plasmalemma (Fig. 4). Each of these elements may contribute to the overall limited vascular response. First, it appears that the junction width for cerebral vessels may be greater than that of peripheral arteries.[4] This has two consequences: (1) It effectively limits the concentration of released transmitter at postjunctional sites and (2) promotes the relative influence of prejunctional mechanisms. Prejunctional factors include uptake mechanisms, inhibitory autoreceptors, and the influence of other inhibitory transmitters. Although uptake blockers have minimal impact on the response to exogenous NE, it is not clear what influence uptake has on neurally released NE. There are indications that uptake may be greater in cerebral vessels than in peripheral arteries, and this may yet prove to be a significant factor. There is ample evidence of negative feedback mechanisms in cerebral vessels: Neurally released NE, NPY, and acetylcholine all act to reduce transmitter release from adrenergic nerves.[28] Given the improbability of NPY uptake mechanisms, neurally released NPY will likely have long-lasting prejunctional effects. Several aspects of the postjunctional receptors may contribute to the limited responsiveness of cerebral vessels. First, functional antagonism may arise from mixed α/β, and β/NPY receptor populations. Second are the receptor characteristics of affinity and receptor density. As was discussed above, cerebrovascular α adrenoceptors probably resemble other α adrenoceptors. However, they are somewhat less sensitive to norepinephrine, and reduced receptor density may be a limiting factor. Cerebrovascular NPY receptors are very sensitive to NPY. However, as with NE, the maximal response

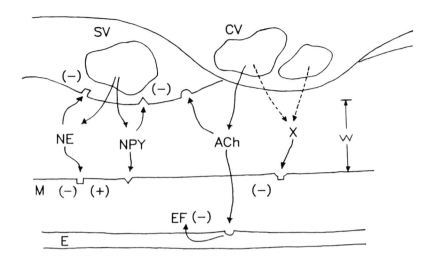

Fig. 4. Diagram of postulated neuroeffector mechanisms of cerebral artery. Norepinephrine (NE) and neuropeptide Y (NPY) are released from sympathetic neural storage sites (SV). They occupy postjunctional sites on the plasmalemma (M)—causing vasoconstriction (+) or relaxation (−) and prejunctional sites to inhibit transmitter release (−). Acetylcholine (ACh) is released from parasympathetic cholinergic neural storage sites (CV) and occupies sites on the vascular endothelium (E) causing vasorelaxation (−) (presumably through the release of endothelial-derived relaxing factor (EF), and prejunctional sites causing decreased adrenergic transmitter release. Noncholinergic transmitter (X) may be released from either cholinergic or other nonadrenergic storage sites to occupy sites on the plasmalemma causing relaxation (−). Junction width (W).

is only modest. In terms of receptor coupling, it is apparent that NE and NPY do not augment each other's responses in cerebral vessels, and this probably arises from a lack of interacting coupling mechanisms.

The elucidation of NPY's participation in the sympathetic neuroeffector mechanism has clarified the functioning of that system, but has only modestly advanced our understanding of certain key questions viz. what mechanisms limit sympathetic influence on vascular tone and what is the role, if any, of the sympathetic nervous system in modulating cerebral blood flow. The buffering of sympathetic influence in cerebral arteries is a vital mechanism. It would be of clinical significance if, in an individual, cerebral adrenergic sensitivity and vascular responsiveness were comparable to the peripheral adrenergic mechanism. This situation might, for example, participate in the diminished regional blood flow associated with the early phases of classical migraine.

References

[1] Tsai, S.-H., Tew, J. M., and Shipley, M. T. (1989) *J. Comp. Neurol.* **279**, 1–12.

[2] Van Riper, D. A. and Bevan, J. A. (1991) *J. Pharmacol. Exp. Ther.* **257**, 879–886.

[3] Duverger, D., Edvinsson, L., McKenzie, E. T., Oblin, A., Rouquier, L., Scatton, B., and Zivkovic, B. (1987) *J. Cereb. Blood Flow Metab.* **7**, 497–501.

[4] Bevan, J. A. and Van Riper, D. A. (1989) *Neurotransmission and Cerebrovascular Function, vol. II.* (Seylaz, J. and Sercombe, R., eds.), Exerpta Medical International Congress Series 870, Amsterdam/New York/Oxford, pp. 65–86.

[5] Gaw, A. J. and Wadsworth, R. M. (1989) *Br. J. Phamacol.* **98**, 741–746.

[6] Pearce, W. J., Hull, A. D., Long, D. M., and Longo, L. D. (1991) *Am. J. Physiol.* **261**, R458–R465.

[7] Wagerle, L. C., Kurth, C. D., and Roth, R. A. (1990) *Am. J. Physiol.* **258**, H1432–H1438.

[8] Toda, N. (1991) *Am. J. Physiol.* **260**, H1443–H1448.

[9] Oriowo, M. A., Bevan, J. A., and Bevan, R. D. (1987) *J. Pharmacol. Exp. Ther.* **241**, 239–244.

[10] Bevan, J. A. (1984) *Trends Pharmacol. Sci.* **5**, 234–236.

[11] Usui, H., Kurahashi, K., Shirahase, H., Fukui, K., and Fujiwara, M. (1987) *Jap. J. Pharmacol.* **44**, 228–231.

[12] Nakagomi, T., Kassell, N. F., Sasaki, T., Lehman, R. M., Torner, J. C., Hongo, K., and Lee, H. (1988) *J. Neurosurg.* **68**, 757–766.

[13] Sercombe, R., Verrechia, C., Oudart, N., Dimitriadou, V., and Seylaz, J. (1985) *J. Cereb. Blood Flow Metab.* **5**, 312–317.

[14] Hayashi, S., Park, M. K., and Kuehl, T. J. (1985) *J. Pharmacol. Exp. Ther.* **235**, 113–121.

[15] Laher, I. and Bevan, J. A. (1985) *J. Pharmacol. Exp. Ther.* **233**, 290–297.

[16] Usui, H., Fujiwara, Y., Tsukahara, T., Tamiguchi, T., and Kurahashi, K. (1985) *J. Cardiovasc. Pharmacol.* **7(Suppl. 3)**, S47–S52.

[17] Shi, A. G., Kwan, C. Y., and Daniel, E. E. (1989) *J. Pharmacol. Exp. Ther.* **250,** 1119–1124.

[18] Brayden, J. E. and Conway, M. A. (1988) *Reg. Peptides* **22,** 253–256.

[19] Lundberg, J. M., Saria, A., Franco-Cereceda, A., Hokfelt, T., Terenius, L., and Goldstein, M. (1985) *Naunyn-Shmiedeberg's Arch. Pharmacol.* **328,** 331–340.

[20] Pernow, J. and Lundberg, J. M. (1989) *Acta Physiol. Scand.* **136,** 507–517.

[21] Edvinsson, L., Emson, P., McCulloch, J., Tatemoto, K., and Uddman, R. (1984) *Acta Physiol. Scand.* **122,** 155–163.

[22] Edvinsson, L., Ekblad, E., Hakanson, R., and Wahlstedt, C. (1984) *Br. J. Pharmacol* **83,** 519–523.

[23] Edvinsson, L. and Goadsby, P. J. (1990) *J. Int. Med.* **228,** 299–304.

[24] Uemura, Y., Sugimoto, T., Okamoto, S., Handa, H., and Mizuno, N. (1987) *J. Neurosurg.* **66,** 741–747.

[25] Edvinsson, L., Alafaci, C., Delgado, T., Ekman, R., Jansen, I., Svengaard, N. A., and Uddman, R. (1991) *Acta Neurol. Scand.* **83,** 103–109.

[26] Pernow, J., Saria, A., and Lundberg, J. M. (1986) *Acta Physiol. Scand.* **126,** 239–249.

[27] Pernow, J. and Lundberg, M. (1989) *Acta Physiol. Scand.* **136,** 507–517

[28] Van Riper, D. A. and Bevan, J. A. (1991) *Circ. Res.* **68,** 568–577.

Chapter 6

Putative Transmitters
In Cerebral Neurogenic Vasodilation

Tony J.-F. Lee

The presence of a vasodilator innervation of the cerebral blood vessels from several species is well established. The exact functional role of these nerves and the nature of transmitters for vasodilation, however, remain undetermined.

The discovery of endothelium-derived nitric oxide (EDNO) has led to the conclusion that NO or a related substance may play a role in cerebral neurogenic vasodilation. Although dense cholinergic and several peptidergic vasodilator nerves are present in cerebral blood vessels, growing evidence indicates that nitric oxidergic nerves may play a predominant role. This communication is centered on recent advances in understanding the synaptic transmission mechanism for cerebral neurogenic vasodilation.

Evidence for the Presence of Vasodilator Nerves

The anatomy and physiology of a vasodilator innervation to the cranial circulation have been demonstrated in some detail for more than 60 yr.[1-4] Results from ultrastructural studies also have provided evidence that cerebral blood vessels are innervated by nonsympathetic vasodilator nerves.[2,5] In vitro pharmacological studies have demonstrated that transmural nerve stimulation (TNS) results in vasodilation of isolated cerebral arteries from several species.[6-11] Although the degree of TNS-induced relaxation is variable among regions and species,[6,9,11,12] it is positively correlated with

From *The Human Brain Circulation*, R. D. Bevan and J. A. Bevan, eds.
©1994 Humana Press

density of nonsympathetic vasodilator nerves.[5,13–16] These dilator fibers innervate mostly the large arteries at the base of the brain. Nerve density decreases as the vessels become smaller, and the vasodilator fibers are usually not seen on the small branches of pial vessels.[5,14,17–19]

Nonadrenergic, Noncholinergic Vasodilator Transmitter

Ample evidence has indicated the presence of cholinergic vasodilator innervation in cerebral blood vessels.[1,2,15,17,19] The proposed role of acetylcholine (ACh) as the vasodilator transmitter, however, has been questioned. This was based on the pharmacological studies in isolated cerebral blood vessels that the TNS-induced cerebral vasodilation was not blocked by atropine, nor was it affected by physostigmine.[6,9] Since similar results were found in cerebral arteries taken from superior cervical ganglionectomized animals, the vasodilator transmitter is therefore considered to be nonadrenergic and noncholinergic (NANC) in nature. This is further supported by results from electrophysiological studies in cat cerebral arteries[20] showing that perivascular nerve stimulation (with a single pulse) elicited transient-membrane hyperpolarizing response, i.e., inhibitory junction potential (IJP) was not affected by atropine (1 µm) and guanethidine (10 µm) (Fig. 1). Atropine and guanethidine at these concentrations have been shown to block the ACh-induced vasodilation and sympathetic nerve-elicited vasoconstriction, respectively.[8,9]

Bevan et al.,[15,16] however, have suggested a direct role for ACh in neurogenic vasodilation of the large cerebral arteries of the cat. A correlation was found between cholineacetyltransferase (ChAT) levels and the capacity of various cerebral and extracerebral arteries to dilate. It was also reported that a component of the TNS-induced dilator response was significantly reduced by atropine. The reason for the contradictory findings remains unclear. Evidence, however, has been presented to indicate that direct stimulation by ACh of smooth muscle cells results in constriction of intracranial arteries,[21,22] which is associated with an increase in phosphatidyl

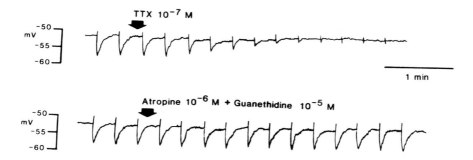

Fig. 1. Typical example of the effect of perivascular nerve stimulation on membrane potentials of cat cerebral vascular smooth muscle cells. Nerve stimulation evoked IJPs, but not EJPs. The IJPs were inhibited by tetrodotoxin (TTX) ($10^{-7}M$) (top), but not by atropine ($10^{-6}M$) and guanethidine ($10^{-5}M$) (bottom).[20]

inositide (PI) turnover.[23] These findings further argue against ACh as a vasodilator transmitter in cerebral arteries.[21]

Since ACh induces endothelium-dependent vasodilation,[21] the possibility remains that ACh transmitters may diffuse across the medial smooth muscle layers to reach the endothelial cells in sufficient concentration to release EDRF and therefore cause relaxation.[9] Although this indirect effect of ACh transmitter in inducing relaxation is unlikely, especially in large arteries, because of the wide distance between the nerve and the endothelium, removal of endothelial cells results in an enhanced relaxation on TNS in pig and cat cerebral arteries (Fig. 2).[8,9] Thus, in the large cerebral arteries, neuronal ACh is very unlikely to elicit an endothelium-mediated relaxation, but this possibility may be feasible in very small arteries or arterioles when fewer medial muscle layers interfere with diffusion of ACh from the adventitia to the intima. The adventitial cholinergic innervation in these distal blood vessels, however, is usually very sparse or not observed.[17,19,24] From a functional point of view, cholinergic nerves seem to play a more direct role in the large cerebral arteries, where they may act as vasoconstrictors.

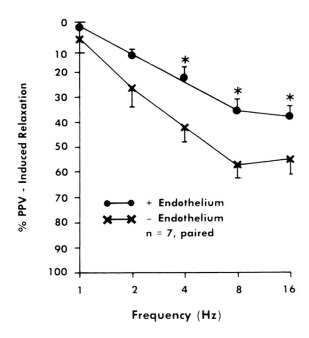

Fig. 2. Frequency–relaxation relationship of the cat cerebral arteries with (+) or without (–) endothelium to transmural nerve stimulation (TNS) at different frequencies (Hz) expressed as a percentage of maximum relaxation induced by papaverine (PPV, $3 \times 10^{-4}M$). The frequency-relaxation relationships were significantly greater at 4, 8, and 16 Hz (paired *t*-test) in arteries without endothelium than those with endothelium. Active muscle tone was induced by serotonin (5HT). Vertical bars represent standard errors. *n* = number of experiments. *$p < 0.05$.[9]

Cerebral Neurogenic Vasodilation is Predominantly Mediated by cGMP Synthesis

We have reported that cerebral neurogenic vasodilation is blocked by hemolysate preparations (membrane-free erythrocyte),[25] hemoglobin (Fig. 3),[26] and methylene blue.[27] Hemoglobin, which is the major component of hemolysate, and methylene blue have been shown to inhibit soluble guanylate cyclase.[28,29] Biochemical mea-

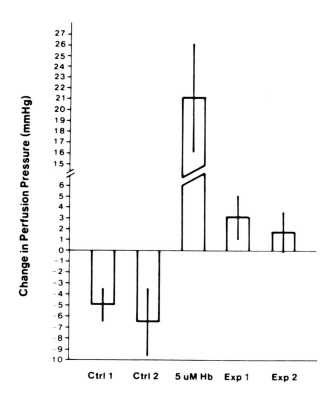

Fig. 3. Effect of hemoglobin (Hb) on perfused arterial preparations. Bars represent mean change in perfusion pressure in response to TNS or 5 μM hemoglobin. Uridine 5'-triphosphate (UTP) or serotonin (5HT) was added to the perfusate prior to TNS to develop active tone in the vessels. Two control relaxation responses to TNS were elicited (Ctrl 1 and Ctrl 2) and were followed by the addition of hemoglobin to the perfusate. The arterial response to 5 μM hemoglobin is indicated. Two responses (Exp. 1 and Exp. 2) were then elicited by TNS in the presence of hemoglobin ($n = 8$).[26]

surement of cyclic nucleotide content in porcine cerebral arteries reveals that both cGMP and cAMP contents were increased during TNS-induced maximum relaxation.[30] Cerebral neurogenic vaso-dilation in isolated preparations, however, was enhanced by block-ing cGMP phosphodiesterase with M&B 22948, but was not affected by blocking cAMP phosphodiesterase with cilostazol.[30] These results suggest that vasodilation of isolated cerebral arteries on TNS is predominantly mediated by cGMP. The increase in cAMP levels seems to play a minor role.

What Are the Dilator Transmitters in Cerebral Blood Vessels?

The variations in types and patterns of vasodilator innervation in cerebral circulation in different regions and species are well recognized.[6,8,10,11,13] The presence of multiple vasodilator transmitters in cerebral circulation has been suggested.[17] Isolated preparations, therefore, provide advantages in examining the nature of the vasodilator transmitters in strategically selected arteries. Accordingly, most published data concerning the nature of vasodilator transmitters were obtained from cerebral arteries of large animals, such as the rabbit, cat, dog, pig, and sheep.[6,8,10,11,13]

As already stated, criteria for a primary vasodilator transmitter in cerebral arteries may include (1) that the potential transmitters should directly relax cerebral smooth muscle—a candidate substance, which induces relaxation only by indirect mechanisms, such as the endothelium-dependent relaxation, is not a primary vasodilator transmitter—and (2) that the primary vasodilator transmitter predominantly increases cGMP synthesis. Accordingly, results from morphological and pharmacological studies of potential transmitters for cerebral vasodilation and constriction are summarized in Fig. 4.

"Purinergic" Transmitter

In isolated vascular preparation, ATP induces endothelium-dependent vasodilation and constriction in arteries without endothelial cells.[31] Similar results were found in cerebral arteries (Lee, unpublished data), suggesting that ATP, like ACh, is not a primary vasodilator transmitter, but acts more like a vasoconstrictor transmitter. Indeed, there is strong evidence that ATP is released from sympathetic nerves to induce constriction of peripheral and cerebral arteries from several species, including humans.[32,33,34]

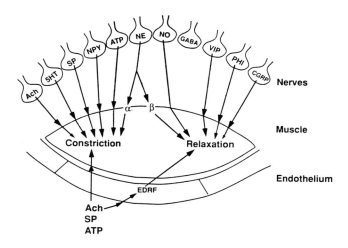

Fig. 4. A schematic illustration of the neurovascular relationship in cerebral arteries. ACh, serotonin (5HT), substance P (SP), neuropeptide Y (NPY), adenosine triphosphate (ATP), and norepinephrine (NE, α action) directly constrict vascular smooth muscle. ACh, SP, and ATP induce vasodilation indirectly by releasing endothelium-derived relaxing factor (EDRF). Nitric oxide (NO), VIP, PHI, CGRP, and NE (β action) directly relax vascular smooth muscle. The potential role of GABA as a transmitter or modulator remains to be clarified.

Peptidergic Innervation

Cerebral blood vessels from various species receive dense vasoactive intestinal polypeptide (VIP)-, peptide histidine isoleucine (PHI)-, and calcitonin gene-related peptide (CGRP)-immunoreactive (I) fibers.[20,35,36–40] Evidence for VIP as a potential vasodilator transmitter in cerebral circulation has been presented. This includes the presence of VIP immunoreactivities in nonsympathetic axonal granular vesicles,[41] the release of neuronal VIP on TNS,[42] the presence of VIP receptors on cerebral vascular smooth muscle cells,[43] activation of these receptors resulting in endothelium-independent vasodilation in vivo and in vitro,[35,41,44–46] and blockade of transmural nerve stimulation (TNS)-induced vasodilation by VIP antiserum.[47] PHI is also a potential vasodilator transmitter. It induces an endothelium-independent relaxation of cerebral arteries.[37] PHI and VIP are fragments of the same precursor molecule, prepro-VIP,[48] and have 13 amino acid residues in identical position.[49] VIP-I and PHI-I fibers have an identical distribution pattern in cerebral blood vessels.[37]

Exogenously applied CGRP also induces a potent cerebral vasodilator response that is independent of the endothelium. After depletion of endogenous CGRP with capsaicin, both TNS-induced vasodilation and inhibitory junction potential (IJP) were attenuated. These results suggest that CGRP or the trigeminal nerve is involved in the TNS-induced vasodilator responses of the cerebral arteries.[20]

Evidence against VIP, PHI, and CGRP as the dilator transmitters in cerebral blood vessels, however, has been presented. VIP-induced vasodilation in the cat cerebral artery was suggested to be mediated by prostaglandin synthesis.[45] The TNS-induced vasodilation of isolated cerebral arteries from several species, however, was not affected by blocking prostaglandin synthesis.[7,50] VIP-receptor antagonists, (Tyr^1, D-Phe^2) GRF (1-29)-NH$_2$ and (D-P-chloro Phe^6, Leu^{17}) VIP, blocked exogenous VIP-induced dilation of isolated cerebral arteries, but failed to affect the TNS-induced relaxation in the same preparation.[27] When cerebral arteries developed significant tachyphylaxis to dilator responses on repeated application of VIP, PHI, and CGRP, TNS-induced relaxation in the same preparation remained unchanged.[11,20,27,37] An alternative interpretation of this negative evidence is that VIP, PHI, and CGRP play a very small role in neurogenic dilation in cerebral blood vessels. It has been shown that TNS-induced cerebral vasodilation is predominantly accompanied by an increase in cGMP synthesis. Also, cAMP content was significantly enhanced during TNS-induced maximum relaxation.[30] Cerebral vasodilations induced by VIP, PHI, and CGRP have been shown to be accompanied by an increase in cAMP synthesis.[23,27,30,51,52] This finding suggests that the increase in vascular cAMP content during TNS-induced maximum relaxation is very likely owing to release of endogenous VIP, CGRP, and/or PHI. Thus, failure to affect the vascular tone following blocking cAMP-dependent phosphodiesterase[30] suggests that VIP, CGRP, and PHI may play a role, although small under in vitro conditions, in neurogenic vasodilation in cerebral blood vessels.

Other Neuropeptides

There is evidence that substance P (SP) and neurokinin A (NKA) relax cerebral arteries.[53,54] The dilator response, however, is dependent on endothelial cells.[41,55] This finding suggests that SP or other tachykinins, such as NKA and neurokinin B (NKB), like ACh, are not primary vasodilator transmitters in cerebral arteries.[41] Several other neuropeptides, such as neurotensin,[56] cholecystokinin (CCK),[57] dynorphin B,[58,59] and galanin,[60] have been demonstrated in cerebral blood vessels. These peptides, however, failed to exert any significant vascular effect in vitro or *in situ*.[59,61–63] The transmitter role of GABA[64] is not determined either.

Nitric Oxidergic Innervation

Pharmacological Evidence

Endothelium-mediated dilation in cerebral arteries is well established.[21] The characteristics of endothelium-mediated relaxation and those induced by TNS are found to be very similar.[12,26,29,65] Both are associated with an increase in vascular cGMP synthesis, and are blocked by hemoglobin (Fig. 3) and NO synthase inhibitors[66–68] (Fig. 5). These results suggest that NO or a NO-related substance may be the principal mediator for vasodilation-induced by TNS. In ring preparations of porcine cerebral arteries without endothelial cells, TNS-induced relaxations were blocked by Nw-nitro-L-arginine (NLA; to 30 μM). At $10^{-5}M$, NLA blocked 90% of the dilator response induced by TNS at 4 Hz and 75% of the response at 8 Hz 30 min after its application. In parallel studies, NLA at 30 μM converted the TNS-induced relaxation to vasoconstriction in some cerebral arteries in the absence of guanethidine.[68] This result suggests that NLA blocks neurogenic vasodilation and unmasks neurogenic vasoconstriction in these particular segments of arteries. Furthermore, the blockade of neurogenic vasodilation at 4 and 8 Hz by NLA was completely reversed 15 min after administration of L-arginine, but not D-arginine. These results indicate that NO or an NO-releasing substance mediates a major component of the NANC neurogenic vasodilation in porcine cerebral arteries.[68] Similar results were obtained in cat[69] and dog.[66,70]

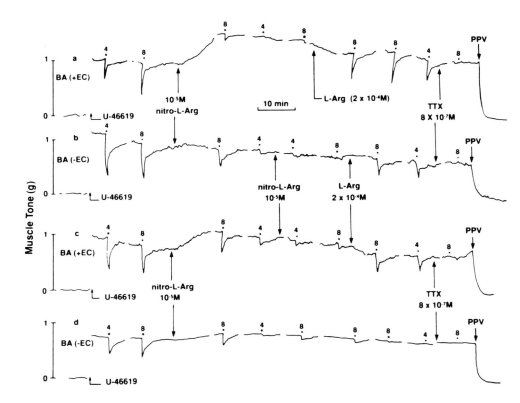

Fig. 5. Evidence for the involvement of NO or an NO-releasing substance in NANC neurogenic vasodilation in basilar arteries (BA) of the pig. In the presence of guanethidine ($3 \times 10^{-7}M$) and atropine ($10^{-6}M$) and in the presence of active muscle tone induced by U-46619, TNS at 4 and 8 Hz induced vasodilations in arteries with (+EC) **(A,C)** or without (−EC) **(B,D)** endothelial cells. Nw-nitro-L-arginine (nitro-L-Arg; 10^{-5}–$2 \times 10^{-5}M$), which increased basal tone in arteries with intact endothelial cells (A,C), but did not effect that in arteries without endothelial cells (B,D), significantly blocked the neurogenic vasodilation. The blockade became greater with time (D) and was reversed by L-arginine (L-Arg) (A–C). L-Arg also decreased the rise in tone induced by nitro-L-Arg in the artery with endothelial cells (A,C) to the original level, but did not affect that in the artery without endothelial cells (B). The degree of reversal by L-Arg depends on the concentration of nitro-L-Arg in the bath; the reversal is almost complete within 15 min in the artery receiving $10^{-5}M$ nitro-L-Arg (A), but is only partial in the artery pretreated with $2 \times 10^{-5}M$ nitro-L-Arg (B,C). In (D), the blockade of neurogenic vasodilation by one application of $10^{-5}M$ nitro-L-Arg persisted throughout the

Chemical Properties of the NANC Vasodilator Transmitters

The biological properties of both NO and vasodilating substance released on TNS in porcine cerebral arteries were examined using a superfusion bioassay cascade method.[71] Porcine pial arteries were used as donor tissue and two rabbit aortic rings as detector tissues. In the presence of adrenergic and cholinergic receptor antagonists, transmural nerve stimulation (TNS) of the denuded cerebral arteries resulted in a frequency-dependent relaxation of the denuded rabbit aortic rings, which were precontracted with phenylephrine. The relaxation of the aortic rings was consistently abolished by tetrodotoxin (TTX) superfused onto the cerebral arteries and by cold-storage denervation of the cerebral arteries. Relaxation was also significantly inhibited by NLA superfused onto the cerebral arteries. This inhibition was reversed by L-arginine, but not D-arginine, a result similar to that found in the ring preparations.[68] These results further support the hypothesis that a vasodilating factor of neuronal origin in the cerebral arteries was released on TNS to relax the aortic rings.

Exogenously applied NO directly onto the cerebral arteries also induced dilations of the aortic rings in a concentration-dependent manner. The transient dilations of the aortic rings induced by the vasodilating factor and by exogenous NO were completely blocked by hemoglobin (Hb) and were markedly enhanced by superoxide dismutase (SOD). Moreover, the relaxations of rabbit aortic rings induced by both the vasodilating factor and NO had similar time-courses and declined to the same extent down the cascade, indicating that the NANC vasodilating factor and NO possess a similar labile nature and half-life. This result further supports the conclusion that the vasodilating factor or transmitter is NO or a related substance.

Physiological Concentration of NO Released on TNS

Using a similar bioassay method as that described above, the frequency–response curves of TNS (2–16 Hz) and concentration–response curves of NO (10–1000 nM) for relaxations in aortic rings were found to be identical.[71] This result suggests that lower than 1

---

entire experiment (3h). The residual vasodilator responses on TNS were abolished by tetrodotoxin (TTX). All four preparations were adjacent segments from the same animal. PPV: $3 \times 10^{-4}M$; U-46619: $3 \times 10^{-8}M$.[68]

µM of NO was released from the cerebral arteries on TNS at the maximal frequency used. This study demonstrated that NO or an NO-releasing molecule in physiological concentrations was released resulting in neurogenic vasodilation of porcine cerebral arteries (Fig. 6).

Neuronal Origin of NO or Related Substance

Morphological evidence for the presence of authentic nitric oxidergic (NOergic) vasodilator fibers in the cerebral circulation was first reported by Bredt et al.[24] These authors demonstrated the presence of nitric oxide synthase (NOS) immunoreactivities in adventitia, presumably in association with advential neuronal structures in cerebral arteries of the rat. NADPH-diaphorase has been suggested to be identical to NOS.[72] NADPH-diaphorase-containing fibers and ganglionic cells were found in cerebral arteries of the cat (Fig. 7), rat, and rabbit (Lee et al., preliminary study), which further supports the presence of nitric oxidergic fibers in cerebral blood vessels. The presence of adventitial ganglionic cells suggests that some NOergic nerves may originate in intrinsic neurons. These prominent neural localizations of NOS and NADPH-diaphorase provide evidence for a strong association of NO with cerebral vasodilator nerves. This is consistent with results from pharmacological studies that Hb abolished the TNS-induced neurogenic vasodilation.[12,26] Since Hb is not likely to cross the cell membrane because of its large molecular weight, blockade of NANC nerve stimulation-induced vasodilation in isolated cerebral blood vessels by Hb is most likely the result of its "trapping" the extracellular or synaptic NO.[30] This result argues for the possible release of neuronal NO or an NO-related molecule into the synaptic regions and subsequently to induce relaxation of the smooth muscle cells (Fig. 6).

Since NO is unstable and highly lipid soluble, and neurogenic vasodilation is blocked immediately following inhibiting synthesis of NO,[68] the vesicular storage of NO transmitters is debatable. However, the calcium dependency of the neuronal NOS[73] is consistent with the accepted hypothesis that transmitter release is dependent on neuronal influx of calcium. It appears that NOS is activated, and NO is synthesized and released when the NOergic nerves are activated.

Possible Extraneuronal Source
of NO in Cerebral Neurogenic Vasodilation

It has been reported that in sheep cerebral arteries, relaxation induced by exogenously applied vasoactive intestinal polypeptide (VIP) was inhibited by NO synthesis inhibitor L-N^G-monomethyl arginine (L-NMMA) and Hb.[74] These authors suggest that neuronal VIP, on release into the synapses, may initiate release of NO from its site of action. This is not impossible, since each VIP molecule contains two arginine amino acids.[75] This result implies that NO can be generated extraneuronally and extracellularly (since Hb traps only extracellular NO). In porcine and feline pial arteries, however, VIP-induced relaxation is not affected by NLA at concentrations (>30 μM) that abolish TNS-induced relaxation in the same preparations.[76] Although species variation cannot be ruled out, Thomas and Ramwell[77] reported that the inhibitory effect of L-NMMA on VIP-induced relaxation may be attributed to the antagonistic effect of L-NMMA on cytoplasmic cAMP receptors. Furthermore, freshly dissected porcine and feline cerebral arteries without endothelial cells do not respond to L-arginine or NLA following 2 h of incubation in the Krebs solution.[68,69,78] This finding does not support the notion that NO of the myo origin is mediating cerebral neurogenic vasodilation under normal condition.

Gonzalez and Estrada[67] reported that neurogenic vasodilation in bovine cerebral arteries was mediated by endothelium-derived NO based on the observation that TNS-induced relaxation was abolished by denuding the endothelium. An indirect release of NO from endothelial cells to induce vasodilation in response to an unidentified neuronal substance on TNS was therefore postulated by these authors. Denuding endothelial cells in cerebral arteries from several other species, however, did not block the TNS-induced relaxation. On the contrary, removal of endothelial cells has been shown to enhance TNS-induced vasodilation in the cat and pig pial arteries.[5,8] The possible species difference in defining cerebral neurogenic vasodilation cannot be ruled out. However, as has been described earlier, a sufficient concentration of neural transmitters at the endothelial cells following diffusion across a wide vessel wall may be difficult to achieve, especially in large arteries.[9]

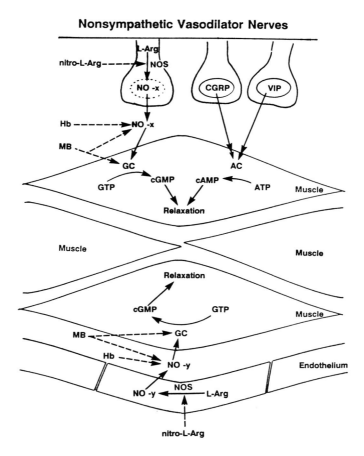

Fig. 6. A simple schematic illustration of neuronal and endothelial nitric oxidergic vasodilator mechanism in cerebral blood vessel wall. There is good evidence that endothelium-derived relaxing factor (EDRF) is nitric oxide (NO) or an NO-releasing substance (NO-y), and the precursor from which it is synthesized is L-arginine (L-Arg). NO or NO-y induces vasodilation by activating soluble guanylate cyclase (GC), and its synthesis is blocked by arginine analogs, such as nitro-L-Arginine (nitro-L-Arg). Hemoglobin (Hb), which traps extracellular NO or NO-y, and methylene blue (MB), which inactivates NO-y and inhibits GC, also diminish the NO-y and endothelium-mediated relaxation. The synthesis of NO or NO-y in the endothelial cells is evidenced by the presence of nitric oxide synthase (NOS) in these cells. NOS-immunoreactive nerve fibers have also been demonstrated in the cerebral arteries, indicating the presence of NOergic innervation in this

Conclusion

Multiple NANC transmitters for vasodilation have been demonstrated in cerebral blood vessels. Among neural peptides, VIP, CGRP, and PHI are likely candidate transmitters for vasodilation, although evidence against their transmitter role has been presented. These peptides increase vascular cAMP synthesis and probably mediate a small component (<10%) of TNS-induced dilator response. Vasodilation in isolated cerebral arteries induced by TNS is predominantly associated with an increase in cGMP synthesis. Results from pharmacological experiments suggest that NO, which increases cGMP synthesis, mediates a major component (>90%) of TNS-induced vasodilator response in cerebral arteries from several species: The synthesizing enzyme for NO is present in perivascular nerves, inhibition of NO synthesis abolishes neurogenic vasodilation, release of NO-like substance using a perfusion cascade system can be detected following TNS, the time-course of dilator response induced by NO is identical to that induced by endogenous NANC transmitters, and drugs similarly inhibit (NLA) or potentiate (superoxide dismutase) the action of NO and the endogenous NANC dilator transmitter. These results support the conclusion that NO or an NO-releasing substance is released from the NOergic nerves to act as a vasodilator transmitter and that NOergic nerves may play a predominant role in neurogenic vasodilation. The exact role of NOergic nerves in regulating cerebral circulation in vivo, however, remains to be determined. The origins of NOergic

---

vasculature. NO or a NO-related substance (NO-x) released from these nerves appears to play a major role in cerebral neurogenic vasodilation, which is mediated by an increase in cGMP synthesis and is nearly abolished by Hb, MB, and nitro-L-Arg. Cerebral blood vessels also receive perivascular neurons containing calcitonin gene related peptide (CGRP), vasoactive intestinal polypeptides (VIP), and peptide histidine isoleucine (not shown). These peptides, however, induce vasodilation by activating adenylate cyclase (AC) and, therefore, increasing synthesis of cAMP. Since cAMP plays a minor role in cerebral neurogenic vasodilaton, the role of these peptides as cerebral vasodilator transmitters remains to be established. The possibility that CGRP and VIP induce relaxation by releasing NO remains to be clarified. —————— Activation, – – – – – – inhibition.

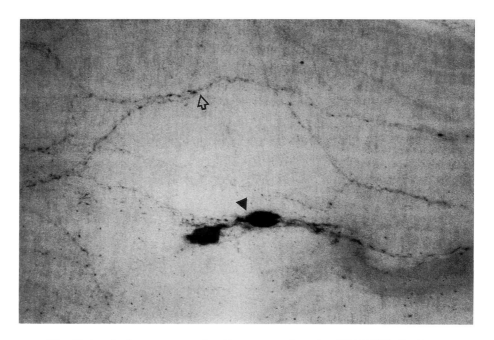

Fig. 7. A whole-mount cat basilar artery showing NADPH-diaphorase-containing fibers (arrow) and ganglionic cells (arrow head). Tissue was fixed by immersion in 4% paraformaldehyde in 0.1M phosphate buffer according to the modified methods of Hope et al.[72] ×200.

nerves like other vasodilator nerves remain to be identified. Evidence presented, however, suggests that some NOergic nerve fibers may originate in intrinsic neurons.

Acknowledgments

This work was supported by grants from NIH (HL27763), American Heart Association (91010850), and SIU SM. We thank Sue Sarwinski for technical assistance and Valerie Beard for typing the manuscript.

References

[1] Forbes, H. S. and Wolff, H. G. (1928) *Arch. Neurol. Psychiat.* **19,** 1057–1080.
[2] Owman, C., Edvinsson, L., and Nielsen, K. C. (1974) *Blood Vessels* **11,** 2–31.

[3] Suzuki, N., Hardebo, J. E., Kahrstrom, J., and Owman, C. H. (1990) *J. Cereb. Blood Flow Metab.* **10**, 383–391.

[4] Seylaz, J., Hara, H., Pinard, E., Mraovitch, S., Mackenzie, E. T., and Edvinsson, L. (1988) *J. Cereb. Blood Flow Metab.* **8**, 875–878.

[5] Lee, T. J.-F. (1981) *Cerebral Blood Flow: Effect of Nerves and Neurotransmitters* (Heistad, D. D. and Marcus, M. L., eds.), Elsevier, North Holland, pp. 431–439.

[6] Lee, T. J.-F., Su, C., and Bevan, J. A. (1975) *Experientia* **31**, 1424–1425.

[7] Lee, T. J.-F., Hume, W. R., Su, C., and Bevan, J. A. (1978) *Circ. Res.* **42**, 535–542.

[8] Lee, T. J.-F., Kinkead, L., and Sarwinski, S. (1982) *J. Cereb. Blood Flow Metab.* **2**, 439–450.

[9] Lee, T. J.-F. (1982) *Circ. Res.* **50**, 870–879.

[10] Duckles, S. P. (1979) *Circ. Res.* **44**, 482–490.

[11] Toda, N. (1982) *Am. J. Physiol.* **243**, H145–H153.

[12] Lee, T. J.-F. (1986) *Neural Regulation of Brain Circulation* (Owman, C. and Hardebo, J. E., eds.), Elsevier, Amsterdam, pp. 285–296.

[13] Lee, T. J.-F., Chiueh, C. C., and Adams, M. (1980) *Eur. J. Pharmacol.* **61**, 55–70.

[14] Lee, T. J.-F. and Saito, A. (1984) *Circ. Res.* **55**, 392–403.

[15] Bevan, J. A., Buga, G. M., Florence, V. M., Gonsalves, A., and Snowden, A. (1982) *Circ. Res.* **48(4)**, 470–476.

[16] Bevan, J. A., Buga, G. M., Jope, C. A., Jope, R. S., and Moritoki, H. (1982) *Circ. Res.* **51(4)**, 421–429.

[17] Lee, T. J.-F. (1985) *Trends in Autonomic Pharmacology* vol. 3 (Kalsner, S., ed.), pp. 187–202.

[18] Edvinsson, L. (1985) *TINS March* 126–131.

[19] Saito, A., Wu, J. Y., and Lee, T. J.-F. (1985) *J. Cereb. Blood Flow Metab.* **5**, 327–344.

[20] Saito, A., Masaki, T., Uchiyama, Y., Lee, T. J.-F., and Goto, K. (1989) *J. Pharmacol. Exp. Ther.* **248**, 455–462.

[21] Lee, T. J.-F. (1980) *Eur. J. Pharmacol.* **68**, 393–394.

[22] Linnik, M. D. and Lee, T. J.-F. (1992) *Chinese J. Pharmacol. Toxicol.* **6**, 19–28.

[23] Miao, F. J.-P. and Lee, T. J.-F. (1991) *J. Cardiovasc. Pharmacol.* **18**, 369–378.

[24] Bredt, D. S., Hwang, P. M., and Snyder, S. (1990) *Nature* **347**, 768–770.

[25] Lee, T. J.-F., McIlhany, M. P., and Sarwinski, S. (1984) *J. Cereb. Blood Flow and Metab.* **4**, 474–476.

[26] Linnik, M. D. and Lee, T. J.-F. (1989) *J. Cereb. Blood Flow Metab.* **9**, 219–225.

[27] Lee, T. J.-F. (1987) *Peptidergic Mechanisms in the Cerebral Circulation* (Edvinsson, L. and McCulloch, J., eds.), Ellis Horwood, Weinheim, pp. 65–74.

²⁸ Gruetter, C. A., Kadowitz, P. F., and Ignarro, L. (1981) *Can. J. Physiol. Pharmacol.* **59,** 150–156.

²⁹ Martin, W., Villani, G. M., Jothianandan, D., and Turchgott, R. F. (1985) *J. Pharmacol. Exp. Ther.* **232,** 708–716.

³⁰ Lee, T. J.-F., Fang, Y. X., and Nickols, G. A. (1989) *Neurotransmission and Cerebrovascular Function* (Seylaz, J. and MacKenzie, E. T., eds.), Elsevier, Amsterdam, pp. 277–280.

³¹ Mathie, R. T., Ralevic, V., Alexander, B., and Burnstock, G. (1991) *Br. J. Pharmacol.* **103,** 1602–1606.

³² Sneedon, P. and Burnstock, G. (1985) *Eur. J. Pharmacol.* **106,** 149–152.

³³ Muramatsu, I. and Kogoshi, S. (1987) *Br. J. Pharmacol.* **92,** 901–908.

³⁴ Taddei, S., Pedrinelli, R., and Salvetti, A. (1990) *Circ. Res.* **82,** 2061–2067.

³⁵ Duckles, S. P. and Said, S. I. (1982) *Eur. J. Pharmacol.* **78,** 371–374.

³⁶ Edvinsson, L., Fahrenkrug, J., Hanko, J., Owman, C., Sundler, F., and Uddman, R. (1980) *Cell Tissue Res.* **208,** 135–142.

³⁷ Edvinsson, L. and McCulloch, J. (1985) *Regul. Peptides* **10,** 345–356.

³⁸ Gibbins, I. L., Brayden, J. E., and Bevan, J. A. (1984) *Neuroscience* **13,** 1327–1346.

³⁹ Larsson, L.-I., Edvinsson, L., Fahrenkrug, J., Hakanson, R., Owman, C., Schaffalitzky de Muckadel, O. B., and Sundler, F. (1976) *Brain Res.* **113,** 400–404.

⁴⁰ Tsai, S.-H., Tew, J. M., McLean, J. H., and Shipley, M. T. (1988) *J. Comp. Neurol.* **271,** 435–444.

⁴¹ Lee, T. J.-F., Saito, A., and Beresin, I. (1984) *Science* **224,** 898–901.

⁴² Bevan, J. A. and Brayden, J. E. (1986) *Neural Regulation of Brain Circulation* (Owmand, C. and Hardebo, J. E., eds.), Elsevier, Amsterdam, pp. 383–391.

⁴³ Suzuki, Y., McMaster, D., Huang, M., Lederis, K., and Rorstad, O. P. (1985) *J. Neurochem.* **45,** 89–899.

⁴⁴ Heistad, D. D., Marcus, M. D., Said, S. I., and Gross, P. M. (1980) *Am. J. Physiol.* **239,** H73–H89.

⁴⁵ Wei, E. P., Raper, A. J., and Kontos, H. A. (1975) *Stroke* **6,** 654–658.

⁴⁶ Wilson, D. A., O'Neill, J. T., Said, S. I., and Traystman, R. J. (1981) *Circ. Res.* **48,** 138–148.

⁴⁷ Bevan, J. A., Moskowitz, M., Said, S. I., and Buga, G. (1984) *Peptides* **5,** 385–388.

⁴⁸ Hoh, N., Obata, K., Yanaihara, N., and Okamoto, H. (1983) *Nature* **304,** 547–549.

⁴⁹ Tatemoto, K. and Mutt, V. (1981) *Proc. Natl. Acad. Sci. USA* **78,** 6603–6607.

⁵⁰ Winquist, R. J., Webb, R. C., and Bohr, D. F. (1982) *Circ. Res.* **51,** 769–776.

⁵¹ Edvinsson, L., Fredholm, B. B., Hamel, E., Jansen, I., and Verrecchia, C. (1985) *Neurosci. Lett.* **58,** 213–217.

⁵² Huang, M. and Rorstad, O. P. (1983) *J. Neurochem.* **40,** 719–726.

53 Dalsgaard, C.-J., Haegerstrand, A., Theodorsson-Norheim, E., Brodin, E., and Hökfelt, T. (1985) *Histochemistry* **83**, 37–39.

54 Edvinsson, L., Brodin, E., Jansen, I., and Uddman, R. (1988) *Regul. Peptides* **20**, 181–197.

55 Edvinsson, L. and Jansen, I. (1987) *Br. J. Pharmacol.* **90**, 553–559.

56 Chan-Palay, V. (1977) *Neurogenic Control of Brain Circulation* (Owman, C. and Edvinsson, L., eds.), Pergamon, Oxford, pp. 39–53.

57 Liu-Chen, L.-Y., Norregaard, T. V., and Moskowitz, M. (1985) *Brain Res.* **359**, 166–176.

58 Moskowitz, M. A., Brezina, L. R., and Kuo, C. (1986) *Cephalalgia* **6**, 81–86.

59 Moskowitz, M. A., Saito, K., Brezna, L., and Dickson, J. (1987) *Neurosci.* **23**, 731–737.

60 Uddman, R. (1987) *Peptidergic Mechanisms in the Cerebral Circulation* (Edvinsson, L. and McCulloch, J., eds.), Ellis Horwood, Chichester, pp. 15–23.

61 McCulloch, J. and Kelly, P. A. T. (1984) *J. Cereb. Blood Flow Metab.* **4**, 625–628.

62 Uddman, R., Edvinsson, L., Owman, C., and Sundler, F. (1983) *J. Cereb. Blood Flow Metab.* **3**, 386–390.

63 Wagner, F. and Wahl, M. (1986) *Arch. Int. Pharmacodyn. Ther.* **282**, 240–251.

64 Imai, I., Okuno, T., Wu, J. Y., and Lee, T. J.-F. (1991) *J. Cereb. Blood Flow Metab.* **11**, 129–134.

65 Ignarro, W., Buga, G. M., Wood, K. S., Byrns, R. E., and Chaudhuri, G. (1987) *Proc. Natl. Acad. Sci. USA* **84**, 9265–9269.

66 Toda, N., Minami, Y., and Okamura, T. (1990) *Life Sci.* **47**, 345–351.

67 Gonzalez, C. and Estrada, C. (1991) *J. Cereb. Blood Flow Metab.* **11**, 366–370.

68 Lee, T. J.-F. and Sarwinski, S. (1991) *Blood Vessels* **28**, 407–412.

69 Lee, T. J.-F., Sarwinski, S., and Chen, F. Y. (1991) *J. Cereb. Blood Flow Metab.* **11**, 5264.

70 Toda, N. and Okamura, T. (1991) *J. Pharmacol. Exp. Ther.* **258**, 1027–1032.

71 Chen, F. Y. and Lee, T. J.-F. (1993) *J. Pharmacol. Exp. Ther.* **265**, 339–345.

72 Hope, B. T., Michael, G. J., Knigge, K. M., and Vincent, S. R. (1991) *Proc. Natl. Acad. Sci. USA* **88**, 2811–2814.

73 Knowles, R. G., Palacios, M., Palmer, R. M. J., and Moncada, S. (1989) *Proc. Natl. Acad. Sci. USA* **86**, 5159–5162.

74 Gaw, A. J., Aberdeen, J., Humphrey, P. P. A., Wadsworth, R. M., and Burnstock, G. (1991) *Br. J. Pharmacol.* **102**, 567–572.

75 Moncada, S., Palmer, R. M. J., and Higgs, E. (1991) *Pharmacol. Rev.* **43**, 109–142.

76 Lee, T. J.-F. and Sarwinski, S. (1993) *FASEB J.* **7**, A529.

77 Thomas, G. and Ramwell, P. W. (1992) *J. Pharmacol. Exp. Ther.* **260**, 676–679.

78 Ueno, M. and Lee, T. J.-F. (1993) *J. Cereb. Blood Flow Metab.* **13**, 712–719.

Chapter 7

Is There a Neurogenic Influence on the Diameter of Human Small Pial Arteries?

Rosemary D. Bevan, John T. Dodge,
Theresa Wellman, Carrie L. Walters,
and John A. Bevan

In vitro studies of neural influences on cerebral arteries have for the most part been carried out on segments of the basilar artery, the Circle of Willis, or the origins of the major cerebral arteries (for example, refs. 1–4). In both animals and humans, constriction on electrical activation of intramural nerves has been observed, whereas dilation has been demonstrated only in nonhuman species. The relative size of neurogenic dilator and constrictor effects, and the variety of putative neurotransmitters and mechanisms, are remarkably different between species.[4–6]

There are several reasons for questioning if the demonstrated neural control of these large arteries and branches extends to the pial vessels. In the rabbit, the constrictor response of the middle cerebral artery (MCA) to perivascular nerve stimulation decreased with increasing branch order. The decrease in responsiveness was paralleled by the size of the contraction to norepinephrine (NE) and 5-hydroxytryptamine, but not histamine.[7] The conclusion to be drawn in this species is that pial artery caliber is probably not normally regulated by perivascular nerves. Quantitative morphometry of the same successive segments of the rabbit cerebral artery (J. Dodge, personal communication) showed that nerve density diminishes significantly in the more distal segments and confirms

From *The Human Brain Circulation*, R. D. Bevan and J. A. Bevan, eds.
©1994 Humana Press

early observations made in the cat[8] that there is a wide range of neuromuscular separation in cerebral pial arteries, with relatively few close contacts.[9]

The influence of the innervation on pial artery tone is not entirely of academic interest. The cerebrovascular innervation has been implicated in the pathophysiology of migraine and cluster headaches (*see also* Chapters 34 and 35),[10] and there is some evidence that the presence or absence of innervation may influence the severity of stroke.[11,12]

The more theoretical question has been raised concerning the role of perivascular nerves in a vascular bed that very effectively autoregulates.[13] In vivo studies suggest that neural control is only efficacious in influencing cerebral blood flow at the limits of autoregulation and then only to a modest degree in the normotensive.[14,15] Stimulation of the sympathetic nerves has relatively little influence on cerebral blood flow when arterial pressure is within normal limits.[16,17] In general, there is support for the conclusion that neural activity is unimportant for the integrated activity of the pial branching system that contributes significantly to the autoregulation of flow when blood pressure changes are not extreme. There are very effective intrinsic local regulating mechanisms, for example, the vascular wall response to changes in pressure and flow, that could account for the efficient regulation of pial caliber.

In this chapter, we will present results of studies of human pial arteries sent to the Totman Laboratory for Human Cerebrovascular Research from various neurosurgical centers. They suggest that perivascular constrictor nerves normally have a negligible influence on the tone of pial arteries. In our studies, the term pial refers to the small arteries on the surface of the cerebral cortex. Other investigators refer to the major arterial branches from the Circle of Willis as pial arteries. In the discussion we have changed their nomenclature to our designation of named major cerebral arteries, branches, and pial.

Experimental Methods

Ring segments of human pial artery (1.5–3.00 mm length) were mounted in a resistance artery myograph using two 20-μm OD tungsten wires (California Fine Wire Co., Grover Beach, CA) inserted through their lumen.[18] One was anchored to a support that could be moved with a micrometer to apply rest force and the other connected to a Minebea force displacement transducer (VL-10GR) for isometric recording of muscle tone. The preparation was submerged in a jacketed tissue bath containing physiologic salt solution (P.S.S.) at 37°C bubbled with either 95% O_2 and 5% CO_2 or 80% N_2, 15% O_2, 5% CO_2, and pH 7.4. Changes in force were recorded on a Soltec Model 1240 recorder. Optimal length for each size of vessel was defined by measuring the contractile response to 30 mM K^+ (equimolar substitution for NaCl in the P.S.S.), which produces a contraction that is 30–50% of tissue maximum applied at different tissue lengths. The length at which maximum active force developed was subsequently used for the balance of the experiment. Drugs were added directly to the bath in small volumes. Cumulative addition was utilized to obtain a concentration–response curve.

Transmural Electrical Field Stimulation (TEFS)

The important component of these experiments is the study of perivascular neural influences on vascular smooth muscle tone. Electrical stimulation of nerves, which are usually situated in the adventitia adjacent to the muscle layer in the artery wall, results in release of neurotransmitters, presumably by the initiation of action potentials. In a number of arteries of the rabbit and other species examined, the "nerve" response specifically identified by the change in tone of the blood vessel or by the release of labeled neurotransmitter is tetrodotoxin (TTX)-sensitive. It is possible to define the parameters of stimulation so that nerve activation can be achieved without changes in tone owing to direct electrical activation of other cell types, such as muscle or endothelium. The latter are TTX-insensitive. TTX is considered to block effectively and selectively neuronal conduction by blockade of the sodium channels in the axonal membrane.

Because the wall thickness of the pial arteries from different patients is not identical, the stimulation voltage for each segment studied was determined experimentally using standard frequencies of 8 and 16 Hz, pulse duration of 0.3 ms, and a train length of 60 s in the presence of TTX. Arterial segments were stimulated at 60 s intervals with increasing voltage until an increase in wall force was recorded. This is termed the breakthrough voltage and is the result of direct activation of nonneural cells, principally the smooth muscle. After TTX was washed out, the voltage was reduced by 1–2 V to ensure selective nerve activation. There is a possibility that this voltage is inadequate to activate all nerves. However, in a number of previous studies, the response elicited by the 1 or 2 V lower than breakthrough voltage was not significantly different from that obtained with 1–4 V higher, reduced by the TTX-insensitive component. There are theoretical reasons for not having complete reliance on this latter technique. The direct activation of smooth muscle cells by electrical pulses could change the response to the neurotransmitter. This, however, has never been demonstrated. Pial artery segments were stimulated at 8 and 16 Hz, pulse duration 0.3 ms, at the predetermined voltage until a maximum response was obtained with a train length of 60 s in the absence of a response, at 10-min intervals.

Catecholamine Histofluorescence

Segments of the pial arteries (2 mm) used for functional studies were opened and processed for examination of catecholaminergic histofluorescence of the perivascular nerves by the glyoxylic acid method,[19] with the addition of pontamine sky blue 0.5% w/v to mask nonspecific background associated with elastin fibers.

Experimental Results

Patient Population

Pial artery segments were obtained from patients between 15–66 yr of age (mean 44 yr). They were taken from normal cortical tissue, removed for access to tumors. The unstretched internal diameters measured between 300–800 μm (mean 530 μm). This chapter includes the result from 25 segments from 16 patients. Tissues were either studied the same day or held at 4°C in P.S.S. for study within 24 h.

Contractile Response
to Transmural Electrical Field Stimulation

In the pial arteries studied, with only two exceptions, no contractile response to TEFS was observed at either 8 or 16 Hz (Figs. 1 and 2). The neurogenic contractile response in the segments from two patients was extremely small, <2% of the maximum norepinephrine (NE) response. In 12 segments in which spontaneous or $PGF_{2\alpha}$-induced tone was present, no additional response to TEFS was seen.

Contractile Response to Norepinephrine

NE (10^{-8}–$10^{-5}M$) was added cumulatively to the tissue bath to obtain a concentration–response curve. The mean maximum response obtained from 15 patients was $13.46 \pm 1.63\%$ of the maximum contractile tissue response (Figs. 1 and 2). The NE ED_{50} was $3.82 \times 10^{-7}M \pm 0.08$, $n = 15$.

Maximum Force Development

At the end of the experiment, the segment was exposed to K^+ 127 mM followed by arginine vasopressin $10^{-6}M$. Responses to NE were normalized by expressing them in relation to this maximum response.

Catecholamine Histofluorescence

The fluorescence of catecholamine-containing nerve processes and varicosities was clearly defined, but there was great variation in their density in segments from different patients. The majority of the segments were pial arteries from the distribution of the MCA, so we do not know if there is a difference in the major cerebral arteries. In a few segments, no fibers were seen; a few had only one or two single fibers; others a variable mixture of fibers in small nerve bundles and single fibers with varicosities. A segment of moderate density is illustrated in Fig. 3. In an adjacent segment, no neurogenic constriction or dilation could be elicited. Endothelial function was well preserved in this artery.

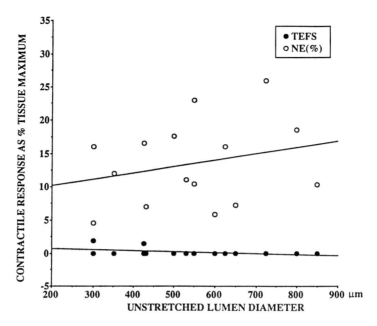

Fig. 1. Relationship between contractile response of segments of human pial arteries to L-norepinephrine ($10^{-5}M$) and to transmural electrical field stimulation (TEFS) expressed as percentage of maximum tissue response (K^+ 127 mM plus arginine vasopressin $10^{-6}M$), and the internal diameter of the unstretched segments (for details of TEFS, *see text*).

Discussion

The goal of this study was to determine if activation of the nerves in the adventitia of human pial arteries increased the tone of the vascular smooth muscle cells in the medial layer. Under the experimental conditions we employed, in 14 of 16 patients, no evidence was found that they did. In two patients, the response was minimal. This conclusion is consistent with the observed poor reactivity of these vessels to norepinephrine, the presumed major neurotransmitter released from the catecholamine-containing nerves visualized in the adventitia. It is also in agreement with a prior in vitro study of the human main middle cerebral artery (MCA) and branches taken within 6 h postmortem, when only a

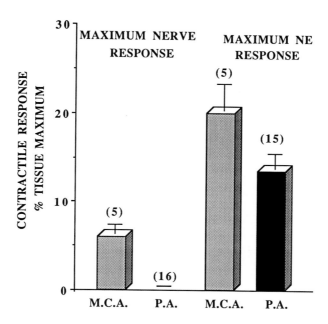

Fig. 2. Magnitude of maximum nerve response of segments of human middle cerebral artery (M.C.A.) and pial arteries (P.A.) elicited by transmural electrical field stimulation and to norepinephrine ($10^{-5}M$)—a maximally effective concentration, expressed as a percentage of tissue maximum (K^+ 127 mM and arginine vasopressin $10^{-6}M$); for nerve stimulation parameters, *see text*. Numbers in brackets refer to segments studied. Data for M.C.A. cited from ref. 4.

small (6%) neurogenic constriction was observed in the MCA.[4] In the rabbit, neurogenic responses were obtained from segments of the MCA taken at its origin from the circle of Willis, but not from branches several orders removed where reactivity was minimal.[7] Hardebo et al.,[20] using various stimulating paradigms causing neurogenic responses in peripheral arteries of cat, rabbit, and rat, have reported that they were unable to demonstrate a neurogenic response in pial arteries of humans and basilar and MCA arteries of cow, dog, cat, rabbit, and rat. The diameters of the human pial arteries they studied were between 300 and 600 μm OD, which is at the lower range of those we examined in the present study.

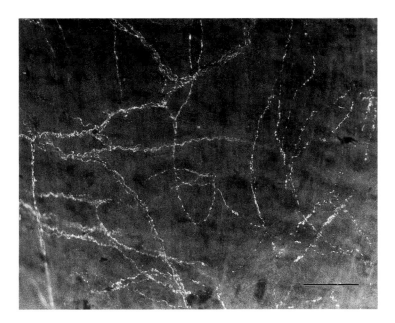

Fig. 3. Fluorescence micrograph of the adventitial surface of an opened human pial artery approx 750 μm internal diameter with a plexus of catecholamine-containing nerve fibers, some in small nerve bundles. Scale bar = 100 μm.

In contrast to human arteries from other sites,[21] attempts to activate vascular smooth muscle cells of the cerebral arteries by electrical stimulation of their perivascular nerves have proven difficult. Compared with animal research, there is a greater time interval between harvesting and study, and the tissues have been exposed to anesthetic and therapeutic agents. There are two reports of successful stimulation of perivascular nerves causing constriction. Shibata et al.[22] found TEFS induced constriction blocked by TTX or the nonspecific α-adrenergic antagonist phentolamine in two of four MCA segments tested. The stimulation parameters used were extremely high (80 V, 100 Hz), pulse duration was long (10 s), and only very small phasic contractions were produced. Edvinsson et al.[23] reported TEFS contraction of human adult pial arteries, illustrated by one frequency–response curve. The parameters used and the consistency of response are not detailed. Others have reported an inability to elicit contraction on TEFS in human arteries, either from the Circle of Willis[24] or from the pial surface.[19]

The parameters of nerve stimulation we used were biphasic pulses of 0.3 ms duration, frequency 8 and 16 Hz, and train length either until a maximum response was obtained or in its absence for 60 s using voltage determined by "breakthrough" values. The pulse duration and frequency are the stimulation characteristics demonstrated to activate perivascular nerves in other arteries in animals[15,25] and humans.[4] These stimulation parameters are blocked by TTX and do not cause changes in recorded wall force after sympathetic denervation. The selection of the pulse duration of 0.3 ms based on extensive prior measurements of animal blood vessels in vitro caused a maximum neurogenic response without concomitant direct muscle activation. In rabbit arteries, when longer pulse durations, for example, 2 ms, were used, a direct muscle response was obtained in addition. When this was small, the size of the TTX-sensitive component of the response at 2 ms was not different from that elicited by 0.3 ms alone. TEFS of 2 ms or greater in these human pial arteries caused a contraction that was not reduced by TTX and was detrimental to function. We did not employ the pattern of stimulation, simulating bursts of sympathetic activity, used by Hardebo,[26] which increased the neurogenic response by approx 50% in the rabbit ear artery and revealed a small phentolamine-resistant component. He did not reveal a neurogenic contractile response by this approach in the rabbit basilar and MCA (although in monkey basilar artery, a neurogenic tonic response was significantly increased with burst stimulation). His observation in the rabbit is not in agreement with others.[7,27,28] A possible reason for this difference is that Hardebo used only 10-s monophasic trains or bursts of pulses. The latency of the vasoconstrictor response in the rabbit following TEFS has been found to be considerably >10 s in the majority of blood vessels examined.[7] In our experiments, biphasic, square wave pulses were used.

Neurogenic cerebral artery constriction has been studied in most detail in the rabbit, and in this species, the constriction of the MCA is blocked only with the combination of phenoxybenzamine and NPY desensitization.[29] The presence of NPY in the perivascular innervation of human cerebral arteries has been observed by immunocytochemistry.[30] In the Duckworth study,[4] the small neurogenic response was entirely sensitive to phentolamine. It is possible that this peptide is rapidly lost in vitro. Hardebo,[28] measuring the fractional release of ^{14}C NE from a variety of vascular segments, found no difference between the major cerebral arteries of monkey and rat, rabbit basilar and ear arteries with stimulation for 3 min with 10 V at 0.3-ms impulse duration at 6 Hz. Only in the rabbit central ear artery was the release significantly increased with burst stimulation at 10 V. At 30 V, the mean release from the monkey arteries was only one-fifth to one-sixth that of the rabbit ear artery, whereas values for rat major cerebral and rabbit basilar were not different from the ear vessel. Human cerebral arteries were not studied. These findings, admittedly rather sparse, contain no reason to consider that the properties of catecholamine-containing nerves of pial arteries are functionally different from those of other blood vessels.

One feature of the adrenergic (and also nonadrenergic innervation) of cerebral arteries, as noted in cat[8] and rabbit,[9] is the wide range of separation of nerve varicosities with Schwann cell-free areas from the closest smooth muscle cells. Studies made in the peripheral circulation indicate that this separation diminishes with arterial diameter.[31] In the cerebral arteries examined, this distance is considerably greater than that of arteries from other regional beds of comparable size. For example, in the rabbit study,[9] comparisons were made of the distribution and density of innervation of comparable-sized ear and cerebral artery segments. The mean separation of nerve varicosities and nearest smooth muscle of segments of diameter 105–400 µm in the ear is 1.18 µm, and in the cerebral for equivalent segments, is 4.95 µm. Varicosities within 500 nm of the smooth muscle, which qualify for the designation "close neuromuscular contact," were 25% of the total in the ear and only 3% in the cerebral arteries. The latter were only found in the main MCA and first-order branch. Varicosity density per unit of adventitial-medial junction in all segments was similar if all the varicosities throughout the adventitial thickness were considered. However, the distribution in the adventitia was quite different. In the ear, the majority of varicosities were within 1–2 µm of the smooth muscle cells, but in the cerebral, they were distributed fairly evenly throughout the entire adventitial thickness of 10 μm. Within 1 μm, the density of varicosities is only one-sixth in the cerebral compared to that of the ear artery. In the cerebral, in contrast to the ear arteries, there is known to be a progressive diminution of response to TEFS with successive branching.[7] No comparable morphometric study has been made of the human pial arteries, but preliminary electromicroscopy of one section from each of nine pial arteries shows the innervation limited to the adventitia, the varicosity density low, and considerable nerve varicosity–muscle separation (J. Dodge, personal communication). These studies are being continued.

After release of the neurotransmitter, it must traverse the tissue space between the nerve and the smooth muscle cells of the tunica media. Human pial arteries do not show evidence of β-adrenoceptor-mediated relaxation and only contract to NE, an effect that is blocked by α-adrenoceptor antagonists, such as phentolamine. Thus, if an effect of sympathetic adrenergic nerve transmission were to be evident, it would be mediated through the α-adrenoceptor. Our results show that when there is no tone present, the maximum force development of the pial artery segments to NE is $13.46 \pm 1.63\%$ (mean $\pm$ SE) of the maximum force of which the tissue is capable. In human main MCA, the NE maximum response was only 20% of tissue maximum.[4] Other reports state that NE causes only a weak response of human and animal cerebral vessels.[30-37] Rose and Moulds[32] reported that the constriction to NE of large human cerebral vessels was 27.42% of that elicited by potassium chloride (80 mM), whereas in human digital arteries, this value was 136.77%. The rabbit main MCA shows a similar small response to NE, being only 25–30% of tissue maximum, and this falls progressively, so that by the second- and third-order branches, no response to NE can be elicited.

In the rabbit basilar artery, the α-adrenoceptor has a low affinity (pK_a 4.6) for NE,[36] and there is no receptor reserve. The maximum response is associated with complete receptor occupancy.[36,37] The inference is that responsiveness is limited by receptor number, and there is evidence based on agonist potency ratios that the α-adrenoceptor is not typically α_1 or α_2. Although the K_b for prazosin is the same as for other rabbit arteries, imidazolines are not effective agonists. There is some suggestion that there may be ineffective coupling between receptor occupation and response.[40,41] Parallel information is not available for the human.

To summarize, the low nerve density, wide neuromuscular separation, low sensitivity of the α-adrenergic receptor, and the possible weak coupling combined with absence of receptor reserve make the adrenergic innervation ineffectual in influencing tone in rabbit cerebral arteries. The human pial α-adrenoceptor is more sensitive, but it remains to be shown whether the other features are present in human pial arteries.

There is an experimental problem in demonstrating that a response is minimal or absent, especially when human tissues may be compromised during harvesting and have been exposed to anesthetic agents. It is unlikely that all human pial segments would be equally affected. We consider that our results are consistent with response patterns seen in animal studies not subject to these problems. The method of nerve excitation is indirect, but this technique has revealed neurogenic responses in human middle cerebral arteries (postmortem), and superficial temporal and omental arteries (unpublished results) obtained under comparable circumstances. Furthermore, the same experimental procedure has provided consistent responses from many different arteries of varied species, including animal cerebral vessels,[27,28] and has been utilized by a number of laboratories.

We have not yet investigated factors that could modify or inhibit neurogenic and NE-mediated constriction. We did not use blockers to eliminate neuronal and extraneuronal uptake of NE or eliminate the influence of the endothelium. One measure of endothelial function is the release of a relaxing factor(s) by acetylcholine. This response was very variable in the pial artery segments. Some of the patients had diseases, such as diabetes hypertension, or arteriosclerosis, that have been shown to impair endothelial function. It is possible that under some circumstances, such as partial depolarization of the smooth muscle cells by other vasoconstrictor agents, injury, or a change in the pH, potentiation of the NE response and the appearance of a neurogenic constrictor response could occur.

The absence of neurogenic effects is unlikely to be the result of the production of oxygen radicals that might exert an inhibitory effect on vascular smooth muscle, since this was observed by Lamb and Webb[42] only with prolonged field stimulation of up to 5 min. No significant difference in results has been detected with use of gas mixtures with different oxygen contents. It cannot be explained by concomitant activation of dilator nerves. Neurogenic dilator effects were not seen in the studies of Duckworth[4] and in these pial arteries after acute sympathetic denervation with guanethidine. When vascular tone was raised prior to TEFS, in 2 of the 25 segments, however, there was an extremely small dilation that was TTX-sensitive. We have no evidence of β-adrenoceptor activation, since isoproterenol failed to cause relaxation in these vessels after tone was raised (unpublished data). We have commented previously on the results of Hardebo et al.,[20] who obtained responses in many respects consistent with our own. However, our technique did reveal nerve activity in some arteries where they had reported its absence.

The cerebral arterial vasculature efficiently autoregulates, so it is of interest to speculate on the role of vasoconstrictor nerves apparently limited to the larger arteries. In vivo studies suggest that their function is to extend the limits of autoregulation.[45,46] This implies that they are important when arterial pressure is high or low. This is consistent with observations that stimulation of the sympathetic nervous system has little influence on cerebral blood flow.[1,14–16] when blood pressure is within normal levels. Certainly because of the location and distribution of the nerves around the larger cerebral arteries, the innervation would only be expected to have a generalized influence on the distribution of blood to the brain. Within the pial artery network outside the brain parenchyma, adjustments of flow would presumably occur by the action of local regulating mechanisms, such as intravascular pressure and flow. However, activation of the innervation of the cerebral circulation in some species under some circumstances has been observed to alter, although modestly, cerebral blood flow.[45,46] If our in vitro observations in humans and rabbits reflect what takes place in vivo, nerve activity would cause changes in caliber of the larger arteries leading to downstream changes in flow and pressure.

The function of the sympathetic nerves in the adventitia of pial arteries remains to be defined. They may have a trophic or metabolic influence on the cells in their vicinity. Their relevance to the cerebral circulation during growth and maturation is unknown.

Acknowledgments

Arteries were kindly supplied by Paul L. Penar and Carrie L. Walters. This work was supported by the Ray and Ildah Totman Medical Research.

References

[1] Lee, T. J. F., Su, C., Bevan, J. A. (1976) *Circ. Res.* **39**, 120–126.

[2] Lee, T. J. F. (1982) *Circ. Res.* **50**, 870–879.

[3] Duckles, S. P. (1979) *Circ. Res.* **44**, 482–490.

[4] Duckworth, J. W., Wellman, G. C., Walters, C. L., and Bevan, J. A. (1989) *Circ. Res.* **65(2)**, 316–324.

[5] Lee, T. J. F. (1986) *Neural Regulation of Brain Circulation* (Owman, C. and Hardebo, J. E., eds.), Elsevier, New York, pp. 285–296.

[6] Bevan, J. A. and Brayden, J. E. (1987) *Circ. Res.* **60(3)**, 309–326.

[7] Van Riper, D. A. and Bevan, J. A. (1991) *J. Pharmacol. Exp. Ther.* **257(2)**, 879–886.

[8] Lee, T. J. F. (1981) *Circ. Res.* **49**, 971–979.

[9] Dodge, J. T., Bevan, R. D., and Bevan, J. A. (1993) *Circ. Res.*, submitted for publication.

[10] Moskowitz, M. A. (1988) *Headache* **28**, 584–586.

[11] Sadoshima, S., Busija, D. W., and Heistad, D. D. (1983) *Am. J. Physiol.* **244** (*Heart Circ. Physiol.* **13**) H406–H412.

[12] Kano, M., Moskowitz, M. A., and Yokota, M. (1991) *J. Cereb. Blood Flow Metab.* **11**, 620–637.

[13] Bevan, J. A. and Bevan, R. D. (1993) *News in Physiol. Sci.* **8**, 149–153.

[14] Harper, A. M. (1975) *Cerebral Vascular Diseases* (Whisnant, J. P. and Sandok, B. A., eds.), Grune & Stratton, New York, pp. 27–35.

[15] Hernandez, M. J., Raichle, M. E., and Stone, H. L. (1977) *Neurogenic Control of the Brain Circulation* (Owman, C. and Edvinsson, L., eds.), Pergamon Press, New York, pp. 377–386.

[16] Gross, P. M., Heistad, D. D., Strait, M. R., Marcus, M. L., and Brody, M. J. (1979) *Circ. Res.* **44**, 288–294.

[17] MacKenzie, E. T., McGeorge, A. P., Graham, D. I., Fitch, W., Edvinsson, L., and Harper, A. M. (1979) *Pfluegers Arch.* **378**, 189–195.

[18] Bevan, J. A. and Osher, J. V. (1972) *Agents Actions* **2**, 257–260.

[19] Lindvall, O. and Björklund, A. (1974) *Histochemistry* **39**, 97–127.

[20] Hardebo, J. E., Hanko, J., Kahrstrom, J., and Owman, C. (1987) *J. Auton. Pharmacol.* **6**, 85–96.

[21] Bevan, J. A. (1983) *Gen. Pharmacol.* **14**, 21–26.

[22] Shibata, S., Cheng, J. B., and Morakami, W. (1975) *Blood Vessels* **14**, 356–365.

[23] Edvinsson, L., Owman, C., and Sjoberg, N. O. (1976) *Brain Res.* **11**, 377–393.

[24] Toda, N. and Fujita, Y. (1973) *Circ. Res.* **33**, 98–104.

[25] Bevan, J. A., Bevan, R. D., and Duckles, S. P. (1980) *Handbook of Physiology, Sec. 2: The Cardiovascular System, vol. 2: Vascular Smooth Muscle* (Bohr, D. F., Somlyo, A. P., and Sparks, H. V., eds.), American Physiological Society, Baltimore, pp. 515–566.

[26] Hardebo, J. E. (1992) *Acta. Physiol. Scand.* **144**, 333–339.

[27] Bevan, J. A. and Bevan, R. D. (1973) *Stroke* **4**, 760–763.

[28] Lee, T. J. F., Su, C., and Bevan, J. A. (1976) *Circ. Res.* **39**, 120–126.

[29] Van Riper, D. A. and Bevan, J. A. (1991) *Circ. Res.* **68**, 568–577.

[30] Edvinsson, L., Copeland, J. R., Emson, P. C., McCulloch, J., and Uddman, R. (1987) *J. Cereb. Blood Flow Metab.* **7(1)**, 45–57.

[31] Rowan, R. A. and Bevan, J. A. (1983) *Vascular Neuroeffector Mechanisms—IV*, Proceedings of the 4th International Symposium on Vascular Neuroeffector Mechanisms, July 28–30, Kyoto, Japan (Bevan, J. A., Maxwell, R. A., Fujiwara, M., Shibata, S., Toda, N., and Mohri, K., eds.), Raven, New York, pp. 75–84.

[32] Rose, G. A. and Moulds, R. F. W. (1979) *Stroke* **10**, 736–741.

[33] Allen, G. S. (1976) *J. Neurosurg.* **44**, 594–600.

[34] Shibata, S. (1977) *Factors Influencing Vascular Reactivity* (Carrier, O., Jr. and Shibata, S., eds.), Igaku-Shoin Ltd., Tokyo, pp. 132–155.

[35] Toda, N. (1977) *Am. J. Physiol.* **232**, H267–274.

[36] Toda, N. (1983) *J. Pharmacol. Exp. Ther.* **226**, 861–868.

[37] Medgett, I. C. and Langer, Z. (1983) *Arch. Pharmacol.* **323**, 24–32.

[38] Duckles, S. P. and Bevan, J. A. (1976) *J. Pharmacol. Exp. Ther.* **197**, 371–378.

[39] Bevan, J. A., Oriowo, M. A., and Bevan, R. D. (1986) *Science* **234**, 196–197.

[40] Laher, I. and Bevan, J. A. (1985) *J. Pharmacol. Exp. Ther.* **233**, 290–297.

[41] Laher, I. and Bevan, J. A. (1985) *Eur. J. Pharmacol.* **119**, 17–21.

[42] Lamb, F. S. and Webb, R. C. (1984) *Am. J. Physiol.* **247**, H709–H714.

[43] Baumbach, G. and Heistad, D. (1983) *Circ. Res.* **52**, 527.

[44] Bill, A. and Linder, J. (1976) *Acta. Physiol. Scand.* **96**, 114–121

[45] D'Alecy, L. G. and Feigl, E. O. (1972) *Circ. Res.* **31**, 267–283.

[46] Traystman, R. J. and Rapela, C. E. (1975) *Circ. Res.* **36**, 620–630.

Chapter 8

Autonomic Receptors in Human Brain Arteries

Jan Erik Hardebo and Christer Owman

Adrenergic Receptors

Pial and brain parenchymal arteries down to the arteriolar level are richly innervated by sympathetic nerves. The main transmitter in these nerves appears to be norepinephrine (NE). The smooth muscle membranes in pial and parenchymal vessels are equipped with α- and β-adrenergic receptors. The effect on cerebrovascular tone of NE depends on which segment along the vascular tree is studied, and whether the monoamine reaches the vessel wall from the adventitial side (owing to release from the sympathetic nerves and, during pathological conditions, possibly also from NE neurons in the brain parenchyma) or from the intimal side (i.e., via the blood stream). During physiological conditions, the morphological and enzymatic blood–brain barrier (BBB) effectively prevents circulating catecholamines from reaching beyond the endothelial lining and thus to the outer layer of the smooth musculature, where the majority of receptors for catecholamines are present.

In vitro studies of isometric changes in tone on isolated segments of vessels have been widely used to define their receptor equipment. Studies with exogenous NE have revealed that the smooth muscle cell membranes of most large pial arteries, including the intracranial segment of the internal carotid artery from various species, including humans, are equipped with vasocontractile

From *The Human Brain Circulation*, R. D. Bevan and J. A. Bevan, eds.
©1994 Humana Press

(postjunctional) α-adrenergic receptors, with little or no contribution from β-adrenergic receptors, except in rat basilar and pig large pial arteries, where only β-receptors are found.[1-4] As in other vessels, the β-receptor-induced relaxation involves an increase in the activity of adenylate cyclase. The sensitivity of α-receptors in cerebral arteries is up to 10 times lower than that found in noncerebral arteries, and in the rabbit, the sensitivity is even lower.[5,6] The contractile response to NE is fairly homogenous in the various main pial arteries, as studied in the cat.[7] The contractile reactivity to NE is similar, but the dilatory response to the β-stimulating agent isoprenaline is greater in the distal compared to the proximal end of the middle cerebral artery, as studied in the dog.[8,9] High NE concentrations (above $10^{-4}M$) produce further contraction, not involving α-receptor activation.[6]

Studies in isolated pial arteries on changes in tone on electrical-field-stimulated release of neurotransmitters, such as NE, have not revealed any large vasocontractile response. In fact, in most species, including humans, it has not been possible to demonstrate a clear neurogenic response without a direct electrical activation of the smooth muscle cells.[9a,b]

Studies where the effect of exogenous NE on tone in large pial arteries is blocked by specific receptor antagonists have revealed that the α_1-receptor subtype predominates in humans, which is also the case in the monkey, baboon, rabbit, and rat.[6,10-14] In the cow, dog, and cat, α_2-receptors predominate.[10,13-16] Similar conclusions about α_1 predominance in human large and small pial vessels have been reached from radioligand binding and autoradiography studies,[17,18] although one group studying large arteries found α_2-receptor predominance.[19] Based on findings in noncerebral vessels, it has been postulated that α_2-receptors are preferentially located extrajunctionally on the smooth muscle cells, perhaps on the cells located near the intima.[20]

As elsewhere in the body, α_2-receptors are also located prejunctionally to control the neuronal release of NE. Radioligand binding studies have revealed that β_2-receptors are more numerous than β_1-receptors in human large and small pial vessels.[17,21]

The effect on tone of exogenous NE in isolated pial arterial segments, although clearly indicative of the presence of adrenergic receptors, provides little information to elucidate the importance of their effect in the intact vasculature under physiological conditions. To meet these objectives, the vasomotor response of pial arteries has been examined following perivascular microapplication or superfusion of the brain surface *in situ* with exogenous NE. Also, these studies in the mouse, rat, and cat have revealed predominant α-receptor-induced constrictions by NE.[3,4]

The contraction on exposure to α-receptor-stimulating substances, such as NE, is more dependent on influx of extracellular calcium in cerebral arteries—but not veins—than is the case in noncerebral arteries.[22,23] Such dependence is higher in pial arteries from dogs and humans than in rabbits and monkeys.[24] It is possible, however, that the response to neurally released NE is less dependent on extracellular calcium, as demonstrated in noncerebral arteries.[25]

Adrenergic receptors in isolated segments of small-surface (pial) and penetrating intracerebral arteries (with a diameter around 100 μm) and arterioles (diameter about 20–40 μm), branching off from the middle cerebral artery, have been studied in the rat and rabbit in vitro, and expressed as changes in isometric tone and perfusion pressure on exposure to NE.[1,26,27] Because of the BBB, isolated vessel segments cannulated at both ends can be used for differentiation between an effect of NE applied extraluminally onto smooth muscle receptors and intraluminally onto endothelial receptors. A primarily extraluminal effect can also be elucidated through perivascular microapplication to pial vessels *in situ* or by stimulation of their sympathetic nerves. The intraluminal effect can be demonstrated in vessels before and after removal of endothelium. The studies have revealed that small-surface and penetrating arteries are weakly contractile—via activation of α-receptors—or unresponsive, and arterioles are either unresponsive or dilate through activation of β-receptors to extraluminally applied NE.[1]

The tonic response to NE in the isolated rabbit and cat middle cerebral artery involves an endothelium-dependent dilatory component.[28,29] This may comprise activation of endothelial α_2-receptors[30] leading to a release of an endothelial factor attenuating NE-induced α-adrenergic smooth muscle contraction. On the occasion that serotonin is released together with NE from the cerebrovascular sympathetic nerves, serotonin will add to the contraction of pial vessels through an action on serotonin$_{1D}$-like receptors, as studied in the human internal carotid artery, pial arteries, and arterioles.[2,31,32]

Cerebral veins from animals and humans are equipped with more sensitive contractile α-receptors than the cerebral arteries.[22,23] Because of the BBB and the presence of adrenergic receptors on the endothelium down to the microvascular level, the effect on CBF by circulating NE may be fundamentally different from that of sympathetically released NE. Systemic or intracarotid administration of NE, during controlled blood pressure and blood gas levels, results in a minor decrease in cerebral blood flow or, particularly in primates, in no response.[3,4,34,35]

At enhanced perfusion pressure and alkaline pH, the sensitivity of the contractile α-receptor is augmented, as studied in large pial arteries and penetrating arterioles from animals.[1,3] At pH 7.80, a contractile α-response to NE predominates over the dilatory β-response in rat penetrating arterioles, starting at very low NE concentrations. There is reason to believe that the tonic effect of NE is stronger in vessels with only one smooth muscle cell layer, as in penetrating cerebral arterioles, provided a sensitive α/β-receptor is present.

The predominance of adventitial contractile α-receptors in the pial arteries, and of adventitial β-receptors in small-surface and penetrating arteries and arterioles, is in agreement with the view that the perivascular sympathetic nerves, activated during acute stress conditions, constrict only proximal cerebral arteries (with little flow-regulating capacity), while dilating or leaving small distal vessels unaffected. This prevents a harmful overdistension of the small vessels by the wave of acutely raised blood pressure, while still ensuring an adequate blood supply to the brain in this acute situation.

Cholinergic Receptors

Pharmacological studies in various animal species on tonic changes on ACh application in vitro and *in situ* have revealed the presence of muscarinic receptors mediating relaxation in pial arteries and arterioles as well as penetrating cortical arterioles (30–70 μm). This has also been demonstrated in isolated human pial arteries.[1,4,36,37] Radioligand binding studies in various species have confirmed the presence of muscarinic receptors in pial arteries and arterioles, and identified them into subclasses.[36] In some species, a contractile muscarinic receptor in pial arteries is also revealed at high ACh concentrations or at lower concentrations after removal of the endothelium.[5,36,37]

The cholinergic receptor on the smooth muscle cell has been identified as an M_1 receptor.[38] The contraction involves an increase in intracellular phosphoinositide hydrolysis.[39] The M_3 receptor is located on the smooth muscle and/or endothelial cell; activation causes relaxation.[40,41] M_1, M_2, and M_3 receptor sites in human pial arteries account for 40, 0, and 20%, respectively, of the total number of receptor sites. Comparative figures in cat pial vessels are 20, 35, and 40%.[42] The remaining 40% in humans appears to be of the M_5 type.

Interaction with M_3 receptors on the endothelial cells is central for inducing the dilatation, as is also the case in noncerebral vessels.[36] The interaction elicits the release of an endothelium-derived relaxing factor, i.e., nitric oxide or a nitric oxide-containing compound.[43,44] It is not known to what extent the M_3 receptors are located on the smooth muscle cells and on the abluminal endothelial cell membrane, the latter receptors being reached by ACh after diffusion through the musculature from the adventitial nerves.

ACh is poorly penetrable across the luminal endothelial membrane. Despite this, ACh and muscarinic cholinomimetic agents increase CBF on intravenous, intracarotid, or intravertebral administration.[1,4,35,37,45] This indicates that muscarinic receptors are present also on the luminal endothelial membrane, as demonstrated in human cortical arteries by autoradiography.[46] Although one study has indicated concomitant increase in cerebral oxygen consumption, it is likely that the flow effect of ACh is primarily caused by direct activation of endothelial cholinergic receptors.

The ACh-induced dilatation is less pronounced in pial arterioles from aged rats,[47] and the response is more pronounced at alkaline pH.[48] In pial veins, ACh causes only contraction, and at fairly high concentrations.[22]

These biochemical and pharmacological findings suggest a role in tone regulation for ACh stored in cerebrovascular nerves. However, findings on transmural nerve stimulation of isolated pial vessel segments are contradictory. Some authors have found a tetrodotoxin-sensitive atropine-blockable dilatation, particularly in vessels with high ChAT activity,[49] whereas others find no such response.[50,51] Further, the flow increase on stimulation of postganglionic parasympathetic fibers to the brain circulation in the rat is not affected by muscarinic blockade, and thus, is probably attributable to release of VIP or some other cotransmitter alone.[52] In addition to its possible postjunctional effect on tone, evidence has been presented that ACh may be involved in prejunctional blockade of noradrenaline released from the cerebrovascular sympathetic nerves, by stimulating muscarinic receptors on these nerves.[36,53]

References

1 Hardebo, J. E. (1989) *Neurotransmission and Cerebrovascular Function*, vol. II (Seylaz, J. and Sercombe, R., eds.), Elsevier, Amsterdam, pp. 193–210.
2 Hardebo, J. E. (1992) *Cephalalgia* **12**, 280–283.
3 Kuschinsky, W. and Wahl, M. (1978) *Pharmacol. Rev.* **58**, 656–689.
4 Sercombe, R., Lacombe, P., and Seylaz, J. (1984) *Neurotransmission and the Cerebral Circulation* (MacKenzie, E. T., Seylaz, J., and Bès, A., eds.), Raven, New York, pp. 65–89.
5 Hardebo, J. E., Hanko, J., and Owman, C. (1983) *Gen. Pharmacol.* **14**, 135–136.
6 Bevan, J. A., Duckworth, J., Laker, I., Oriowo, M. A., McPherson, G. A., and Bevan, R. D. (1987) *FASEB J.* **1**, 193–198.
7 Hamel, E., Edvinsson, L., and MacKenzie, E. T. (1988) *Br. J. Pharmacol.* **94**, 423–436.
8 Toda, N. and Miyazaki, M. (1984) *J. Cereb. Blood Flow Metab.* **6**, 1230–1237.
9 Toda, N., Okamura, T., and Miyazaki, M. (1985) *Eur. J. Pharmacol.* **106**, 291–299.
9a Hardebo, J. E., Hanko, J., Kåhrström, J., and Owman, C. (1986) *J. Auton. Pharmacol.* **6**, 85–96.
9b Hardebo, J. R., Chang, J. Y., and Owman, C. (1989) *Arch. Int. Pharmacodyn. Ther.* **300**, 94–106.
10 Toda, N. (1983) *J. Pharmacol. Exp. Ther.* **226**, 861–868.
11 Högestätt, E. D. and Andersson, K. E. (1984) *J. Auton. Pharmacol.* **4**, 161–173.

12 Hayashi, S., Park, M. K., and Kuehl, T. J. (1985) *J. Pharmacol. Exp. Ther.* **235,** 113–121.

13 Sasaki, T., Kassell, N. F., Torner, J. C., Maixner, W., and Turner, D. M. (1985) *Stroke* **16,** 482–489.

14 Usui, H., Fujiwara, M., Tsukahara, T., Taniguchi, T., and Kurahashi, K. (1985) *J. Cardiovasc. Pharmacol.* **7(Suppl. 3),** S47–S52.

15 Skärby, T. V. C., Andersson, K. E., and Edvinsson, L. (1983) *Acta Physiol. Scand.* **117,** 63–73.

16 Medgett, I. C. and Langer, S. Z. (1983) *Naunyn-Schmiedebergs Arch. Pharmacol.* **323,** 24–32.

17 Alexander, E. III and Friedman, A. H. (1990) *Neurosurg.* **27,** 52–59.

18 Nakai, K., Itakura, T., Naka, Y., Nakakita, K., Kamei, I., Imai, H., Yokote, H., and Komai, N. (1986) *Brain Res.* **381,** 148–152.

19 Tsukahara, T., Taniguchi, T., Fujiwara, M., Handa, H., and Nishikawa, M. (1985) *Stroke* **16,** 53–58.

20 Langer, S. Z and Shepperson, N. B. (1982) *Trends Pharmacol. Sci.* **5,** 440–444.

21 Tsukahara, T., Taniguchi, T., Shimohama, S., Fujiwara, M., and Handa, H. (1986) *Stroke* **17,** 202–207.

22 Hardebo, J. E., Kåhrström, J., Owman, C., and Salford, L. G. (1987) *J. Cereb. Blood Flow Metab.* **7,** 612–618.

23 Skärby, T., Högestätt, E. D., and Andersson, K. E. (1985) *Acta. Physiol. Scand.* **123,** 445–456.

24 Nosko, M., Krueger, C. A., Weir, B. K. A., and Cook, D. A. (1986) *J. Neurosurg.* **65,** 376–381.

25 Skärby, T. V. C. and Högestätt, E. D. (1990) *Br. J. Pharmacol.* **101,** 961–967.

26 Sercombe, R., Hardebo, J. E., Kährström. J., and Seylaz, J. (1990) *J. Cereb. Blood Flow Metab.* **10,** 808–818.

27 Sercombe, R., Hardebo, J. E., Kåhrström, J., and Seylaz, J. (1989) *J. Cereb. Blood Flow Metab.* **9(Suppl. 1),** S686.

28 Sercombe, R., Verrecchia, C., Oudart, N., Dimitriadou, V., and Seylaz, J. (1985) *J. Cereb. Blood Flow Metab.* **5,** 312–317.

29 Sercombe, R. and Verrecchia, C. (1986) *Neural Regulation of Brain Circulation* (Owman, C. and Hardebo, J. E., eds.), Elsevier, Amsterdam, pp. 27–41.

30 Vanhoutte, P. M. (1989) *Hypertension* **13,** 658–667.

31 Jansen, I., Edvinsson, L., and Olesen, J. (1993) *Acta. Physiol. Scand.* **147,** 141–150.

32 Hamel, E. and Bouchard, D. (1989) *Br. J. Pharmacol.* **102,** 227–233.

33 Auer, L. M. and MacKenzie, T. T. (1984) *The Cerebral Veins and Its Disorders* (Kapp, J. P. and Schmidek, H. M., eds.), Grune & Stratton, London, pp. 169–227.

[34] Edvinsson, L. and MacKenzie, T. T. (1977) *Pharmacol. Rev.* **28**, 275–348.

[35] MacKenzie, E. T. and Scatton, B. (1987) *CRC Crit. Rev. Clin. Neurobiol.* **2**, 357–419.

[36] Hamel, E. and Estrada, C. (1989) *Neurotransmission and Cerebrovascular Function,* vol. II (Seylaz, J. and Sercombe, R., eds.), Elsevier, Amsterdam, pp. 151–173.

[37] Wahl, M. (1985) *J. Cardiovasc. Pharmacol.* **7(Suppl. 3)**, S36–S46.

[38] Dauphin, F., Ting, V., Payette, P., Dennis, M., and Hamel, E. (1991) *Eur. J. Pharmacol.* **207**, 319–327.

[39] Galrcia-Villalon, A. L., Ehlert, F. J., Krause, D. N., and Duckles, S. P. (1990) *Life Sci.* **47**, 2163–2169.

[40] Dauphin, F. and Hamel, E. (1990) *Eur. J. Pharmacol.* **178**, 203–207.

[41] Garcia-Villalon, A. L., Krause, D. N2., Ehlert, F. J., and Duckles, S. P. (1991) *J. Pharmacol. Exp. Ther.* **258**, 304–310.

[42] Dauphin, F. and Hamel, E. (1992) *J. Pharmacol. Exp. Ther.* **260**, 660–667.

[43] Faraci, F. M. (1991) *Am. J. Physiol.* **261**, H1038–H1042.

[44] Parsons, A. A., Schilling, L., and Wahl, M. (1991) *J. Cereb. Blood Flow Metab.* **11**, 700–704.

[45] Pinard, E. (1989) *Neurotransmission and Cerebrovascular Function*, vol. II (Seylaz, J. and Sercombe, R., eds.), Elsevier, Amsterdam, pp. 175–191.

[46] Tsukahara, T., Kassell, N. F., Hongo, K., Vollmer, D. G., and Ogawa, H. (1989) *J. Cereb. Blood Flow Metab.* **9**, 748–753.

[47] Mayhan, W. G., Faraci, F. M., Baumbach, G. L., and Heistad, D. D. (1990) *Am. J. Physiol.* **258**, H1138–H1143.

[48] Dacey, R. G., Jr. and Bassett, J. E. (1987) *Am. J. Physiol.* **253**, H1253–H1260.

[49] Bevan, J. A., Buga, G. M., Florence, V. M., Gonsalves, A., and Snowden, A. (1982) *Circ. Res.* **50**, 470–476.

[50] Lee, T. J. F., Hume, W. R., Su, C., and Bevan, J. A. (1978) *Circ. Res.* **42**, 535–542.

[51] Hardebo, J. E., Kåhrström, J., and Owman, C. (1989) *Quart. J. Exp. Physiol.* **74**, 475–491.

[52] Suzuki, N., Hardebo, J. E., Kåhrström, J., and Owman, C. (1990) *J. Cereb. Blood Flow Metab.* **10**, 383–391.

[53] Sercombe, R. and Wahl, M. (1982) *J. Cereb. Blood Flow Metab.* **2**, 451–456.

Chapter 9

Cholinergic Receptors in Human Brain Arteries and Microvessels

Alterations in Alzheimer's Disease

Edith Hamel, François Dauphin, Donald Linville, Vincent Ting, and Nadim Zamar

Introduction

Cholinergic mechanisms have long been known to be implicated in the regulation of cerebral blood flow (CBF). The parasympathetic control of brain superficial vessels and the intracerebral cholinergic regulation of cerebral cortex microvasculature are well described. In vivo administration of acetylcholine (ACh) or cholinomimetics, as well as stimulation of specific neuronal structures, result in CBF increase[1-3] sensitive to muscarinic and/or nicotinic blockade.[4-6] In vitro administration of ACh to human isolated brain arteries results almost exclusively in an endothelium-dependent relaxation.[7,8] This prominent dilatory effect contrasts with the dual vasomotor response (dilatation followed by constriction at higher doses of ACh) observed in such species as the dog[7] and cat.[9] At the level of the intraparenchymal microvessels, ACh induces vasodilatation[10] and could mediate functions such as the fine tuning of local CBF[1-3] and possibly blood–brain barrier permeability.[11] Recent evidence indicates that ACh is

From *The Human Brain Circulation*, R. D. Bevan and J. A. Bevan, eds.
©1994 Humana Press

not a direct smooth muscle vasodilatory agent, but rather interacts with specific cholinergic receptors strategically located on nerve terminals and/or endothelial cells to modulate the synthesis and release of a relaxing factor, corresponding to nitric oxide (NO).[12–15] ACh has also been implicated in the release of other vasoactive neurotransmitters.[9,16,17] However, a direct effect on the cerebrovascular smooth muscle cannot be totally excluded, at least in species in which cerebral blood vessels constrict in response to ACh.[12]

In most cerebrovascular cholinergic-related functions, muscarinic receptors have been implicated, although nicotinic receptors also seem to be involved.[4,6,14] Muscarinic receptors are highly heterogeneous, and five different receptor genes have recently been cloned (m_1–m_5) (for review, *see* ref. 18). A pharmacological profile has been described for the five cloned receptors,[19,20] but unequivocal identification can only be achieved by the use of molecular biology techniques wherein the expression of a given receptor can be assessed. Using pharmacological approaches, multiple muscarinic receptor subtypes have been identified at the cerebrovascular level,[21,22] but little is known in the human, although such information is essential for our understanding of cholinergic regulation of CBF at both the extra- and intracerebral level. Moreover, perfusion of the cerebral cortex is governed by the combined action of pial and the intracortical vessels, which are under the influence of cholinergic parasympathetic[23,24] and intracerebral nerves,[1–3] respectively. In view of the known dysfunction of the intracerebral (mainly basal forebrain) cholinergic system in Alzheimer's disease[25] (AD) and of the most likely alterations of peripheral cholinergic nervous systems in this pathology (*see* Cholinergic Pial Vessel Functions in Alzheimer's Disease), it is possible that the parasympathetic control of cerebral blood vessels is affected in AD.

In the present study of human brain vessels and microvessels, we report on the pharmacological and molecular identification of cerebrovascular muscarinic receptor subtypes. In addition, parasympathetic cholinergic neuronal and receptor functions were assessed in pial vessels from histopathologically confirmed cases of Alzheimer's disease and compared to age-matched nondemented subjects. Parts of these results have been published[22] or have appeared as abstract presentations.[26,27]

Materials and Methods

Vascular Specimen

Human brains were obtained at autopsy (postmortem delay: 5–72 h) from subjects with Alzheimer's disease (confirmed by histopathological analysis) or with nonneurological or neurological pathologies without associated dementia (control subjects). Pial vessels were carefully removed from the cortical surface, and individual vessels were separated from the pia-arachnoid membrane under a dissecting microscope (for molecular biology experiments only). They were frozen and stored (–80°C). The subjacent cortical gray matter was then scooped gently from the underlying white matter and used for preparation of microvessel fractions (*see* next section).

Microvessel Fractions

Cortical microvessels (MV) were prepared based on previously described methods.[28] Cerebral cortices were minced, hand-homogenized, and centrifuged (1000g, 10 min) in phosphate-buffered saline (PBS). The pellet (P_1) was washed and spun a second time under the same conditions. The resulting pellet (P_2) was washed and centrifuged (1500g, 20 min) in PBS + Dextran 15%. The pellet (P_3) was washed and centrifuged as P_2. The final pellet (P_4) was resuspended in PBS, poured over a nylon mesh (150 μm), and rinsed strongly with PBS. The large microvessels remaining on the mesh were collected, frozen, and stored (–80°C). Purity of the MV fraction was determined by light microscopy and quantification of alkaline phosphatase and γ-glutamyl transpeptidase activities as compared to their respective cortical activities.

Radioligand Binding Studies

Membrane Preparations

Membrane from pial vessels and MVs were prepared as described.[22] Shortly after homogenization in 50 mM Tris-HCl buffer (4°C, pH = 7.4) and centrifugation (1000g, 10 min), the supernatants were ultracentrifuged (100,000g, 90 min), and the resulting pellet recovered in a small volume of Tris-HCl. The protein concentration of each vascular preparation was standardized to obtain approx 3.2 mg/mL and then frozen at –80°C. Proteins were determined according to Lowry and colleagues (1951).[29]

Muscarinic Binding Studies

Binding was performed with [³H]-*N*-methyl scopolamine ([³H]-NMS; 85 Ci/mmol; Amersham; Canada) in 50 mM Tris-HCl buffer (pH 7.4) at 25°C in a final vol of 250 µL (pial vessels) or 125 µL (MV fraction). After 90 min of incubation, the reaction was stopped by vacuum filtration. The filters were washed (3 × 5 mL Tris-HCl) and counted for radioactivity. Nonspecific binding was determined with 1 µM atropine. Saturation of specific binding sites was examined by increasing the concentration of [³H]-NMS from 0 to 6000 pM. The total number of sites (B_{max}) and binding site affinity (K_D) were determined with the program LIGAND. Competition studies were performed against 150 pM [³H]-NMS using various concentrations of the unlabeled drug under study. Antagonists selected were shown to exhibit a certain degree of selectivity at the various muscarinic receptor subtypes.[19,20] The affinity of the unlabeled drug is expressed as -log of the equilibrium dissociation constant (K_D) or pK_D as determined with LIGAND for both the high (H) and low (L) affinity sites when applicable.

The following antagonists were used and kindly donated: AF DX 116, AF DX 384, and AQ-RA 741 (H. N. Doods, Dr. Karl Thomae GmbH, Biberach, Germany); DAU 6202 (M. Turconi, Instituto de Angeli, s.p.A., Milano, Italy); HHSiD (G. Lambrecht, University of Frankfurt/Main and R. Tacke, University of Karlsruhe, Germany). The other antagonists, pirenzepine, 4-DAMP methiodide, methoctramine hydrochloride, and scopolamine hydrochloride, were obtained at Research Biochemicals, Inc. (Natick, MA).

Binding Site Analysis

Discrimination among models (one-site, two-site) was performed with the partial F test implemented in the program LIGAND. Linear regression lines and correlation coefficients were calculated in order to detect and quantify correlations between vascular and cloned receptor binding potencies of various compounds.

Northern Blot Hybridization

Human pial vessels, individually cleaned of the pia-arachnoid membrane, were frozen in liquid nitrogen, powdered, and total RNA extracted in a $4M$ guanidinium thiocyanate solution. Total RNA (5–10 µg) was electrophoresed on denaturing agarose gel (1%), transferred to nitrocellulose filter, and permanently bound by UV irradiation using a Stratalinker (for details, *see* ref. 30). The filter was then hybridized using a specific human m_1 (Hm_1) antisense full-length RNA probe[31] or a muscarinic receptor subtype-specific cDNA probe. The cDNA corresponds to a 726-bp *Bal*I fragment of the nonconserved third intracellular (i_3) loop of the Hm_1 clone.[31]

Parasympathetic Cholinergic Functions in Alzheimer's Dementia

Pial vessels obtained postmortem from eight histopathologically proven cases of AD and eight nondemented elderly subjects (C) were matched for age (AD: 75 ± 4 and C: 78 ± 4 yr old), postmortem delay (AD: 27 ± 8 h; C: 27 ± 6 h) and, whenever possible, sex (M/F ratio: 2/6 [AD] and 4/4 [C]). Total muscarinic binding sites were determined with [³H]-NMS as described above (Muscarinic Binding Studies) or in the presence of 75 nM pirenzepine in order to block the m_1 site population, which corresponds to approx 50% of total muscarinic binding sites in human pial vessels.[22] ChAT activity was determined in pial vessels from elderly nondemented controls and Alzheimer's patients according to the radiochemical assay of Fonnum.[32] Proteins were determined according to Lowry et al. (1951).[29] Comparisons between Alzheimer's patients and elderly controls were determined by Student's t-test for independent observations. In all cases, P was significant when ≤ 0.05.

Results

Muscarinic Binding Sites in Human Pial Vessels

Specific binding of [³H]-NMS to membrane preparations from human pial vessels was saturable and of high affinity (*see* Table 1 for details of binding parameters). When subtype-specific muscarinic antagonists were tested as inhibitors of [³H]-NMS binding in

Table 1
[³H]-NMS Specific Binding Parameters in Human Pial Vessels
and Cortical Microvessels

	Pial vessels[a]	Cortical microvessels[b]
B_{max} (fmol/mg protein)	67 ± 7	27 ± 1.3
K_D (pM)	125 ± 12	183 ± 27

Data are means ± SEM of at least four different experiments (pial vessels) or triplicate determinations (microvessels).

[a]Values are taken from Dauphin and Hamel, 1992.[22]

[b]Values were obtained from triplicate determinations on one microvascular preparation resulting from the pooling of cortical microvessels isolated from seven human cerebral cortices.

human pial membranes (Fig. 1), a heterogeneous population of muscarinic binding sites was identified. Pirenzepine delineated a population of high-affinity sites (pK_D = 8.34) that comprised approximately half of the total receptors. The residual sites were of lower affinity (pK_D = 7.28). The rather selective m_3 antagonist, HHSiD, was best fitted to a single population of sites with a pK_D of 7.59, and the m_2/m_4 compounds AF DX 116, methoctramine, and AQ-RA 741 were poor inhibitors of [³H]-NMS binding to human pial vessel membranes (see Table 2). Correlation analyses performed between the antagonist cerebrovascular potencies (pK_D) determined by binding competition of [³H]-NMS and their published affinities (pK_i) at the five cloned receptors revealed highly significant correlations with the m_1, m_3, and m_5 ($p < 0.001$ in all cases) receptor subtypes, whereas correlations with m_2 and m_4 subtypes were not significant (Fig. 2).

Muscarinic Receptor mRNA Expression in Human Pial Vessels

Northern blot hybridization to total RNA extracted from pia-arachnoid-free human pial vessels showed that mRNA transcripts for the Hm_1 receptor subtype were present in human postmortem pial vessels. Similar results were obtained whether a full-length Hm_1 riboprobe (Fig. 3), or a cDNA probe corresponding to the Hm_1 i_3 loop was used. Specificity of the probes was demonstrated by

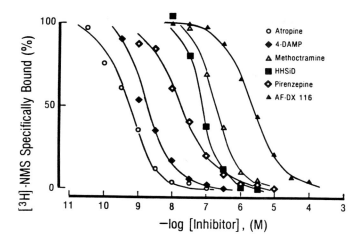

Fig. 1. Inhibition of specific [^{3}H]-NMS binding to human pial vessel membranes by atropine and subtype-selective muscarinic antagonists. Modified from ref. 22.

slot-blot hybridization against Hm_1, Hm_2, and rat m_5 full-length clones (data not shown).

Muscarinic Binding Sites in Human Cortical Microvessels

The isolated microvessels from human cerebral cortex were found to be highly enriched in vessels containing smooth muscle with few attached capillaries as observed under light microscopy. The relative purity of the MV fraction was further confirmed by its enrichment over cortical gray matter in marker enzymes alkaline phosphatase and γ-glutamyl transpeptidase (37- and 33-fold, respectively).

Analysis of the specific binding of [^{3}H]-NMS as determined by saturation experiments in human microvascular membranes revealed an affinity similar to that described in pial vessels, whereas the total amount of specific sites was slightly less (Table 1). In competition studies with subtype-specific antagonists, all compounds including pirenzepine were best fitted to a single-site model (Table 2). Correlation analysis performed as described above for pial ves-

Table 2
Affinity of Subtype-Specific Antagonists to Muscarinic Binding Sites
in Human Pial Vessels and Cortical Microvessels Determined
by Inhibition of [³H]-NMS Specific Binding[a]

Antagonists	Pial vessels[b] pK_D or $pK_{DH'}$ pK_{DL}	Cortical microvessels pK_D
Pirenzepine	8.34 (54%) 7.28 (46%)	7.87
AF DX 116	5.78	NT
AF DX 384	NT	7.44
Methoctramine	7.04	6.89
AQ-RA 741	6.88	6.91
HHSiD	7.59	7.47
4-DAMP	8.88	NT
DAU 6202	NT	8.62

[a]The binding affinity of the unlabeled ligand, expressed as -log of the equilibrium dissociation constant (K_D) or pK_D, is given at the high (H) and low (L) affinity sites when applicable. When present, the percentages of these two sites are given within parentheses.

[b]Data are means from 3–5 experiments and are taken from Dauphin and Hamel (1992).[22] In microvessels, values are means ± SEM of triplicate determinations from a single experiment. Except for pirenzepine in pial vessels (n Hill = 0.74 ± 0.03), Hill coefficients were not significantly different from unity, and binding parameters were best fitted to a one-site model.

NT: not tested.

sels (*see* Muscarinic Binding Sites in Human Pial Vessels) gives the best correlation with the m_1 receptor subtype ($r = 0.96$; $p < 0.005$) followed by m_2 ($r = 0.69$; ns) and m_3 ($r = 0.69$; ns), whereas the m_4 and m_5 receptor subtypes were excluded (r of -0.18 and 0.42, respectively) as putative sites in human cortical microvessels.

Parasympathetic Cholinergic Functions in Pial Vessels from Alzheimer's Patients

The activity of the ACh-synthesizing enzyme choline acetyltransferase (ChAT) was slightly, although not significantly,

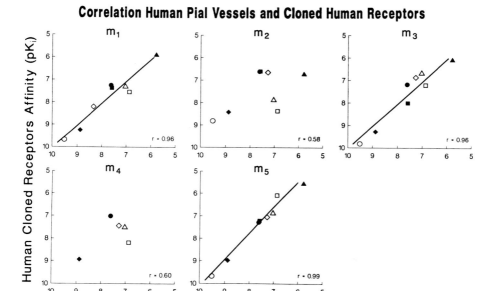

Fig. 2. Correlation between cerebrovascular potencies (pK_D, Table 2) of subtype-specific antagonists in inhibiting the binding of [³H]-NMS to human pial vessel membranes and their affinities (taken from refs. 19,20; and personal communication from H. N. Doods) at the five cloned muscarinic receptors. For pirenzepine at the m_1 receptor, the pK_{DH} value was used (Table 2), whereas the pK_{DL} was used for correlation with the four other subtypes.

lower in pial vessels from AD as compared to controls (Table 3). The specific binding site capacity (B_{max}) for [³H]-NMS in pial vessel membranes from AD patients was, however, significantly decreased (43%, $p < 0.05$) as compared to control values, whereas the affinity was unaltered (Table 3). When the [³H]-NMS binding was performed in the presence of 75 nM pirenzepine in order to block all m_1 and a fraction of putative, although unlikely (*see* Muscarinic Binding Sites in Human Pial Vessels), cerebrovascular m_4 sites, the remaining muscarinic binding sites were still significantly decreased in AD as compared to controls.

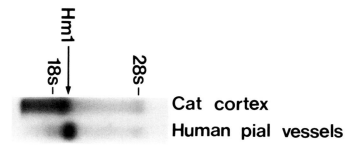

Fig. 3. Radioautogram produced by hybridization of a full-length Hm_1-specific ribonucleoprobe to total RNA (5–10 µg) extracted from cat cortex or human pial vessels. The positions of the 18S and 28S ribosomal RNA species are indicated.

Discussion

The present results on human cerebrovascular muscarinic receptors suggest that multiple subtypes exist in pial arteries (m_1, m_3, and possibly m_5), whereas only a homogeneous population of m_1 sites could be clearly identified in cortical microvessels. The detection of mRNA transcripts for the cloned Hm_1 receptor in pia-arachnoid-free human pial vessels unequivocally attests to the presence of m_1 receptor in this cerebrovascular bed. Furthermore, the results show a severe decrease in pial vessels' muscarinic binding sites in Alzheimer's patients that was accompanied by a slight deficit in cholinergic perivascular innervation.

Localization of Cerebrovascular Muscarinic Receptors

In our study, pial vessels comprised within the pia-arachnoid membrane were used for characterization of muscarinic binding sites. Although a vast proportion of this tissue contains vascular elements, several other cell types as well as nerve terminals are present. Therefore, it is most probable that the receptors identified are not exclusive to vascular elements.[33] However, in Northern blot analysis of vessels isolated from the pia-arachnoid, expression of

Table 3
ChAT Activity and Muscarinic Binding Sites in Pial Vessels
from Alzheimer's Patients and Elderly Controls[a]

	Alzheimer's patients	Elderly controls
ChAT activity		
nmol/mg protein/h	2.1 ± 0.7 (30%)	3.0 ± 0.9
[^{3}H]-NMS specific binding		
B_{max} (fmol/mg protein)	50.2 ± 7[b] (43%)	88.7 ± 18
K_D (pM)	147 ± 43	195 ± 49

[a]Values are means ± SEM of determinations from eight histologically confirmed cases of AD or eight nondemented controls. The percentage of decreased binding site capacity (B_{max}) is indicated within parentheses.
[b]$p < 0.05$ by Student's t-test, as compared to controls.

the m_1 receptor was detected, which is indicative of an association with vascular cells. Similar caveats also apply to MVs and hamper a definitive association of a given receptor to a specific cell type. However, the receptors identified in the MVs most likely are located on cells intimately related to microvascular functions. Indeed, electron microscopic observation of similar fractions showed the presence of perivascular nerves, astrocytes, and pericytes,[34] all of which are believed to form the functional microvascular unit.

Possible Roles
for Cerebrovascular Muscarinic Receptors

Pial Vessel Functions

One major problem in trying to relate a specific role for a given subtype of muscarinic receptor in human cerebrovascular regulation is the lack of parallel information in in vitro or in vivo functional studies. In fact, besides the known vasodilatory effect of intracerebral[1-5] or parasympathetic[23,24] stimulation, virtually no information is available on the pharmacology of the receptor subtypes implicated or the cellular mechanisms involved. Nevertheless, three muscarinic receptor subtypes (m_1, m_3, and m_5) were identified in human pial vessels. Although it may be illegitimate to project results in animals to humans, looking at the role of cerebrovascular muscarinic receptors in other species could provide some insights into their putative functions in humans. The ACh-induced relaxation in human cerebral arteries is mediated by EDRF,[8,13] or NO, which can have an endothelial and/or neuronal origin.[35,36] It is believed that endothelial muscarinic receptors generate the synthesis and release of NO, which then diffuses to the smooth muscle to activate guanylate cyclase.[13] In other species, an m_3 receptor subtype has been associated with this endothelium-dependent, ACh-induced cerebral dilatation.[37] The weak proportion of m_3 receptors in human pial vessels[22] ($\approx 17\%$) could be compatible with an endothelial localization. Indeed, the monolayer endothelium contributes to a small fraction of the cellular elements in the pial vascular fraction.

In contrast, the m_1 subtype appears to represent approximately half of total human cerebrovascular muscarinic receptors. This subtype has been associated with cerebral constriction,[30,38] a response not readily detectable in isolated human arteries. Nevertheless, Northern blot studies indicate that vascular cells express this receptor subtype, and the smooth muscle cells (being the major cellular component in pial vessels) may be the site of localization. However, all the binding site subtypes identified in the human pial vessels may be on more than one cell type as well as on perivascular nerve terminals. The recently described multiplicity of muscarinic receptor expression by peripheral vessel endothelial and smooth muscle cells[39] clearly supports such a statement.

Recent studies have shown that chemical and/or electrical stimulation of perivascular nonadrenergic noncholinergic vasodilator nerves release NO, which causes cerebroarterial relaxation.[40,41] Further, ACh liberated from perivascular cholinergic nerves may act on muscarinic receptors located on these nonadrenergic, noncholinergic terminals to interfere with the release of the vasodilator transmitter, NO.[14] It thus appears that presynaptic muscarinic receptors have a regulatory role in neurally induced cerebroarterial vasodilatation and the increase in cortical CBF noted after electrical stimulation of the parasympathetic pathways, by directly controlling the release of NO. Such a role for cerebrovascular muscarinic receptors might be important in autoregulation of brain circulation as suggested following lesion of perivascular parasympathetic fibers.[42] In addition, presynaptic muscarinic receptors have also been found to modulate noradrenaline release from perivascular sympathetic nerves. The three receptor subtypes identified in human pial vessels may be involved in some or all of these effects, but clearly more functional studies need to be done.

Microvascular Functions

The neurogenically induced cholinergic increase in cerebral cortical blood flow is partly mediated by muscarinic receptors,[2,4,5] although a precise subtype has not been implicated. There is evidence that NO may play a critical role in the mediation of intracerebral neurogenic vasodilatation induced by basal forebrain stimulation.[43] The possibility that muscarinic receptors regulate the release of the vasodilator transmitter, as described in pial arteries,[14] remains to be ascertained.[10] In human cortical microvessels, a homogeneous population of m_1 binding sites was identified, although the m_2 and m_3 correlation analyses were close to being significant as well. These results would favor the m_1 subtype as the best candidate for cholinergic regulation of CBF by intrinsic pathways. As discussed above, the receptor could be located at several steps in the neurovascular pathway, including neuronal, vascular, and possibly astrocytic cells, all of which are compatible with the regulation of intracortical blood flow by muscarinic mechanisms.[44-46] Although not conclusive, our data may suggest a weak proportion of m_2 and m_3 receptors in MVs. The possible existence of an m_2 subtype in MVs contrasts with its clear exclusion from the pial vessels. Interestingly, in peripheral blood vessels, m_2 mRNA transcripts were present in endothelial, but not smooth muscle cells.[39] Would the enrichment of endothelial cells in microvascular as opposed to pial fractions have allowed its detection by binding studies or, alternatively, could the receptor be an exclusive constituent of intraparenchymal microvasculature? Characterization of muscarinic receptor subtypes in human brain capillaries is clearly needed to better define the endothelial-associated muscarinic receptor subtypes. Indeed, MVs contain few attached capillaries branching off the arterioles, and muscarinic receptors involved in regulation of blood–brain barrier functions, such as fluid and protein exchange,[11] could form a small proportion of overall MV receptors.

Cholinergic Pial Vessel Functions in Alzheimer's Disease

Electrical stimulation of parasympathetic cholinergic pathways causes vasodilatation and increases in CBF,[23,24] to which the small pial resistance vessels are a major contributor. In confirmed cases of Alzheimer's dementia, we observed a low perivascular ChAT activity and marked decrease in pial vessel muscarinic bindingsites. These findings suggest that a failure in parasympathetic cerebrovascular functions, although probably not a first degree causality of this disease, may contribute to the severe cortical vascular deficit in AD (for review, *see* ref. 47). The recently described protective role for autonomic parasympathetic fibers in the pathophysiology of focal cerebral ischemia[42] would favor such a contention. Furthermore, these findings suggest that AD is a generalized disorder affecting not only brain neurons, but other structures within and outside the brain as well. Together with the reported changes in human lymphocytic muscarinic binding sites,[48] adrenergic and cholinergic skin vessels reactivity,[49] and cholinergic sweat responses[50] in AD, our results are indicative of a peripheral decline of cholinergic mechanisms in AD.

Conclusion

The identification of the functional importance of cholinergic muscarinic binding sites or receptors in the human cerebral vasculature awaits further physiological study. Nevertheless, a more detailed pharmacological and molecular characterization of the subtypes present in muscular and endothelial compartments would help clarify a role for these receptors in vasomotor and/or permeability functions. In addition to the muscarinic component of neurovascular cholinergic mechanisms, the participation of nicotinic receptors in modulating CBF[6,51] could provide a complementary mechanism through which ACh may affect brain perfusion and deserves further exploration. Finally, our study implies that autonomic parasympathetic dysfunction could contribute to the involvement of severe cortical vascular alterations in AD.

Acknowledgments

These studies were supported by the Medical Research Council (MRC) of Canada, the Canadian Heart and Stroke Foundation, a Pharmacology-Pharmaceutical Network from the Fonds de la Recherche en Santé du Québec (FRSQ), and Karl Thomae, GmbH. The authors thank the Douglas Hospital Brain Bank, and we are most grateful to Y. Robitaille for the neuropathological examination of human brain specimen. We are also thankful to Linda Michel for preparation of the manuscript, Susan Kaupp for graphics, and Charles Hodge for photographic work.

References

[1] Arneric, S. P., Iadecola, C., Underwood, M. D., and Reis, D. J. (1987) *Brain Res.* **411**, 212–225.

[2] Scremin, O. U., Allen, K., Torres, C., and Scremin A. M. E. (1988) *Neuropsychopharmacology* **1**, 297–303.

[3] Lacombe, P., Sercombe, R., Verrecchia, C., Philipson, V., MacKenzie, E. T., and Seylaz, J. (1989) *Brain Res.* **491**, 1–14.

[4] Biesold, D., Inanami, O., Sato, A., and Sato, Y. (1989) *Neurosci. Lett.* **98**, 39–44.

[5] Dauphin, F., Lacombe, P., Sercombe, R., Hamel, E. and Seylaz, J. (1991) *Brain Res.* **553**, 75–83.

[6] Arneric, S. P. (1989) *J. Cereb. Blood Flow Metab.* **9(Suppl. 1)**, S502.

[7] Tsukahara, T., Usui, H., Taniguchi, T., Shimohama, S., Fujiwara, M., and Handa, H. (1986) *Stroke* **17**, 300–305.

[8] Tsukahara, T., Kassell, N. F., Hongo, K., Vollmer, D. G., and Ogawa, H. (1989) *J. Cereb. Blood Flow Metab.* **9**, 748–753.

[9] Edvinsson, L., Falck, B., and Owman, C. (1977) *J. Pharmacol. Exp. Ther.* **200**, 117–126.

[10] Dacey, R. G., Jr. and Bassett, J. E. (1987) *Am. J. Physiol.* **253**, H1253–H1260.

[11] Tucker, V. L. and Huxley, V. H. (1990) *Circ. Res.* **66**, 517–524.

[12] Lee, T. J. F. (1980) *Eur. J. Pharmacol.* **68**, 393–394.

[13] Moncada, S. (1990) *Blood Vessels* **27**, 208–217.

[14] Toda, N. and Okamura, T. (1990) *Am. J. Physiol.* **259**, H1511–H1517.

[15] Toda, N. Ayajiki, K. (1990) *Am. J. Physiol.* **258**, H983–H986.

[16] Duckles, S. P. and Kennedy, C. D. (1982) *J. Pharmacol. Exp. Ther.* **222**, 562–565.

17 Ferrer, M., Galván, R., Marín, J., and Balfagón, G. (1992) *Naunyn-Schmiedeberg's Arch. Pharmacol.* **345**, 619–626.

18 Bonner, T. I. (1989) *TIPS* **(Suppl.)**, 11–15.

19 Buckley, N. J., Bonner, T. I., Buckley, C. M., and Brann, M. R. (1989) *Mol. Pharmacol.* **35**, 469–476.

20 Dörje, F., Wess, J., Lambrecht, G., Tacke, R., Mutschler, E., and Brann, M. R. (1991) *J. Pharmacol. Exp. Ther.* **256**, 727–733.

21 Garcia-Villalon, A. L., Krause, D. N., Ehlert, F. J., and Duckles, S. P. (1991) *J. Pharmacol. Exp. Ther.* **258**, 304–310.

22 Dauphin, F. and Hamel, E. (1992) *J. Pharmacol. Exp. Ther.* **260**, 660–667.

23 Seylaz, J., Hara, H., Pinard, E., Mraovitch, S., MacKenzie, E. T., and Edvinsson, L. (1988) *J. Cereb. Blood Flow Metab.* **8**, 875–878.

24 Goadsby, P. J. (1990) *Brain Res.* **506**, 145–148.

25 Whitehouse, P. L., Struble, R. G., Hedreen, J. C., Clark, A. W., and Price, D. L. (1985) *Crit. Rev. Clin. Neurobiol.* **1**, 319–339.

26 Zamar, N., Robitaille, Y., Kravitz, E., and Hamel, E. (1992) Cholinergic Neurotransmission: Function and Dysfunction meeting, Montreal, July 26–30.

27 Linville, D. G. and Hamel, E. (1992) *Neuroscience Absracts* **18(Part 1)**, 117.1.

28 Estrada, C., Hamel, E., and Krause, D. N. (1983) *Brain Res.* **266**, 261–270.

29 Lowry, O. H., Rosebrough, N. J., Farr, A. L., and Randall, R. J. (1951) *J. Biol. Chem.* **193**, 265–275.

30 Dauphin, F., Ting, V., Payette, P., Dennis, M., and Hamel, E. (1991) *Eur. J. Pharmacol.—Mol. Pharmacol. Sec.* **207**, 319–327.

31 Payette, P., Gossard, F., Whiteway, M., and Dennis, M. (1990) *FEBS Lett.* **266**, 21–25.

32 Fonnum, F. (1975) *J. Neurochem.* **24**, 407–409.

33 Lasbennes, F., Verrecchia, C., Philipson, V., and Seylaz, J. (1992) *J. Neurochem.* **58**, 2230–2235.

34 White, F. P., Dutton, G. R., and Norenberg, M. D. (1981) *J. Neurochem.* **36**, 328–332.

35 Palmer, R. M. J., Ashton, D. S., and Moncada, S. (1988) *Nature* **333**, 664–666.

36 Vincent, S. R. and Hope, B. T. (1992) *TINS* **15**, 108–113.

37 Dauphin, F. and Hamel, E. (1990) *Eur. J. Pharmacol.* **178**, 203–213.

38 Armstead, W. M., Mirro, R., Leffler, C. W., and Busija, D. W. (1988) *J. Pharmacol. Exp. Ther.* **247**, 926–933.

39 Tracey, W. R. and Peach, M. J. (1992) *Circ. Res.* **70**, 234–240.

40 Toda, N. and Okamura, T. (1991) *J. Pharmacol. Exp. Ther.* **258**, 1027–1032.

41 González, C. and Estrada, C. (1991) *J. Cereb. Blood Flow Metab.* **11**, 366–370.

42 Kano, M., Moskowitz, M. A., and Yokota, M. (1991) *J. Cereb. Blood Flow Metab.* **11**, 628–637.

43 Raszkiewicz, J. L., Linville, D. G., Kerwin, J. F., Jr., Wagenaar, F., and Americ, S. P. (1992) *J. Neurosci. Res.* **33**, 129–135.

44 Ferrari-Dileo, G., Davis, E. B., and Anderson, D. R. (1991) *Blood Vessels* **28**, 542–546.

45 Ishizaki, Y., Ma, L., Morita, I., and Murota, S. (1991) *Neurosci. Lett.* **125**, 29–30.

46 Prado, R., Watson, B. D., Kuluz, J., and Dietrich, W. D. (1992) *Stroke* **23**, 1118–1124.

47 Rapoport, S. I. (1991) *Cerebrovasc. Brain Metab. Rev.* **3**, 297–335.

48 Rabey, M., Shenkman, L., and Gilad, G. M. (1986) *Ann. Neurol.* **20**, 628–631.

49 Hörnqvist, R., Henriksson, R., Bäck, G., Buchot, G., and Winblad, B. (1987) *Gerontology* **33**, 374–379.

50 Lamb, K., Bradshaw, C. M., and Szabadi, E. (1983) *Eur. J. Clin. Pharmacol.* **24**, 55–62.

51 Linville, D. G. and Americ, S. P. (1991) *J. Cereb. Blood Flow Metab.* **11(Suppl. 2)**, S25.

Chapter 10

Peptide Receptors
in Human Brain Arteries

*Jan M. Lundberg, Gunvor Ahlborg, Annette Hemsén,
Anders Rudehill, and Eddie Weitzberg*

Introduction

Human cerebral arteries respond to a variety of peptide mediators with either contraction or relaxation. As summarized in Table 1, peptides originating from endothelial cells or perivascular nerves can influence cerebral vascular tone, at least when given exogenously in pharmacological doses. It should be emphasized from the start that the involvement of endogenous peptides as agonists for these perivascular receptors is not yet clear, partly because of lack of specific receptor antagonists and because of ethical problems in human experiments on the cerebral circulation. Furthermore, peptides administered via the circulation generally do not cross the blood–brain barrier. Therefore, peptides released from perivascular nerves or abluminally from endothelial cells may still have profound vascular effects.

Examples of Peptide Receptors
on Human Cerebral Vessels

The powerful vasoconstrictor peptide endothelin 1 (ET-1) is produced by endothelial cells of the cerebral vasculature. In fact, the Circulus Willis has the highest content of ET-1 in peripheral

From *The Human Brain Circulation*, R. D. Bevan and J. A. Bevan, eds.
©1994 Humana Press

Table 1
Examples of Peptide Receptors on Human Cerebral Vessels[a]

Peptide receptor	Agonist source	Contractile effect	Second messenger
Endothelin A	Endothelium	+	IP3, Ca^{2+}
NPY	Symp. nerves	+	Ca^{2+}
VIP/PHI	Parasymp. nerves	-	cAMP
CGRP	Sensory nerves	-	cAMP
NK-1	Sensory nerves	-	NO, cGMP

[a]+ = contraction, - = relaxation, IP3 = inositol trisphosphate, cAMP = cyclic adenosine monophosphate, NO = nitric oxide, and cGMP = cyclic guanosine monophosphate.

vessels.[1] So far, at least two types of vascular receptors have been cloned for ET, namely ET_A[2] and ET_B[3], whereby ET_A mediates vasoconstriction via an action on vascular smooth muscle and ET_B mediates vasodilation indirectly via endothelial cell formation of NO or prostacyclin.[4] Recent development of selective receptor antagonists for the ET_A receptors mediating vasoconstriction, such as BQ123[5,6] (Fig. 1), opens up further possibilities to characterize ET mechanisms in the human cerebral circulation, at least in vitro. Furthermore, ET-1 has been given systemically in vivo to human volunteers, and vascular effects have been recorded.

Neuropeptide Y (NPY) is colocalized with noradrenaline (NA) in sympathetic perivascular nerves, and this peptide is present in high concentrations around human cerebral vessels.[7] NPY is a powerful vasoconstrictor on human cerebral arteries,[8,9] probably acting on specific receptors. Vasoactive intestinal polypeptide (VIP) and peptide histidine isoleucine (PHI) are present in perivascular nerves of parasympathetic origin, whereby VIP is usually most potent as a vasodilator acting on VIP receptors on vascular smooth muscle[8,10] stimulating cAMP formation. Furthermore, the perivascular VIP nerves in the cerebral circulation most probably also contain nitric oxide synthase, suggesting that they may also release NO as a mediator.[11] Calcitonin gene related peptide (CGRP) and tachykinins (such as substance P, SP) are coreleased from capsai-

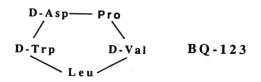

Fig. 1. Amino acid composition of endothelin-1 and the ET_A receptor antagonist BQ123.

cin-sensitive afferent nerves.[12] CGRP mainly acts directly on vascular smooth muscle via specific receptors linked to cAMP formation, whereas SP activates endothelial cells,[13] causing formation of NO,[14] and subsequently activating cGMP. Therefore, it is not surprising that CGRP rather than SP has been considered the main mediator of capsaicin-evoked vasodilation.[9,13,15] Recently, selective receptor antagonists for CGRP and tachykinins have been developed. Thus, the fragment αCGRP (8–37) can antagonize the vasodilation by αCGRP 1-37.[16] Furthermore, the specific nonpeptide NK-1 and NK-2 antagonists, CP96345[17] and SR48968,[18] respectively, may be used further to study the involvement of tachykinins in cerebrovascular sensory control.

Effects of ET-1 on Human Pial Arteries in Vitro

ET-1 caused powerful contractions of isolated human pial arteries with a threshold effect at 1 p*M* (Fig. 2A), which is even

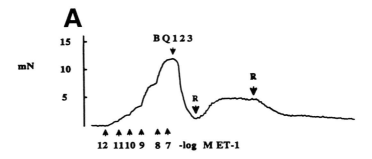

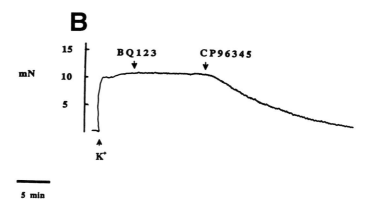

Fig. 2. **(A)** Contractile effects (mN) of ET-1 on an isolated human pial artery (diameter about 1 mm), given in increasing concentrations in a cumulative manner (arrows). The relaxant influence of adding the ET_A receptor antagonist BQ123 (5 μM) at the maximal ET-1 spasm is also illustrated. R = rinsing. **(B)** Influence of BQ123 (5 μM) or the NK-1 antagonist CP96345 (10 μM) on K+ (127 μM)-evoked contraction of an isolated human pial artery (diameter about 1 mm). Note the relaxant action of CP96345, whereas BQ123 was without effect. Time scale for 5 min is indicated by bar.

lower than earlier reported values from larger human cerebral blood vessels.[19] The maximum contractile response was almost 130% of high K+ (127 mM) (Fig. 3). After rinsing, the ET effect was extremely

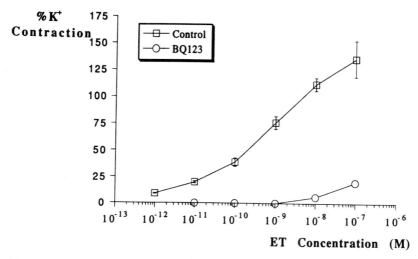

Fig. 3. Concentration–response curve for the contractile effects of ET-1 on isolated human pial arteries (diameter 0.5–1 mm) in the absence (squares) or presence (circles) of 5 µM BQ123. Note the marked inhibition of the ET-1 effect by BQ123. Data (means ± SEM) are expressed as percentage of the contraction evoked by 127 mM K^+ in each preparation ($n = 4$).

long-lasting (not shown). Preincubation with 5 µM of the ET_A receptor antagonist BQ123 caused a marked inhibition of the ET-1 effect, shifting the concentration–response curve to the right without influencing basal tone *per se* (Fig. 3).

Furthermore, even in a maximal precontracted state with ET-1 ($10^{-7}M$), BQ123 caused relaxation (Fig. 2A). After subsequent rinsing, the ET-1 contraction partly returned (Fig. 2A). In contrast, BQ123 did not relax pial arteries that were precontracted with high K^+ (127 mM) (Fig. 2B), suggesting some specificity of action.

Effects of ET-1 Infusion on Human Cerebral Circulation

In contrast to the short half-life of circulating ET-1 (1–2 min) in humans stands the prolonged vasoconstrictor effect (up to hours) in tissues like the kidney.[20] This has been explained by an almost irreversible binding of ET-1 to its human receptor.[21]

In vivo studies on animals have interestingly shown that ET-1 given via the circulation does not cause vasoconstriction in cerebral circulation. Thus, when given iv or ia, ET-1 has no vasoconstrictive effect, and on squirrel monkeys, ET-1 actually increases blood flow in the brain.[22] However, when given intracisternally in vivo, ET-1 causes extremely long-lasting (up to 12 h) contraction of the basilar artery, which indicates that the smooth muscle of cerebral arteries is quite sensitive to ET-1.[23]

To investigate the effects and clearance of ET-1 in the human brain, four healthy subjects were given a continuous infusion of ET-1 (4 pmol/kg/min) for 20 min. Catheters were inserted in the internal jugular venous bulb, a renal vein, an antecubital vein, and the brachial artery for measurements of ET-1-like immunoreactivity (ET-1-LI) in plasma,[1] oxygen content in whole blood, and estimation of renal blood flow. Furthermore, blood pressure was recorded continuously.[20] The recovery period was 1 h after the end of infusion.

The mean arterial blood pressure increased slightly during the ET-1 infusion by 7% ($p < 0.05$). At the end of the 20-min infusion, arterial plasma ET-1-LI had increased from 4.8 ± 0.4 pmol/L to 64.8 ± 10.4 pmol/L (Fig. 4A). The corresponding value for jugular vein plasma ET-1-LI at 20 min was 68.0 ± 11.8 pmol/L (Fig. 4A), indicating absence of clearance of ET-1 in the brain circulation, which in Fig. 4B is expressed as no significant fractional extraction (F). In contrast, the F (arterial-venous difference/arterial concentration) of ET-1-LI in the kidney was $60 \pm 2\%$ ($p < 0.05$). These results indicate that the permeability of the endothelium may be important in the clearance of ET-1 in an organ. The endothelium in the brain vessels participates in creating the blood–brain barrier, and it is difficult for the peptide to pass over to the abluminal side of the vessels, whereas in the kidney, the vascular endothelium is much more prone to allow passage of ET-1.

As shown in Fig. 5A, the arterial-jugular venous oxygen difference ([a-jv]O2) was reduced from 80.6 ± 3.4 mL/L at basal state to 70.1 ± 4.4 mL/L at the end of the infusion ($p < 0.05$). This reduction remained significant up to 1 h of recovery after ET-1 infusion.

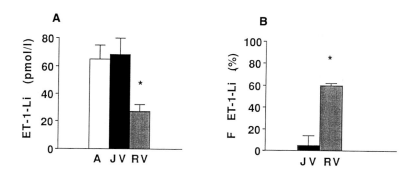

Fig. 4. **(A)** Arterial (A, open bar), jugular vein (JV, filled bar), and renal vein (RV, hatched bar) plasma concentrations of ET-1-LI after 20 min of infusion of ET-1 (4 pmol/kg/min) in four healthy subjects. Antiserum E1 was used.[1] Data are given as means ± SEM,* $p < 0.05$ using Student's t-test. **(B)** Fractional extraction (F) of ET-1-LI in the brain (filled bar) and kidney (hatched bar) in the same subjects. F was calculated as the arterial-venous difference in the organ divided by the arterial concentration. Data are presented as means ± SEM.* Indicates $p < 0.05$.

In the kidney, the corresponding arterial–renal vein oxygen difference ([a-rv]02) was increased, and the estimated renal blood flow (ERBF) was reduced by ET-1 (Fig. 5B and C). Hence, the reduction in renal blood flow was followed by an increased (a-rv)O_2 resulting in an unchanged renal O_2 uptake during the infusion. This allows us to assume that the brain oxygen consumption is stable during the ET-1 infusion, which indicates a slight cerebral vasodilatory response to elevated plasma levels of ET-1 in humans. This vasodilation can again be explained by the specific structure of the endothelium in the brain vessels, creating the blood–brain barrier. It has been suggested that the ET_B receptor, which in response to ET-1 produces vasodilation, is located on the endothelium, whereas the ET_A receptor, which mediates vasoconstriction, is situated on the vascular smooth muscle cell.[2-4] The difficulty of ET-1 in reaching the muscular side of the vessel might hinder the vasoconstriction, but allows an action on the vasodilatory, endothelium-located ET_B receptor. This is in accordance with the results

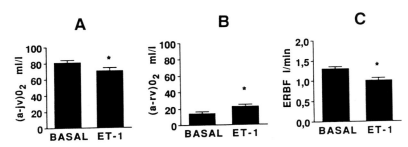

Fig. 5. Arterial-venous oxygen difference (a-v)O$_2$ in the brain (artery-internal jugular vein, jv) **(A)** and kidney (artery-renal vein, rv) **(B)** in the basal state and after 20 min of ET-1 infusion (4 pmol/kg/min) in four healthy male subjects. **(C)** Estimated renal blood flow (ERBF), determined by a constant iv infusion of paraaminohippuric acid at basal and after 20 min of ET infusion. Data are presented as means ± SEM. * Indicates $p < 0.05$.

that intracisternally, but not iv or ia, administration of ET-1 elicits vasoconstriction in the cerebral arteries of experimental animals.[22,23] Furthermore, the isolated human pial arteries, as seen in the present study, were very responsive to the contractile action of ET-1 in vitro, even in much lower concentrations (1 pM) than those reached in plasma on the systemic iv infusion (50 pM).

ET-1 has been suggested as a participant in the pathogenesis of cerebral vasospasm that follows subarachnoid hemorrhage.[24] It can be speculated that the disruption of the endothelium allows ET-1 to act on the smooth muscle in the vessel involved, causing long-lasting vasoconstriction. The local production of ET-1 may also be enhanced, supporting the vasospasm.[25] It is therefore of interest that the ET$_A$ receptor antagonist BQ123 could not only prevent ET-1-induced cerebral vasoconstriction, but even reversed the maximal spasm evoked by a high ET-1 concentration (10^{-7}M). This novel antagonist may therefore represent an interesting tool to study the possible involvement of ET-1 in the vasospasm seen on cerebral hemorrhage further. Furthermore, the observation that the ET-1 effect could be reversed by BQ123 is of interest considering that the cold ligand cannot displace the ^{125}I-ET-1 binding to the membrane receptor of human tissues.[21]

Influence of the NK-1 Antagonist CP96345 on Human Pial Arteries In Vitro

CP96345 relaxed K^+ (127 mM) precontracted human pial arteries with a threshold concentration of $10^{-6}M$. At $10^{-5}M$, CP96345 evoked a slowly developing, virtually complete relaxation (Fig. 2B). These findings are in agreement with recent data from studies on other vascular beds of experimental animals where the NK-1 receptor blocking activity could be dissociated from the vaso-relaxant effect of CP96345.[26] Furthermore, the vasodilatory effect of CP96345 can most likely be attributed to Ca^{2+} antagonistic properties.[26,27] Therefore, this compound is not suitable for studies on characterization of NK-1 receptor mechanisms, which are likely to be present in human cerebral vessels.[9,28] Finally, it has been suggested that αCGRP(8–37) can inhibit the relaxant effect of αCGRP(1–37) of human cerebral arteries, although the effect of βCGRP(1–37) was not inhibited.[29]

Acknowledgments

The present data have been supported by grants from the Swedish Medical Research Council (14X-6554). For expert secretarial help, we are grateful to Ylva Jerhamre.

References

[1] Hemsén, A. and Lundberg, J. M. (1991) *Regul. Peptides* **36**, 71–83.

[2] Arai, H., Hori, S., Aramori, I., Ohkubo, H., and Nakanishi, S. (1990) *Nature* **348**, 730–732.

[3] Sakurai, T., Yanagisawa, M., Takuwa, Y., Miyazaki, H., Kimura, S., Goto, K., and Masaki, T. (1990) *Nature* **348**, 732–735.

[4] Hemsén, A., Larsson, O., and Lundberg, J. M. (1991) *Eur. J. Pharmacol.* **208**, 313–322.

[5] Ihara, M., Noguchi, K., Saeki, T., Fukuroda, T., Tsuchida, S., Kimura, S., Fukami, T., Ishikawa, K., Nishikibe, M., and Yano, M. (1991) *Life Sci.* **50**, 247–255.

[6] Nakamichi, K., Ihara, M., Kobayashi, M., Saeki, T., Ishikawa, K., and Yano, M. (1992) *Biochem. Biophys. Res. Commun.* **182,1**, 144–150.

[7] Lundberg, J. M., Terenius, L., Hökfelt, T., and Goldstein, M. (1983) *Neurosci. Lett.* **42**, 167–172.

[8] Edvinsson, L., Ekman, R., Jansen, I., Ottosson, A., and Uddman, R. (1987) *Ann. Neurol.* **21**, 431–437.

9   Armando-Mejia, J., Pernow, J., von Holst, H., Rudehill, A., and Lundberg, J. M. (1988) *J. Neurosurg.* **69,** 913–918.

10 Lundberg, J. M., Fahrenkrug, J., Hökfelt, T., Martling, C.-R., Larsson, O., Tatemoto, K., and Änggård, A. (1984) *Peptides* **5,** 593–606.

11 Ceccatelli, S., Lundberg, J. M., Fahrenkrug, J., Bredt, D. S., Snyder, S. H., and Hökfelt, T. (1992) *Neuroscience* **51(4),** 769–772.

12 Lundberg, J. M., Franco-Cereceda, A., Hua, X.-Y., Hökfelt, T., and Fischer, J. (1985) *Eur. J. Pharmacol.* **108,** 315–319.

13 Franco-Cereceda, A., Rudehill, A., and Lundberg, J. M. (1987) *Eur. J. Pharmacol.* **142,** 235–243.

14 Palmer, R. M. J., Ferrige, A. G., and Moncada, S. (1987) *Nature* **327,** 524–526.

15 Jansen, I., Alafaci, C., Uddman, R., and Edvinsson, L. (1990) *Regul. Peptides* **31,** 167–178.

16 Chiba, T., Yamaguchi, A., Yamatani, T., Nakamura, A., Morishita, T., Inui, T., Fukase, M., Noda, T., and Fujita, T. (1989) *Am. J. Physiol.* **256,** 331–335.

17 Snider, R. M., Constantine, J. W., Lowe, J. A. III, Longo, K. P., Lebel, W. S., Woody, H. A., Drozda, S. E., Desai, M. C., Vinick, F. J., Spencer, R. W., and Hess, H.-J. (1991) *Science* **251,** 435–438.

18 Edmonds-Alt, X., Vilain, P., Goulaouic, P., Proietto, V., van Broeck, D., Advenier, C., Naline, E., Neliat, G., Le Fur, G., and Breliere, J. C. (1992) *Life Sci.* **50,** 101–106.

19 Martin de Agilera, E., Irurzun, A., Vila, J. M., Aldasoro, M., Galeote, M. S., and Lluch, S. (1990) *Br. J. Pharmacol.* **99,** 439–440.

20 Weitzberg, E., Ahlborg, G., and Lundberg, J. M. (1991) *Biochem. Biophys. Res. Commun.* **180,3,** 1298–1303.

21 Hemsén, A., Franco-Cereceda, A., Matran, R., Rudehill, A., and Lundberg, J. M. (1990) *Eur. J. Pharmacol.* **191,** 319–328.

22 Closel, M. and Closel, J.-P. (1989) *J. Pharmacol. Exp. Ther.* **250,** 1125–1131.

23 Mima, T., Takakura, K., Shigeno, T., Yanagisawa, M., Saito, A., Goto, K., and Masaki, T. (1989) *Stroke* **20,** 1553–1556.

24 Goto, K., Yanagisawa, M., Kimura, S., and Masaki, T. (1992) *Jpn. Circ. J.* **56,** 162–169.

25 Papadopoulos, S. M., Gilbert, L. L., Webb, R. C., and d'Amoto, C. J. (1990) *Neurosurgery* **26,** 810–815.

26 Delay-Goyet, P., Franco-Cereceda, A., Gonsalves, S. F., Clingan, C. A., Lowe, J. A. III, and Lundberg, J. M. (1992) *Eur. J. Pharmacol.* **222,** 213–218.

27 Schmidt, A. W., McLean, S., and Heym, J. (1992) *Eur. J. Pharmacol.* **215,** 351–353.

28 Jansen, I., Alafaci, C., McCulloch, J., Uddman, R., and Edvinsson, L. (1991) *J. Cereb. Blood Flow Metab.* **11,** 567–575.

29 Jansen, I., Nilsson, L., Mortensen, A., and Edvinsson, L. (1992) *Neuropeptides* **22-1,** 34–35.

Chapter 11

Ion Channels in Cerebral Arteries

John M. Quayle and Mark T. Nelson

Introduction

Ion channels form ion selective pores in cell membranes, which, when open, allow movement of ions down their electrochemical potential gradient. A channel may be selective for a particular ion, for example, potassium, calcium, or chloride ions. Channel activation results in the membrane potential approaching the equilibrium potential for that ion, at which there is no net electrochemical driving force for ion movement. In vascular smooth muscle, the equilibrium potential is approx –90 mV for potassium, –20 mV for chloride, +50 mV for sodium, and >+150 mV for calcium ions.[1] Channel activity may be highly regulated, for example, by membrane potential, membrane stretch, intracellular substances (e.g., Ca^{2+}, ATP, pH), vasoconstrictors, or vasodilators. In this chapter, we will present evidence for the role of dihydropyridine-sensitive calcium channels and of potassium channels in the regulation of membrane potential and calcium influx into cerebrovascular smooth muscle cells.

Calcium Channels

Activation of voltage-dependent calcium channels, either by membrane depolarization or by agonists, allows calcium entry into smooth muscle cells, triggering muscle contraction. For example, tone induced by depolarization from elevated extracellular potassium, pressurization, or vasoconstrictors is reduced or abolished

From *The Human Brain Circulation*, R. D. Bevan and J. A. Bevan, eds.
©1994 Humana Press

by removing extracellular calcium, organic calcium entry blockers, or membrane hyperpolarization.[2-4] Although other processes are clearly important in regulating vascular tone (for example, regulation of intracellular calcium release, calcium extrusion, or the calcium-force relationship), these results strongly suggest that calcium entry through dihydropyridine-sensitive calcium channels is necessary for maintenance of tone development in many cases, and that the membrane potential dependence of arterial tone arises from the voltage-dependence of the calcium channel.[4]

Calcium entry into a single smooth muscle cell, measured as the whole-cell calcium current, shows a characteristic bell-shaped dependence on membrane potential. As the cell is depolarized, a calcium current is first measured around −50 mV and increases to a peak around 0 mV in physiological calcium gradients because of voltage-dependent channel activation (Fig. 1, refs. 5,6). Current declines at more positive potentials; channels are maximally activated, but the driving force for calcium entry and, therefore, the single-channel current, falls as the membrane potential approaches the electrochemical reversal potential for the calcium channel (Fig. 1).

Whole-cell calcium current is the product of the single-channel current (i), the number of active channels (N), and the single-channel open probability (P_{open}). The study of single calcium channel properties in arterial smooth muscle cells, as in other cells, has been limited by the small single-channel currents and short-lived openings of the calcium channel. Barium ions pass through calcium channels at eightfold higher rate than calcium ions, and many single-channel studies have used a high concentration of barium as charge carrier to maximize the single-channel current amplitude (e.g., Fig. 2, refs. 2,3,7,8). In addition, a dihydropyridine calcium channel agonist (e.g., Bay K 8644 or Bay R 5417) is often present to prolong single-channel openings. In these recording conditions, the single-channel conductance lies in the range of 18–28 pS (e.g., Fig. 2, refs. 2,3,8,9), similar to that reported for the channel in other muscle preparations.[7,10] Calcium passes through the channel less freely than barium. For example, the single-channel conductance in rabbit basilar arteries (negative to −20 mV) is 24.6 pS in 80 mM Ba^{2+} and 15.1 pS in 80 mM Ca^{2+}.[9]

A Whole cell calcium currents

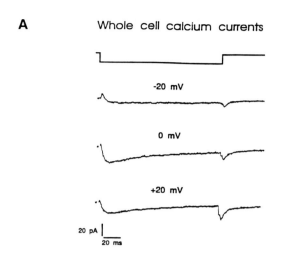

B Calcium current-voltage relationship

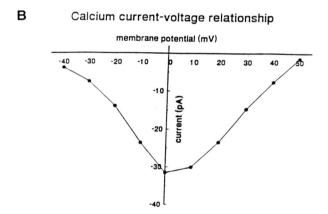

Fig. 1. Whole-cell calcium currents in a rabbit cerebellar artery smooth muscle cell. **(A)** Calcium currents recorded on depolarization form a holding potential of –70 mV to the potentials indicated. The voltage protocol is shown in the upper trace. The amphotericin permeabilized patch technique was used. Pipet solution (in mM): 75 Cs_2SO_4, 55 CsCl, 7 $MgCl_2$, 10 HEPES/ NaOH, pH 7.2. Bathing solution (in mM): 2.6 $CaCl_2$, 137 NaCl, 5.6 KCl, 1 $MgCl_2$, 20 TEACl, 1 4-aminopyridine, 10 HEPES/NaOH, pH 7.4. Series resistance was 36.4 Mohms; cell capacitance was 18.4 pF. **(B)** Peak calcium current–voltage relationship for the cell in A.

A 80mM Ba, SHRSP, +BayR

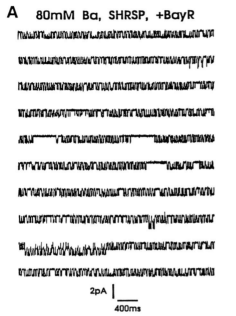

2pA |

400ms

B 80mM Ba,SHR-SP, +BayR

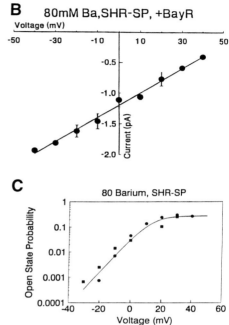

Fig. 2. Single calcium channel currents in a smooth muscle cell from the posterior cerebral artery of a spontaneously hypertensive stroke-prone rat (SHRSP). **(A)** A continuous recording of single calcium channels in the steady state at a membrane potential of 0 mV. Channel currents are inward (opening downward). Pipet solution (in mM): 80 $BaCl_2$, 10 HEPES, adjusted to pH 7.4 with NaOH. Extracellular solution (in mM): 120 KCl, 1 $MgCl_2$, 10 HEPES, adjusted to pH 7.4 with NaOH. The extracellular solution contained the dihydropyridine calcium channel agonist Bay R 5417 (500 nM) to prolong channel openings. **(B)** Single-channel current–voltage relationship. Mean unitary currents (±SEM) from five patches with 80 mM Ba^{2+} as charge carrier and 500 nM Bay R 5417 present. Fitted by linear regression between −40 and +40 mV with a slope conductance of 19.9 pS. **(C)** Voltage dependence of open-state probability. Two patches, SHRSP rats, 80 mM Ba^{2+}, 500 nM Bay R 5417. The solid line is a Blotzman function fitted to the data with a midpoint of the activation curve at 13.7 mV, and open probability changing 2.7-fold for a 6.5 mV depolarization negative to −20 mV (for details, *see* ref. 8).

Early studies of unitary calcium currents through the dihydropyridine-sensitive calcium channel in heart cells indicated the presence of a single saturable binding site for calcium in the channel, with a half-saturation constant of 13.9 mM. This led to predictions of unitary calcium currents at physiological calcium concentrations of <0.1 pA, immeasurably small with available techniques.[7] However, more recent data indicated that currents through the cardiac channel were surprisingly large at low barium concentrations (conductance was 7 pS with 1 mM Ba^{2+}).[11] Recently, we have recorded single calcium channel currents in cerebral arteries at low divalent cation concentrations and were able to resolve single channels in 2 mM calcium at physiological membrane potentials (between –60 and –30 mV) of between 0.3 and 0.1 pA.[12]

Although the single calcium channel current declines on depolarization (Fig. 2), calcium entry into the cell increases because the dihydropyridine-sensitive calcium channel is very sensitive to membrane potential, channel open probability (P$_{open}$) increasing exponentially with membrane depolarization over the physiological range of membrane potentials (Fig. 2C). Thus, any physiological variable causing a depolarization (e.g., vasoconstrictors or pressurization) will open the channel, and any agent causing membrane hyperpolarization (e.g., vasodilators) will cause channel closure. The activity of dihydropyridine-sensitive calcium channels in cerebral arteries can also be modulated by vasoactive agents independently of changes in the membrane potential. Serotonin increases calcium currents by shifting the voltage dependence of activation of calcium channels in the hyperpolarizing direction in rabbit basilar arteries.[9]

To gain insight into the voltage dependence of arterial smooth muscle tone, we have recently analyzed the voltage dependence of calcium channels in rat and rabbit cerebral arteries (Fig. 2, refs. 8,9). Channel properties (80 mM barium, 0.5 μM Bay R 5417) were studied using a conventional approach, in response to depolarizing steps from a negative holding potential, and also in the steady state at different membrane potentials, which is presumably more relevant to conditions of steady-state tone development in arteries (Fig. 2). In response to voltage steps, channel open probability increases approximately 2.7-fold for a 4.5 mV depolarization at membrane potentials negative to –20 mV. Channel activity was also recorded in the steady state, and channels showed similar voltage dependence for pulsed and steady-state data, although absolute levels of open probability were lower in the steady state (because of voltage-dependent inactivation).

The calcium channel can be considered to reside in a number of states, with rate constants governing transitions between states. Our single-channel data in rat cerebral arteries are consistent with a simple linear scheme comprising two closed states, an open state, and an inactivated state.

$$C_r \underset{k_{-1}}{\overset{k_1}{\rightleftharpoons}} C_s \underset{k_{-2}}{\overset{k_2}{\rightleftharpoons}} O \underset{k_{-3}}{\overset{k_3}{\rightleftharpoons}} I$$

The voltage dependence of channel activation arises mainly from transitions k_1 and k_{-1}. Inactivation is not inherently voltage-dependent, but does increase with depolarization, as a result of the voltage dependence of channel activation (i.e., the channel must open before it can inactivate). Although such a scheme is clearly an oversimplification and describes channel gating under unphysiological conditions, it is similar to that proposed in a recent review of calcium channels in muscle cells based on data from a wide variety of techniques.[10]

These observations represent a first step in understanding the steady-state properties of calcium current in arterial smooth muscle cells, an issue of obvious importance for steady-state tone development. However, a better knowledge of the steady-state properties of calcium current in more physiological conditions is required. Whole-cell calcium currents have been recorded in the steady state in single smooth muscle cells, but the exact relationship between membrane potential and calcium current in more physiological conditions remains to be determined.[13]

Calcium channels in smooth muscle cells, as in other cells, have been subdivided into a number of classes by voltage dependence of channel gating, single-channel properties (e.g., conductance), and sensitivity to calcium channel antagonists. Dihydropyridine-sensitive calcium channels have a pharmacology that allows them to be distinguished from other classes of calcium channel, being inhibited by organic calcium entry blockers belonging to the dihydropyridine, phenylalkylamine, and benzothiazipine classes, and by certain divalent cations (e.g., cadmium).[10]

The calcium current in cerebral arteries at the whole-cell and single-channel level is inhibited by the dihydropyridines.[5,6,9] Single channels (80 mM Ba^{2+}, 1 μM Bay K 8644, or 500 nM Bay R 5417) are blocked by nimodipine with high affinity; 20 nM inhibit currents by 95% (holding potential = –30 mV; test potential = 0 mV).[9] Channel inhibition by dihydropyridines is membrane-potential-dependent. Dihydropyridines bind the inactivated state of the calcium channel with highest affinity, and depolarization favors entry into the inactivated state and therefore channel inhibition.[3,9]

The dihydropyridine calcium channel agonist Bay R 5417 activates calcium channels in cerebral arteries.[8,9] Bay R 5417 (0.5 μM) has little effect on single-channel amplitude, increases channel open times, shifts the voltage dependence of channel activation by about 15 mV in the hyperpolarizing direction, and increases maximum channel open probability at depolarized potentials.[8,9]

There are at least two components of dihydropyridine-sensitive calcium current in cerebral artery cells. In rabbit basilar, in addition to the most frequently observed single-channel conductance level (25 pS negative to –10 mV, 80 mM Ba^{2+} as charge carrier), a single-channel conductance level of about 12 pS is seen.[9] This smaller channel shows similar voltage dependence and dihydropyridine sensitivity to the dominant form.[9] Two components of current have also been observed in guinea pig and rat cerebral arteries.[5,6] Cloning studies also indicate the presence of multiple isoforms of the dihydropyridine-sensitive calcium channel in arterial smooth muscle.[14]

Potassium Channels

Activation of a potassium channel will allow potassium ions to leave the cell, causing the membrane potential to approach the equilibrium potential for potassium ions, around –90 mV. This will cause membrane hyperpolarization, thus closing voltage-dependent calcium channels and causing arterial relaxation. Four classes of potassium channels have been identified in cerebral artery myocytes: inward rectifiers, calcium-activated potassium channels, delayed rectifiers, and ATP-sensitive potassium channels.

Inward Rectifier Potassium Channels (K_{IR})

The resting potassium conductance of small cerebral arteries allows potassium ions to pass more easily into the cell than out of it.[15] This inwardly rectifying potassium channel may be important in determining the resting membrane potential in cerebral arteries. (Although electrophysiological measurements show that the K_{IR} allows potassium ions to move more easily into the cell than outward, it is important to note that the membrane potential is normally positive to the potassium equilibrium potential, so potassium ions will leave the cell, and an outward and hyperpolarizing current will flow through the K_{IR}.)

Small cerebral arteries dilate in response to moderate increases in the extracellular potassium concentration (0–14 mM; higher concentrations cause constriction.[16] Release of potassium ions from neurons may have a role in linking neuronal activity to local increases in blood flow. On elevating extracellular K^+ in the range of 0–7 mM, pressurized rat cerebral arteries undergo a transient, ouabain-sensitive dilation, attributable to extracellular K^+ activating the electrogenic Na/KATPase. At higher potassium concentrations (7–14 mM), there is a sustained, barium-sensitive dilation attributable to the K_{IR}.[16] An increase in extracellular K^+ results in the potassium equilibrium potential becoming more positive, which would be predicted to cause membrane depolarization (if membrane potential follows the potassium equilibrium potential). However, extracellular K^+ activates the K_{IR} channel, and so can result in an increase in outward current, membrane hyperpolarization, and arterial dilation. In support of this hypothesis, barium ions, which block the K_{IR} in other tissues, reverse the potassium-induced hyperpolarization and dilation.[1,16]

Calcium-Activated Potassium Channels (K_{Ca})

Calcium-activated potassium channels in cerebral arteries, as in other cells, are activated by membrane depolarization and/or by an increase in the intracellular Ca^{2+}.[17] Tone development, for example, in response to vasoconstrictors, increasing extracellular K^+ or pressurization, is usually associated with membrane depolarization and a rise in the intracellular Ca^{2+}. Both of these are predicted to activate K_{Ca}, which could therefore provide a negative feedback on membrane potential, opposing further depolarization and stabilizing the membrane potential. In support of this, charybdotoxin, iberiotoxin, and tetraethylammonium ions depolarize and constrict pressurized cerebral arteries at concentrations shown to block the K_{Ca} channel.[17]

Delayed Rectifier Potassium Channels (K_{DR})

Delayed rectifier potassium channels are activated by membrane depolarization. In voltage-clamped segments of rat middle cerebral artery, the K_{DR} provides the main repolarizing current activated in response to membrane depolarization.[5] Regenerative action potentials seen in the presence of 10 mM TEA are probably owing to the ability of this compound to inhibit the K_{DR}.[5] As with the K_{Ca}, conditions resulting in membrane depolarization and tone generation would be predicted to activate the K_{DR}, which may therefore act to stabilize the membrane potential.

ATP-Sensitive Potassium Channels (K_{ATP})

Cerebral arteries dilate to compounds belonging to the class of pharmacological agents termed potassium channel openers[18] (rat cerebral arteries appear to be exceptional in being insensitive to these compounds; *see* ref. 19). There is now considerable evidence that these agents activate potassium channels that are inhibited by intracellular ATP (K_{ATP}). The hyperpolarizations and dilations are abolished by inhibitors of K_{ATP} channels, such as the sulfonylureas glibenclamide and tolbutamide, and by barium ions (100 μM) (e.g.,

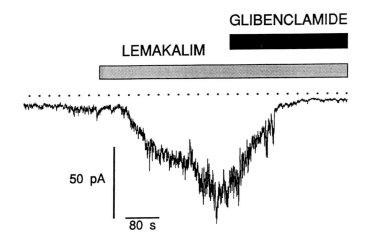

Fig. 3. Whole-cell, ATP-sensitive potassium current activated by lemakalim (10 μM) and inhibited by glibenclamide (10 μM) in a rabbit basilar artery cell. The extracellular solution contained 60 mM K+, and the intracellular solution 140 mM K+, so inward current (downward) was flowing through the membrane at the holding potential of –70 mV. Currents were recorded with the permeabilized patch method using the antibiotic amphotericin. Pipet solution (in mM): 70 K$_2$SO$_4$, 55 KCl, 8 MgCl$_2$, 10 HEPES/NaOH, pH 7.2. Extracellular solution (in mM): 60 KCl, 80 NaCl, 4 MgCl$_2$, 0.1 CaCl$_2$, 10 HEPES/NaOH, pH 7.4.

ref. 20). We have recently confirmed these observations by recording currents activated by the potassium channel opener lemakalim in rabbit basilar artery cells, and found that they are inhibited by glibenclamide (Fig. 3).

In addition to pharmacological agents, endogenous substances may also activate K$_{ATP}$ in cerebral arteries. For example, in rabbit middle cerebral arteries, the endothelium releases endothelial-derived hyperpolarizing factor (chemical identity unknown) in response to acetylcholine, which causes membrane hyperpolarization and arterial dilation.[21] These effects are inhibited by the K$_{ATP}$ channel blockers glibenclamide and barium.[21] Because K$_{ATP}$ channel activity is regulated by intracellular [ATP], the channel may also be involved in linking local blood flow to neuronal metabolism.

Conclusions

Regulation of membrane potential is an important determinant of cerebrovascular smooth muscle tone. Many vasodilators activate potassium channels, causing membrane potential hyperpolarization and relaxation (e.g., extracellular acidification, potassium channel openers, increases in extracellular K^+ in the 7–14 mM range, EDHF). Many vasoconstrictors cause membrane depolarization and constriction (e.g., pressurization, serotonin, extracellular potassium in the 20–80 mM range). We propose that the voltage dependence of arterial smooth muscle tone results from the steep voltage dependence of the dihydropyridine-sensitive calcium channel.

Acknowledgments

This work was supported by grants to MTN from the National Science Foundation (DCB-8702476 and DCB-90195663) and the National Institutes of Health (HL44455). We would like to thank Tomoko Kamishima and Blair Robertson for helpful comments on the manuscript.

References

[1] Hirst, G. D. S. and Edwards, F. R. (1989) *Physiol. Rev.* **69**, 546–604.

[2] Nelson, M. T., Standen, N. B., Brayden, J. E., and Worley, J. F. (1988) *Nature* **336**, 382–385.

[3] Nelson, M. T. and Worley, J. F. (1989) *J. Physiol.* **412**, 65–91.

[4] Nelson, M. T., Patlak, J. B., Worley, J. F., and Standen, N. B. (1990) *Am. J. Physiol.* **259**, C3–C18.

[5] Hirst, G. D. S., Silverberg, G. D., and van Helden, D. F. (1986) *J. Physiol.* **371**, 289–304.

[6] Simard, J. M. (1991) *Pfluegers Arch.* **417**, 528–536.

[7] Hess, P., Lansman, J. B., and Tsien, R. W. (1986) *J. Gen. Physiol.* **88**, 293–320.

[8] Quayle, J. M., McCarron, J. G., Asbury, J. R., and Nelson, M. T. (1993) *Am. J. Physiol.* **264**, H470–H478.

[9] Worley, J. F., Quayle, J. M., Standen, N. B., and Nelson, M. T. (1991) *Am. J. Physiol.* **261**, H1951–H1960.

[10] Pelzer, D., Pelzer, S., and McDonald, T. F. (1990) *Rev. Physiol. Biochem. Pharmacol.* **114,** 107–207.

[11] Yue, D. T. and Marban, E. (1990) *J. Gen. Physiol.* **95,** 911–939.

[12] Gollasch, M., Hescheler, J., Quayle, J. M., Patlak, J. B., and Nelson, M. T. (1992) *Am. J. Physiol.* **263,** C948–C952.

[13] Imaizumi, Y., Muraki, K., Takeda, M., and Watanabe, M. (1989) *Am. J. Physiol.* **256,** C880–C885.

[14] Koch, W. J., Ellinore, P. T., and Schwartz, A. (1990) *J. Biol. Chem.* **265,** 17786–17791.

[15] Edwards, F. R., Hirst, G. D. S., and Silverberg, G. D. (1988) *J. Physiol.* **404,** 455–466.

[16] McCarron, J. G. and Halpern, W. (1990) *Am. J. Physiol.* **259,** H902–H908.

[17] Brayden, J. E. and Nelson, M. T. (1992) *Science* **256,** 532–535.

[18] McPherson, G. A. and Stork, A. P. (1992) *Br. J. Pharmacol.* **105,** 51–58.

[19] McCarron, J. G., Quayle, J. M., Halpern, W., and Nelson, M. T. (1991) *Am. J. Physiol.* **261,** H287–H291.

[20] Standen, N. B., Quayle, J. M., Davies, N. W., Brayden, J. E., Huang, Y., and Nelson, M. T. (1989) *Science* **245,** 177–180.

[21] Brayden, J. E. (1990) *Am. J. Physiol.* **259,** H668–H673.

Chapter 12

A Comparison of the Properties of EDRF, Nitric Oxide, and S-Nitrosocysteine

Robert F. Furchgott

Introduction

It is by now well established that the synthesis of endothelium-derived relaxing factor (EDRF) in endothelial cells of systemic arteries depends on the oxidation of a guanidinium nitrogen of L-arginine to nitric oxide (NO) by the constitutive enzyme nitric oxide synthase, an oxygenase for which NADPH is a cosubstrate with L-arginine, and L-citrulline is a coproduct with NO.[1] The enzyme is dependent on Ca^{2+}/calmodulin for activation, and agonists that stimulate synthesis and release of EDRF from endothelial cells do so by acting on receptors that mediate an increase in the concentration of intracellular Ca^{2+} ions.[1] With the use of arginine analogs that competitively inhibit the enzyme, such as N^G-monomethyl-L-arginine (L-NMMA), evidence has now been obtained that the endothelial cells of peripheral resistance vessels also generate EDRF via the nitric oxide synthase.[1] Findings with these arginine analog inhibitors also indicate that nitric oxide synthase is responsible for formation of EDRF in isolated canine cerebral arteries.[2] On cat cerebral arterioles observed under cranial windows, recent work with arginine analog inhibitors also indicates that the nitric oxide synthase is responsible for the synthesis

From *The Human Brain Circulation*, R. D. Bevan and J. A. Bevan, eds.
©1994 Humana Press

of EDRF released in response to stimulation by topical acetylcholine (ACh).[3]

On rings of cat basilar and other cerebral arteries, ACh at low concentrations produces endothelium-dependent relaxation;[4] however, on rings of dog basilar artery, ACh generally produces an endothelium-dependent contraction.[5] Bradykinin is a reliable agent for producing endothelium-dependent relaxation of rings of dog basilar artery. In studies on this artery, with cyclooxygenase blocked by indomethacin to avoid the production of vasoactive prostanoids, endothelium-dependent relaxation by bradykinin has properties similar to relaxation produced by solutions of NO—namely, augmentation by superoxide dismutase (SOD) plus catalase and inhibition by methylene blue (a superoxide generator) and hemoglobin.[6] In contrast, dilation of pial arterioles of the cat by topical bradykinin appears not to involve NO, since it is inhibited by indomethacin and by SOD plus catalase.[7] However, it should be pointed out that this reported difference in mechanism of bradykinin-induced relaxation of cerebral arteries and cerebral arterioles probably arises not from the difference in the type of vessel studied, but rather from the difference in species used. A number of years ago, we demonstrated that rings of arteries from dogs and humans exhibit endothelium-dependent relaxation to bradykinin even when cyclooxygenase was inhibited, whereas rings of arteries (celiac and superior mesenteric) from cats and rabbits, with or without endothelium present, exhibited relaxation to bradykinin, which is completely blocked by cyclooxygenase inhibitors.[8] Thus, if cerebral arteries and arterioles of these different species behave like the respective noncerebral arteries, then the difference in mechanism of relaxation by bradykinin of cat cerebral arterioles and of dog cerebral arteries is to be expected.

Comparison of EDRF, NO, and *S*-Nitrosocysteine (NC) as Relaxants

Background

Even though there is now general agreement that the synthesis of EDRF in endothelial cells is directly related to the synthesis of NO from L-anginine by nitric oxide synthase, there is still considerable controversy as to whether EDRF on release from endothelial cells is simply NO or is some nitrosyl compound (incorporating newly synthesized NO) that readily generates NO on interacting with the subjacent smooth muscle cells (for reviews, *see* refs. 1,9,10). Meyers et al.,[11] using perfusion-bioassay experiments to compare properties of EDRF (released from cultured bovine endothelial cells by bradykinin), NO, and S-nitrosocysteine (NC), reported that all three had the same half-life (about 30 s), but that the relaxing potency of EDRF on the basis of its NO content (as estimated by chemiluminescence) was much greater than that of NO, but matched that of NC. Also, Wei and Kontos,[12] in studies on cat cerebral arterioles observed through cranial windows, reported that EDRF (released by topical ACh applied in the donor window and transferred to the assay window) behaved more like NC than like NO. In the experiments of Wei and Kontos, as in those of Myers et al., the apparent usually low potency of NO as a relaxant probably reflects a major degradation of NO (largely to nitrite) during the course of sampling, diluting, and infusing the NO solution (*see* refs. 9 and 10 for discussion of this subject).

In view of the reports that the properties of EDRF as a relaxant are matched better by those of NC than by those of NO, we carried out experiments comparing the properties of NO, NC, and EDRF in both organ chamber and perfusion-bioassay experiments. The experiments were carried out on preparations of rabbit thoracic aorta. Some of our results have already been reported.[13] They will be summarized and discussed here along with some new results. The reader is referred to the earlier paper for details of methods and procedures.

Organ Chamber Experiments
Effects of SOD[13]

In tests in organ chambers of endothelium-free rings of rabbit aorta bathed in regular Krebs solution and precontracted with phenylephrine, NC and NO are about equal in potency as relaxants, (ED_{50}, 10–15 nM). The relaxations are transient, and the kinetics of development of and recovery from relaxation is usually only slightly slower for NC than for NO (Fig. 1). Superoxide dismutase (SOD) markedly potentiates the relaxation (especially the duration) induced by both NO and NC, and reduces the ED_{50} for both to about 5 nM. The potentiation by SOD results from its removal of superoxide (O^-_2), which is always being generated in biological test systems and which rapidly inactivates NO.[1,9] The similarity in the kinetics of the relaxation of NC and NO and the potentiation of both by SOD provide evidence that NC undergoes rapid breakdown to yield NO and cystine when it is added to oygenated Krebs solution in organ chambers at pH 7.4, and that the relaxation of the aortic ring is mainly the result of this extracellularly liberated NO rather than of direct actions of NC itself in or on the muscle cells. Evidence for the rapid breakdown of NC in Krebs solution also has been obtained by recording the decay of the 336-nm absorption peak of NC spectrophotometrically.[13] At 37°C in regular Krebs solutions (containing 0.03 mM EDTA), the half-life of NC is about 25 s, and in Krebs solution without EDTA, it is only about 5 s.

On freshly prepared aortic rings with endothelium present, SOD does not significantly shift the log concentration–relaxation curve for ACh. This does not mean that the EDRF released by ACh is not NO or NC, for there may well be enough ectocellular SOD present in the tissue to protect EDRF effectively from inactivation by endogenous superoxide during short diffusion of EDRF from endothelial to smooth muscle cells.

Effects of EDTA and Other Iron Binding Agents[13]

On aortic rings in organ chambers, the responses to low concentrations of both NO and NC (10–75 nM) are usually considerably greater in our regular Krebs solution, which contains EDTA (30 µM), than in Krebs solution without EDTA. This potentiating effect of EDTA can be matched by transferrin (0.1–0.5 µM) or deferoxamine (10–30 µM) (Fig. 1). The potentiation by these agents is not as great at that produced by SOD, and in the presence of SOD, they give no additional potentiation of NO or NC. Since EDTA, transferrin, and deferoxamine are all very powerful binding agents for the ferric ion, the results suggest that in the usual organ chamber experiment, superoxide is being generated continuously in reactions involving traces of ferric ion present in the

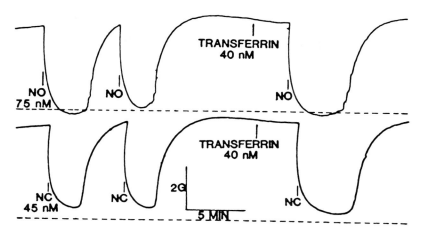

Fig. 1. Potentiation by 40 n*M* transferrin of relaxation of rings of rabbit aorta in response to nitric oxide and to *S*-nitrosocysteine when no EDTA was present in the bathing Krebs solution. Raising the concentration of transferrin to 400 n*M* (not shown) gave maximum potentiation, only slightly greater than at 40 n*M*. Transferrin (400 n*M*) gave the same degree of potentiation of NO- and NC-induced relaxation as did the standard concentration of EDTA (0.03 m*M*) used in our regular Krebs solution, and gave no potentiation when added to such a solution (not shown). The rings were endothelium-free and were precontracted with phenylephrine. Dashed lines show level of basal tone before contraction.

system, and the binding agents, by removing the ferric ion, reduce the rate of superoxide generation and thus the rate of inactivation of NO (either added to or generated from NC). However, even after the ferric ion is removed, there still must be some generation of superoxide, since SOD can still further potentiate NO- or NC-induced relaxation even after addition of one or more of the binding agents.

ACh-induced relaxation of endothelium-containing aortic rings in EDTA-free Krebs solution is not altered by additions of EDTA (30 μ*M*), transferrin (0.1–0.5 *M*), or deferoxamine (10–30 μ*M*). Ach-induced relaxation is somewhat inhibited by high concentrations of deferoxamine (0.3–1.0 m*M*). It should also be noted that at such high concentrations, deferoxamine begins to inhibit rather than potentiate NO- and NC-induced relaxation.

Effects of Serum Albumin

Serum albumin (1–2 μM), when added to EDTA-free Krebs solution, potentiates both the degree and duration of relaxation of aortic rings in response to NO to the same degree as EDTA or transferrin, probably by also binding ferric ions. Similar results are obtained with bovine and human albumin, free or not free of fatty acids. Albumin does not have any significant effect on ACh-induced endothelium-dependent relaxation. However, in the presence of albumin, the relaxation to NC (10–100 μM) on endothelium-free rings is markedly altered, with the degree of relaxation being considerably less, but with the duration being very prolonged (Fig. 2). The nature of the interaction between NC and albumin leading to this change in the relaxation pattern of NC is not yet clear.

Effects of Hemoglobin[13]

Hemoglobin (Hb), which has long been recognized as a very potent inhibitor of relaxation by NO and of endothelium-dependent relaxation by ACh, is also a very potent inhibitor of relaxation by NC. However, at high concentrations of NC (around 1 μM), the blockade of relaxation by Hb (10 μM) is usually not as complete as in the case of a similar concentration of NO.

Effects of Xanthine Plus Xanthine Oxidase[13]

On endothelium-denuded rings of aorta, addition of xanthine (X, 0.1 mM) plus xanthine oxidase (XO, 0.0008 U/mL) to generate O_2^- completely or almost completely inhibits relaxation to NO (10–100 nM). X + XO also strongly inhibits relaxation to NC, but to a somewhat lesser extent than to NO. On precontracted intact rings, pretreatment with X + XO produces some increase in tone (apparently by inactivating basally released EDRF) and a small degree of inhibition of ACh-induced endothelium-dependent relaxation. On the other hand, when X + XO is added during the course of relaxation produced by 1 μM ACh, it rapidly produces an appreciable degree of reversal of the relaxation. This reversal usually ranges from about 25 to 75% of the relaxation, and appears to become larger in tests made late in experiments. In experiments with X + XO, it is important to have catalase present to prevent accumula-

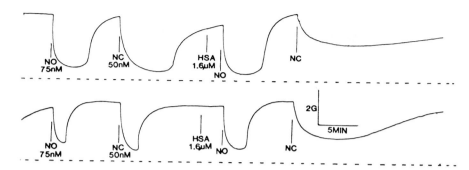

Fig. 2. Human serum albumin (HSA) potentiates relaxation of aortic rings by nitric oxide, but depresses and prolongs relaxation by S-nitrosocysteine. Similar results were obtained with bovine serum albumin.

tion of H_2O_2 resulting from spontaneous dismutation of the O^-_2, since H_2O_2 can cause endothelial cells to release EDRF.[14] The partial reversal of ACh-induced relaxation by X + XO can in turn be reversed by adding SOD, confirming that X + XO acts by generating O^-_2.

Effects of H_2O_2 and Horseradish Peroxidase[13]

H_2O_2 at 10–100 μM only slightly inhibits relaxation induced by NO (10–100 nM), but a combination of H_2O_2 and horseradish peroxidase (HRP, 30 U/mL) completely inhibits NO-induced relaxation (Fig. 3). The H_2O_2 + HRP combination partially inhibits relaxation induced by NC. However, H_2O_2 + HRP fails to inhibit ACh-induced endothelium-dependent relaxation of intact aortic rings. In the course of testing HRP used in these experiments, it was found to have considerable SOD activity as well as peroxidase activity, but the strong inhibitory action of H_2O_2 + HRP against relaxation by NO probably results from the peroxidase rather than the SOD activity.

Perfusion-Bioassay Experiments[13]

In perfusion-bioassay experiments in which endothelium of perfused aorta is the source of EDRF and an endothelium-free ring downstream is the bioassay tissue, the properties of EDRF (released

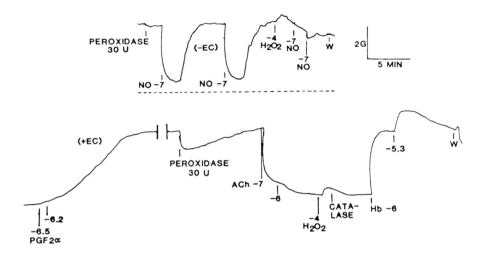

Fig. 3. Horseradish peroxidase plus hydrogen peroxide inhibits nitric oxide-induced relaxation, but not ACh-induced relaxation of rabbit aorta. Peroxidase was added at 30 U/mL. The contracting agent was $PGF_{2\alpha}$ instead of phenylephrine because the latter is inactivated by the peroxidase plus H_2O_2. The upper ring was endothelium-free, and the lower ring had endothelium. ACh-induced relaxation was not inhibited by H_2O_2 in the presence of the peroxidase whether it was added before (not shown) or after ACh. On the lower ring after H_2O_2 failed to reverse the ACh relaxation, catalase was added to remove excess hydrogen peroxide. Finally, the ability of hemoglobin to reverse completely the relaxation showed that the relaxation was the result of EDRF and not of any damage to the smooth muscle.

by ACh) and of NO and NC (both infused) were compared. The rate of decay of activity in transit was much slower for NC than for EDRF and NO. Infusion of H_2O_2 + HRP (below the aorta) almost completely inhibited relaxation by EDRF and NO, but only weakly inhibited relaxation by NC. Thus, the behavior of EDRF released by ACh in the perfusion-bioassay experiments resembled that of NO rather than that of NC.

Discussion

The results of the organ chamber experiments are consistent with the hypothesis that relaxation by NC is mainly produced by

NO, which is released from NC when the latter rapidly decays on being added to the bathing Krebs solution. However, the finding that two NO-inactivating systems, namely X + XO (to generate O^-_2) and H_2O_2 + HRP, which completely or almost completely inhibit relaxation by NO, only partially inhibit relaxation by NC suggests that a small portion of the relaxation by NC on rings in organ chambers results from some of the NC entering the smooth muscle cells before releasing NO. Since the X + XO and the H_2O_2 + HRP inactivating systems only partially or weakly inhibit ACh-induced relaxation of endothelium-containing rabbit aortic rings, the behavior of EDRF released abluminally in organ bath experiments appears to be more like that of NC than of NO. On the other hand, in the perfusion-bioassay experiments, EDRF released into the perfusion stream by ACh acting on the endothelium behaved more like infused NO than infused NC, for the relaxing activity of NO and that of EDRF both decreased much more markedly than that of NC when transit time to the bioassay ring was increased or when H_2O_2 + HRP was added to the perfusion stream below the perfused aorta. Also, addition of serum albumin to the perfusion stream inhibited relaxation by NC much more than that by NO or EDRF.

To explain these somewhat paradoxical results obtained in organ chamber and perfusion bioassay experiments, two hypotheses should be considered. The first is that in the intact aortic ring in an organ chamber, EDRF is released abluminally as NO and that a combination of factors (e.g., short diffusion distances and the presence of SOD and catalase in the tissue) allows it to act on the smooth muscle cells before significant inactivation by O^-_2 generated by X + XO or by H_2O_2 in the presence of HRP. The second hypothesis is that the NO formed from arginine by nitric oxide synthase on stimulation by ACh initially forms some nitrosyl compound by reacting with another cellular constituent(s), and it is this nitrosyl compound that is released abluminally. The compound would be much less sensitive than NO to inactivation by O^-_2 and certain other inactivating systems, but it would release NO spontaneously both extracellularly and intracellularly, and this NO could appear in the perfusion fluid in perfusion-bioassay experiments. The hypothetical nitrosyl compound would not necessarily be NC.

Acknowledgments

The author wishes to acknowledge the expert technical assistance of D. Jothianandan and M. T. Khan in conducting the experiments reported here. The research was supported by USPHS Grant HL21860.

References

1. Moncada, S., Palmer, R. M. J., and Higgs, E. A. (1991) *Pharmacol. Rev.* **43,** 109–142.
2. Katusic, Z. S., Moncada, S., and Vanhoutte, P. M. (1990) *Nitric Oxide from L-Arginine: A Bioregulatory System* (Moncada, S. and Higgs, E. A., eds.), Elsevier, Amsterdam, pp. 69–72.
3. Wei, E. P., Kukreja, R., and Kontos, H. A. (1992) *Stroke* **23,** 1623–1629.
4. Lee, T. J. (1982) *Circ. Res.* **50,** 870–879.
5. Katusic, Z. S., Shepherd, J. T., and Vanhoutte, P. M. (1988) *Stroke* **19,** 476–479.
6. Katusic, Z. S., Marshall, J. J., Kontos, H. A., and Vanhoutte, P. M. (1989) *Am. J. Physiol.* **257,** H1235–H1239.
7. Kontos, H., Wei, E. P., Povlishock, J. T., and Christman, C. W. (1984) *Circ. Res.* **55,** 295–303.
8. Cherry, P. D., Furchgott, R. F., Zawadzki, J. V., and Jothianandan, D. (1982) *Proc. Natl. Acad. Sci. USA* **79,** 2106–2110.
9. Furchgott, R. F., Khan, M. T., and Jothianandan, D. (1990) *Endothelium-Derived Relaxing Factors* (Rubanyi, G. M. and Vanhoutte, P. M., eds.), Karger, Basel, pp. 8–21.
10. Furchgott, R. F., Jothianandan, D., and Freay, A. D. (1990) *Nitric Oxide from L-Arginine: A Bioregulatory System* (Moncada, S. and Higgs, E. A., eds.), Elsevier, Amsterdam, pp. 5–17.
11. Myers, P. R., Minor, R. L., Jr., Guerra, R., Jr., Bates, J. N., and Harrison, D. G. (1990) *Nature* **345,** 161–163.
12. Wei, E. P. and Kontos, H. A. (1990) *Hypertension* **16(2),** 162–169.
13. Furchgott, R. F., Jothianandan, D., and Khan, M. T. (1992) *Jap. J. Pharmacol.* **58(Suppl. II),** 185P–191P.
14. Furchgott, R. F. (1991) *Resistance Arteries, Structure and Function* (Mulvany, M. J., Aalkjaer, C., Hedgerty, A. M., Nyborg, N. C. B., and Strandgaard, S., eds.), Elsevier, Amsterdam, pp. 216–220.

Chapter 13

Endothelium-Dependent Contraction of Cerebral Arteries

Kazuyoshi Kurahashi, Hachiro Usui,
Hiroaki Shirahase, and Hiroshi Jino

Introduction

Vascular tone is regulated by neuronal and humoral factors to maintain appropriate blood flow. Since Furchgott and Zawadzki (1980)[1] found the obligatory role of endothelial cells in the vasodilating action of acetylcholine (ACh) (endothelium-dependent relaxation, EDR), extensive studies on physiological activities of the endothelium in various vascular preparations have been investigated. Palmer et al. (1987)[2] have identified chemically that the endothelium-derived relaxing factor (EDRF) is nitric oxide (NO). In peripheral arteries, EDRF has been considered to play an important role in regulation of vascular tone.

In contrast to EDR, we have found that various vasoactive substances cause endothelium-dependent contraction (EDC) in canine cerebral arteries. In this chapter, EDC and EDCF of cerebral arteries are described, and their pathophysiological implications are discussed.

From *The Human Brain Circulation*, R. D. Bevan and J. A. Bevan, eds.
©1994 Humana Press

Endothelium-Dependent Contraction (EDC)

Features of EDC in Canine Cerebral Artery

In 1983, we found that in canine cerebral artery, ACh-induced contraction is attributed to cholinergic-thromboxane A_2 (TXA_2) synthesis linkage.[3] Later, the involvement of endothelium in the ACh-induced contractions (endothelium-dependent contraction, EDC) in canine cerebral artery was demonstrated.[4-6]

The features of the EDC induced by ACh ($10^{-7}M$) in canine cerebral artery were as follows:

1. The EDC was transient, and the half duration of the EDC was about 4 min.
2. The delay before onset of the EDC was approx 40 s.
3. The administration of ACh ($10^{-7}M$) had to be repeated more than five times (about 4–5 h) to obtain a constant EDC (Fig. 1).

In most experiments, canine basilar artery was used to analyze the EDC, since basilar artery showed more consistent EDC than the other cerebral arteries, anterior, posterior, and middle cerebral arteries. The EDCs of middle, anterior, and posterior arteries were essentially similar to that of basilar artery.

EDCF in Canine Cerebral Artery (Probably TXA$_2$)

As shown in Table 1, ACh,[4] norepinephrine,[5] arachidonic acid,[6] A-23187,[7] ATP,[8] angiotensin I and II,[9] histamine,[10] PGH_2,[11] LTC_4,[12] LTD_4,[12] and transmural stimulation[4] in canine cerebral arteries have been demonstrated to cause EDC in canine cerebral arteries. KCl, 5-hydroxytryptamine, α,β-methylene ATP, and TXA_2 agonist (STA_2) cause endothelium-independent contraction (EIC).[3,4,13]

In canine cerebral arteries, the EDC induced by ACh was attenuated by quinacrine and manoalide (phospholipase A_2, PLA_2 inhibitor), aspirin and indomethacin (cyclooxygenase inhibitor), OKY-046 and RS-5186 (TXA_2 synthetase inhibitor),[14,15] ONO-3708, and S-1452 (TXA_2 antagonist),[16,17] suggesting that the EDCF is probably TXA_2 (Fig. 2). The EDC was not affected by TMK-777 and AA-861 (5-lipoxygenase inhibitor). In addition, arachidonic acid, a precursor of TXA_2, caused EDC and this was attenuated by cyclooxygenase inhibitor, TXA_2 synthetase inhibitor, and TXA_2

Acetylcholine 10^{-7}M

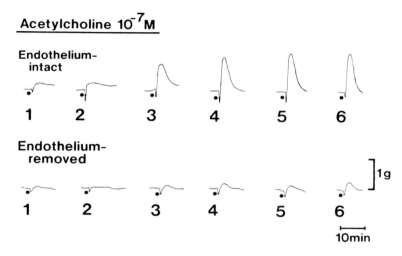

Fig. 1. Characteristic endothelium-dependent contraction (EDC) induced by ACh in canine basilar artery. The numbers indicate the repetitive administration of ACh (10^{-7}M).

antagonist. PGH_2, substrate of TXA_2 synthetase, caused an EDC that was attenuated by TXA_2 synthetase inhibitor, but resistant to a cyclooxygenase inhibitor. Furthermore, the above-described EDCs (norepinephrine, A-23187, ATP, histamine and transmural stimulation, and so forth) were all attenuated by the same enzyme inhibitors and TXA_2 antagonists. These pharmacological results clearly indicate that the EDCF released by various stimuli from cerebroendothelial cells is probably TXA_2 (Fig. 3).

Indeed, canine cerebral arteries released about 10-fold more TXA_2 than the peripheral arteries, and this release was markedly reduced by removal of endothelium, indomethacin, and OKY-046. Arachidonic acid at the concentration that causes the EDC enhanced the release of TXA_2.[7] These facts further support the view that the EDCF is TXA_2.

TXA_2 is a potent vasoconstrictor and is produced mainly in platelets. TXA_2 is produced also by human cerebral arteries. PGI_2 is one of the most potent endothelium-derived relaxing factors. It is assumed that the balance between endothelium- and platelet-

Table 1
EDC and EDCF

Agent	Canine		Monkey	
	Cerebral	Mesenteric	Cerebral	Iliac vein
ACh	EDC (TXA_2)	EDR	EDC (TXA_2)	
NAd	EDC (TXA_2)		EIC	
5-HT	EIC		EIC	EDC (AA met)
Histamine	EDC (TXA_2)		EDR	
Caffeine	EIC	EDC (unknown)		
Nicotine	EDC (TXA_2)			
A-23187	EDC (TXA_2)			
Ionomycin	EDC (TXA_2)			
AA	EDC (TXA_2)		EDC (TXA_2)	EDC (AA met)
PGH_2	EDC (TXA_2)			
PGE_1	EDC (TXA_2)			
LTC_4	EDC (TXA_2)			
LTD_4	EDC (TXA_2)			
ATP	EDC (TXA_2)	EDR		
ADP	EDC (TXA_2)	EDR		
Ang I	EDC (TXA_2)			
Ang II	EDC (TXA_2)			
ET-1	EDC (TXA_2), EIC			

EDC: endothelium-dependent contraction.
(   ): endothelium-derived contracting factor.
EDR: endothelium-dependent relaxation.
EIC: endothelium-independent contraction.
AA met: arachidonic acid metabolite.

derived TXA_2 and endothelium-derived PGI_2 plays an important role in vascular homeostasis. In addition, it has been suggested that TXA_2 is involved in the resting tone of human umbilical arteries, and in arachidonic acid- and ACh-induced contractions of rabbit pulmonary arteries.

The major product from the cyclooxygenase pathway is PGI_2 in endothelial cells, and PGI_2 is a potent relaxant. In fact, canine cerebral arteries produced about 10-fold larger amounts of PGI_2 than TXA_2. However, PGI_2 even at $10^{-6}M$ failed to counteract the TXA_2 agonist ($10^{-9}M$)-induced contraction in canine cerebral

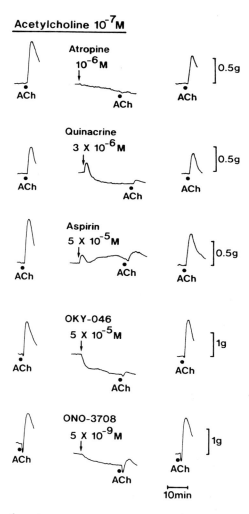

Fig. 2. Effects of various agents on endothelium-dependent contraction (EDC) induced by ACh ($10^{-7}M$) in canine basilar artery. Left column: control. Middle column: under the presence of various agents. Right column: after wash-out.

arteries, suggesting that TXA_2 is at least about 1000-fold more potent than PGI_2. Activation of the cyclooxygenase pathway results in contraction (mediated by TXA_2) rather than relaxation in cerebral arteries.

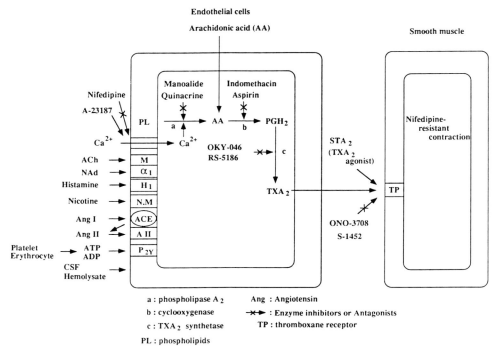

Fig. 3. Schematic presentation of endothelium-dependent contraction (EDC) in canine cerebral artery.

Other EDCFs

At least three distinct EDCFs have been proposed:[18,19] EDCF$_1$, a cyclooxygenase metabolite of arachidonic acid (TXA$_2$;[3–10] unidentified arachidonic acid metabolites[20–22]); EDCF$_2$, a polypeptide (endothelin;[23] unidentified polypeptide[24,25]); EDCF$_3$, an unidentified substance.[26–28]

Endothelial vasoconstrictor metabolites of arachidonic acid have been described in saphenous, splenic, femoral, and pulmonary veins,[20] canine cerebral artery,[3,4] and rabbit pulmonary artery.[29] Evidence for TXA$_2$ as EDCF$_1$ in arteries has been reported in canine basilar artery.[4–7]

There is no general agreement about the precise chemical nature of the EDCF metabolites of arachidonic acid. This factor has been proposed to be probably TXA_2, on the basis of its antagonism by the inhibitors of TXA_2 synthetase, OKY-046 and RS-5186.[3-7] In contrast, other investigators reported that TXA_2 synthetase inhibition by imidazole, BW-149H, dazoxiben, and OKY-046 did not affect the EDC, although the response was susceptible to cyclooxygenase inhibitor. Indeed, the degree of inhibition of EDCs by a specific TXA_2 synthetase inhibitor and PLA_2 inhibitor varied among the various EDCs. ATP-induced and bradykinin-induced EDCs were attenuated by a cyclooxygenase inhibitor, and ATP-induced EDC was nearly abolished by TXA_2 synthetase inhibitor,[8] but the EDC produced by bradykinin was resistant to the agent.[30] These facts suggest that the EDC induced by bradykinin in canine cerebral artery is partly the result of production of something other than TXA_2 (e.g., $PGF_{2\alpha}$, PGE_2, PGD_2).

The EDCF in A-23187-induced EDC in canine basilar artery has been postulated to be a superoxide, since this response was attenuated by the combined treatment of SOD and catalase.[31] In our experiments using the same arteries, A-23187-induced EDC was not affected by SOD and catalase. This contradiction may be attributed to differences in experimental procedures. We started the experiments about 5 h after mounting preparations, since the amplitude of the EDC induced by ACh increased time-dependently (the repetitive applications of ACh) in over 4 h. We have assumed that in addition to TXA_2 production, prostaglandin-mediated contracting process may be activated time-dependently or by the repetitive applications of ACh. Such mechanisms of the delayed activation should be clarified in the near future.

Recently, we observed that in canine mesenteric artery, but not in cerebral arteries, caffeine caused an EDC.[32] The EDCF has not yet been identified (other than arachidonic acid metabolites, radicals, endothelin). It is only known that the EDC was nifedipine-resistant, but sensitive to the deprivation of extracellular Ca^{2+}.

Inhibition of EDC

In canine cerebral artery, EDCF (TXA_2) is primarily released by the activation of cerebroendothelium followed by activation of TXA_2 receptors in vascular smooth muscles. In this context, two types of approaches can be used to inhibit the EDC: One, at the endothelium level, is to inhibit TXA_2 production; the other, at the smooth muscle level, is to inhibit the contraction.

Inhibition of EDCF (TXA₂) Production in Endothelium

As shown in Fig. 3, TXA_2 production in cerebral arteries is triggered by elevation of intracellular Ca^{2+} concentration, which activates PLA_2 and liberates arachidonic acid from membrane phospholipids. Then, arachidonic acid is metabolized to PGH_2 by cyclooxygenase, and then PGH_2 is converted to TXA_2 by TXA_2 synthetase. Exogenously applied arachidonic acid and PGH_2 are considered to be metabolized to TXA_2 by these enzymes. The EDCs were not affected by Gro-PIP (PLC inhibitor), AA-861, and TMK-777 (5-lipoxygenase inhibitor), suggesting that in canine cerebral arteries, EDCFs are not metabolized by these enzymes. The release of stable TXA_2 metabolite, TXB_2, was inhibited by the removal of endothelium, cyclooxygenase inhibitor, and TXA_2 synthetase inhibitor[7] (Table 2). From these, it is clear that in the cerebro-endothelial cells level, Ca^{2+} antagonists (like nifedipine), PLA_2 inhibitors, cyclooxygenase inhibitors, and TXA_2 synthetase inhibitors on the EDCs are effective. Therefore, various selections to inhibit TXA_2 production can be possible.

Inhibition of EDCF (TXA₂ Agonist)-Induced Contraction

STA_2 is a stable TXA_2 agonist. STA_2 (TXA_2 agonist)-induced contraction in canine cerebral arteries was endothelium-independent and was antagonized by TXA_2 antagonist (ONO-3708 and S-1452). The contraction was partly resistant to nifedipine (Table 3). These findings suggest that the nifedipine-resistant Ca^{2+} channel is involved in the EDCF (TXA_2)-induced contraction. STA_2-induced contraction was also resistant to nitroglycerin as reported in the norepinephrine-induced contraction in rabbit ear arteries,[33] and in SHR and WKY tail arteries.[34] In addition to the vascular selective TXA_2 antagonist, agents that antagonize nifedipine-resistant and nitroglycerin-resistant contraction in cerebral artery should be developed.

The newly synthesized vasodilator (LP-805 developed by Pola Cosmetic Ltd. and Nippon Lederle Ltd., Tokyo, Japan) inhibited

Table 2
Effects of Indomethacin and OKY-046
on Spontaneous Release of Thromboxane B$_2$ (TXB$_2$)
from Canine Cerebral Arteries

	TXB$_2$ release, pg/mg wet wt/30 min)	
	Control	Treatment
Indomethacin (10^{-5}M)	46.9 ± 6.6	12.6 ± 1.2[a]
OKY-046 (10^{-4}M)	48.6 ± 12.8	24.1 ± 4.1[b]

[a]$p < 0.01$.
[b]$p < 0.05$, compared with values of TXB$_2$ released from untreated preparations (control) ($n = 4$).

specifically the canine cerebroarterial EDC induced by ACh and the mesenteric arterial EDC induced by caffeine. LP-805 did not affect the endothelium-independent contraction in both preparations.[35] It is assumed that the EDC-inhibitory action of LP-805 may be the result of stabilization of endothelial cells.

Pathological Implications of EDCF (TXA$_2$)

There is a possibility that EDCF is involved in various cerebral vascular diseases as a spasmogen. In the field of neurosurgery, a critical problem is vasospasm after subarachnoid hemorrhage (SAH). Bloody CSF (bCSF) obtained from SAH patients caused contraction, and this response consisted of an EDC and endothelium-independent component.[36] Hemolysate also caused similar EDC. Although substances causing EDC in bCSF have not been identified, hemoglobin is the most possible candidate. However, ATP is also contained in hemolysate, and angiotensins are demonstrated in CSF of SAH patients. Furthermore, platelet-derived ATP, ADP,[37] histamine, and catecholamines seem to cause the EDC. These EDCs may play a role in vasospasm. Anoxia causes an EDC and also enhances EDC owing to other causes. Erythrocyte-derived K$^+$, platelet-derived serotonin and TXA$_2$ may cause endothelium-independent contractions. All of these EDCs and endothelium-independent

Table 3
Effects of Nitroglycerin on Nifedipine-Resistant Ca^{2+}-Induced Contraction
in the Presence of STA_2 in Basilar and Coronary Arteries[a]

	Contractions in normal medium	Nifedipine-resistant Ca^{2+}-induced contractions			
		Control	Nitroglycerin, M		
			10^{-8}	10^{-7}	10^{-6}
Basilar	1.99± 0.16 (42)	1.31± 0.15 (33)	0.90± 0.16 (9)	—	1.08± 0.25 (10)
Coronary	2.63± 0.14 (38)	1.28± 0.17 (20)	0.37± 0.99* (9)	0.04 ± 0.03* (5)	0.05± 0.04* (8)

[a]The nifedipine-resistant Ca^{2+}-contractions (control) were obtained by the addition of Ca^{2+} (2.5 mM) into Ca^{2+}-free medium containing EGTA (0.1 mM), nifedipine ($10^{-6}M$), and STA_2 ($10^{-8}M$). Nitroglycerin was added 10 min after the addition of STA_2. Each value represents the mean ± SE. The number of experiments is shown in parentheses. *$p < 0.01$: significantly different from the control value.

contractions elicited by neuronal and humoral factors after SAH are considered to trigger and maintain vasospasm in a synergic manner at the ischemic area.

The protective effect on cerebral vasospasm of a TXA_2 synthetase inhibitor, which is under clinical trial, may be attributable to its effect on endothelium, and TXA_2 antagonists are also expected to protect against vasospasm. STA_2-induced contraction is rather insensitive to nifedipine and nitroglycerin. This may explain why Ca^{2+} antagonists and nitroglycerin cannot protect against vasospasm effectively. Endothelium-selective TXA_2 synthetase inhibitor, smooth-muscle-selective TXA_2 antagonist, and Ca^{2+} antagonist for both receptor- operated and voltage-operated Ca^{2+} channel are expected to be effective agents in the treatment of cerebral vasospasm.

Recently, endothelin has been focused on as a cerebral vasospasmogen. Indeed, endothelin as well as bCSF caused a biphasic contraction consisting of an EDC and endothelium-independent component.[38] Further study is required to clarify the role of endothelin in cerebral vasospasm after SAH.

Summary and Future Prospects

In canine cerebral arteries, EDCs are commonly observed during both resting and active agonist-induced tone. On the other hand, in monkey cerebral arteries, EDR during active tone or EDC during resting tone is agonist-dependent. Although the role of EDR or EDC in human cerebral arteries is not yet established, we have observed EDC in a few cerebral arteries obtained from autopsy. The proposed EDCF, TXA_2, is an arachidonic acid metabolite, and one of EDRFs, PGI_2, is also. It is assumed that the arachidonic acid metabolites (endothelium-derived factor, negative and positive amplifier) play an important role in maintaining the cerebral blood flow. Further pharmacological characterization of endothelial arachidonate in cerebral arteries would provide an approach to developing effective drug in the treatment for cerebral vascular disease.

References

[1] Furchgott, R. F. and Zawadzki, J. V. (1980) *Nature* **288**, 373–376.

[2] Palmer, R. M., Ferrige, A. G., and Moncada, S. (1987) *Nature* **327**, 524–526.

[3] Usui, H., Kurahashi, K., Ashida, K., and Fujiwara, M. (1983) *Med. Sci. Res.* **11**, 418–419.

[4] Usui, H., Fujiwara, M., Tsubomura, T., Kurahashi, K., Nomura, S., and Mizuno, N. (1986) *Neural Regulation of Brain Circulation* (Owman, C. and Hardebo, J. E., eds.), Elsevier, Amsterdam, pp. 261–272.

[5] Usui, H., Kurahashi, K., Shirahase, H., Fukui, K., and Fujiwara, M. (1987) *Jpn. J. Pharmacol.* **44**, 228–231.

[6] Shirahase, H., Usui, H., Kurahashi, K., Fujiwara, M., and Fukui, K. (1987) *J. Cardiovasc. Pharmacol.* **10**, 517–522.

[7] Shirahase, H., Usui, H., Manabe, K., Kurahashi, K., and Fujiwara, M. (1988) *J. Pharmacol. Exp. Ther.* **247**, 701–705.

[8] Shirahase, H., Usui, H., Manabe, K., Kurahashi, K., and Fujiwara, M. (1988) *J. Pharmacol. Exp. Ther.* **247**, 1152–1157.

[9] Manabe, K., Shirahase, H., Usui, H., Kurahashi, K., and Fujiwara, M. (1989) *J. Pharmacol. Exp. Ther.* **251**, 317–320.

[10] Usui, H., Kurahashi, K., Shirahase, H., Manabe, K., Shibata, S., and Fujiwara, M. (1989) *Med. Sci. Res.* **17**, 1035–1036.

[11] Toda, N., Inoue, S., Bian, K., and Okamura, T. (1988) *J. Pharmacol. Exp. Ther.* **244**, 297–302.

[12] Shirahase, H., Kurahashi, K., Usui, H., Shimaji, H., and Fujiwara, M. (1991) *Role of Adenosine and Adenine Nucleotides in the Biological System* (Imai, S. and Nakazawa, M., eds.), Elsevier, Amsterdam, pp. 423–431.

[13] Shirahase, H., Usui, H., Shimaji, H., Kurahashi, K., and Fujiwara, M. (1991)

[14] Naito, J., Komatsu, H., Ujiie, A., Hamano, S., Kubota, T., and Tsuboshima, M. (1983) *Eur. J. Pharmacol.* **91,** 41–48.

[15] Asai, F., Ito, T., Ushiyama, S., Nagasawa, T., Inagaki, T., Matsuda, K., and Oshima, T. (1988) *Jpn. J. Pharmacol.* **46(Suppl.),** 279p.

[16] Fujioka, M., Nagao, T., and Kuriyama, H. (1986) *Naunyn-Schmiedeberg's Arch. Pharmacol.* **334,** 467–474.

[17] Narisada, M., Ohtani, M., Watanabe, F., Uchida, K., Arita, H., Doteuchi, M., Hanasaki, K., Kakushi, H., Otani, K., and Hara, S. (1988) *J. Med. Chem.* **31,** 1847–1854.

[18] Rubanyi, G. M. (1988) *Endothelial Cells* (Ryan, U. S., ed.), CRC, Boca Raton, FL, pp. 61–70.

[19] Greenberg, S. and Diecke, F. P. J. (1988) *Drug Dev. Res.* **12,** 131–149.

[20] Miller, V. M. and Vanhoutte, P. M. (1985) *Am. J. Physiol.* **248,** H432–H437.

[21] Vanhoutte, P. M. (1987) *Blood Vessels* **24,** 131–144.

[22] Vanhoutte, P. M. (1988) *Cerebral Vasospasm* (Wilkins, R. H., ed.), Raven, New York, pp. 119–128.

[23] Yanagisawa, M., Kurihara, H., Kimura, S., Goto, K., and Masaki, T. (1988) *Nature* **332,** 411–415.

[24] O'Brien, R. F. and McMurtry, I. F. (1984) *Am. Rev. Respir.* **129,** A337.

[25] Hickey, K. A., Rubanyi, G. M., Paul, R. J., and Highsmith, R. F. (1985) *Am. J. Physiol.* **248,** C550–C556.

[26] Rubanyi, G. M. and Vanhoutte, P. M. (1985) *J. Physiol. (Lond.)* **364,** 45–56.

[27] Harder, D. R. (1987) *Circ. Res.* **60,** 102–107.

[28] Jino, H., Usui, H., Shirahase, H., and Kurahashi, K. (1992) *Med. Sci. Res.* **20,** 169–170.

[29] Altierre, R. J., Kiritsy-Roy, J. A., and Catravas, J. D. (1986) *J. Pharmacol. Exp. Ther.* **236,** 535–541.

[30] Usui, H., Suganuma, H., Jino, H., and Kurahashi, K. (1993) *Jpn. J. Pharmacol.* **58(Suppl.),** p. 382.

[31] Katusic, Z. S. and Vanhoutte, P. M. (1989) *Am. J. Physiol.* **257,** H33–H37.

[32] Jino, H., Usui, H., Temma, S., Shirahase, H., and Kurahashi, K. (1994) *Br. J. Pharmacol.,* in press.

[33] Akimoto, Y., Kurahashi, K., Usui, H., Fujiwara, M., and Shibata, S. (1987) *Jpn. J. Pharmacol.* **44,** 506–509.

[34] Kurahashi, K., Akimoto, Y., Usui, H., and Jino, H. (1992) *Life Sci.* **51,** 695–702.

[35] Jino, H., Usui, H., and Kurahashi, K. (1992) *Med. Sci. Res.* **20,** 525–526.

[36] Usui, H., Fujiwara, M., Shirahase, H., and Kurahashi, K. (1987) *Neuronal Messengers in Vascular Function* (Nobin, A., Owman, C., and Arnekro-Nobin, B., eds.) Elsevier, Amsterdam, pp. 537–547.

[37] Shirahase, H., Usui, H., Shimaji, H., Kurahashi, K., and Fujiwara, M. (1990) *J. Pharmacol. Exp. Ther.* **255,** 182–186.

[38] Shirahase, H., Usui, H., Shimaji, H., Kurahashi, K., and Fujiwara, M. (1991) *Life Sci.* **49,** 273–281.

Chapter 14

Myogenic (Stretch-Induced) and Flow-Regulated Tone of Human Pial Arteries

John A. Bevan, Rosemary D. Bevan, Alynn Klaasen, Paul Penar, Tina Poseno, and Carrie L. Walters

The normally functioning cerebral circulation effectively autoregulates, the vascular adjustments responsible for this probably occurring in pial arteries of all sizes. It has been shown that changes in diameter of cerebral blood vessels of several animal species can take place in response to perivascular neural (constrictor or dilator) activity, and through local mechanisms in the vessel wall responsive to intraluminal pressure and flow. A variety of factors, mainly metabolic, influence the intracerebral vasculature (for references, *see* ref. 1). In this chapter, we will describe experimental observations on the pressure and flow-initiated changes in vascular tone of human pial arteries obtained during surgery. These vessels were transported to the Totman Laboratory from various Neurosurgical Centers for experimentation. Only the larger cerebral arteries are influenced by sympathetic nerves. Dilator nerves influence has yet to be observed in human arteries of any size (*see* Chapter 6).[2] Thus, it would seem likely that stretch-induced myogenic contraction and shear stress-initiated changes in tone are the dominant local regulating processes for human arteries.

It has been suggested that blood vessel diameter, the primary variable feature of the vasculature (outside the microcirculation) contributing to short-term circulatory adjustments, reflects a com-

From *The Human Brain Circulation*, R. D. Bevan and J. A. Bevan, eds.
©1994 Humana Press

promise between the power needed to maintain blood flow through a blood vessel and that required by the body to manufacture and maintain the blood. If the arterial diameter were to increase generally, the power required to move the same volume of blood would decrease. However, such an increase in radius would result in an increase in blood volume with added cost to the body.[3] Theoretical considerations suggest that if energy loss is to be minimized, the radii of blood vessels should be proportional to the third power of the blood flow. It might be expected that this would be the diameter that the artery assumes in vivo and there is support for this.[4] If all this is true, and flow change is to be accommodated, then all the arteries that contribute to this adjustment must be capable of constriction and dilation. To achieve this in the resting animal, there must be a basal level of tone allowing both an increase and decrease in diameter, and one that optimizes the energy requirement of flow in the branching system. Although there is little direct evidence, there is reason to entertain the possibility that there is adjustment of the entire pial artery branching system during autoregulation. All these vessels have muscle in their walls and have the capacity to change diameter in response to changes in pressure and flow. Furthermore, the autoregulatory control process is very exact. Only by adjustments in all the consecutive branches can optimality be maintained.

The Stretch-Induced (Myogenic) Response of Human Pial Arteries

Human cerebral pial arteries were transported to the laboratory at 5°C in PSS containing 50 U penicillin/50 µg streptomycin and 20 U heparin/mL. After dissection, the vessel segment, 1.5–3.0 mm in length, was mounted in a pressure-perfusion system arteriograph.[5] The proximal end of the artery was tied onto a cannula, and then it was flushed with bicarbonate (25 mM) PSS (in mM: NaCl, 119; KCl, 4.7; KH$_2$PO$_4$, 1.18; MgSO$_4$, 1.17; NaH$_2$CO$_3$, 24.9; CaCl$_2$, 1.6; EDTA 23 µM; glucose 11). The free end of the artery was then tied onto the distal cannula, and the artery pressurized to 5–10 mmHg, depending on its size. This pressure is just sufficient to remove all the internal corrugations. The vessel was superfused with 25 mM bicarbonate PSS at 2–3.5 mL/min and allowed to heat up from room temperature to 37°C, when the arterial diameter was measured using the video-dimension analyzer. Another diameter measurement was taken after an instantaneous pressure step to 50–60 mmHg, and appropriate longitudinal stretch applied. Stretch-induced myogenic tone developed over the subsequent 60–150 min. Once tone was established, a series of random pressure steps at increments of 10–20 mmHg over the range of 20–120 mmHg were conducted. The initial passive diameter achieved immediately after the change in pressure was measured together with the equilibrium diameter achieved several minutes later. Subsequently, after exposure to a superfusate of K$^+$ (127 mM) PSS, a similar series of pressure steps and observations were made.

Finally, in order to obtain the passive pressure–diameter curve relationship of the perfused vessel, the superfusate was changed to Ca^{2+}-free bicarbonate (25 mM) PSS containing EGTA (1 mM). Once a plateau was reached indicating that all stretch-induced myogenic tone was lost, a sequential order of pressure steps was carried out up to 200 mmHg in increments of 5 or 10 mmHg, vessel diameter measurements being made at each step. All diameters were normalized to those obtained either at 5–10 or 50–60 mmHg during the initial 30-min setup.

In Fig. 1 are shown the three pressure diameter curves used to characterize the myogenic response of the artery wall and its passive wall properties. The middle curve shows the diameter obtained by the segment in normal PSS (bicarbonate 25 mM) when it is free to develop tone and change diameter. Over the pressure range 20–120 mmHg, the measurement in this vessel remained constant. The experimental design, which involves repeating one of the pressure responses during the course of the experiment, allows trends, if any, in the active maintained diameter to be detected during the duration of the experiments. Such changes were found to be minimal. At 50–60 mmHg, the arterial diameter decreased by 18.5 $\pm$ 2.1% ($n = 15$). This assumes that the diameter of the vessel can be reduced to zero. In practice, this is not obtainable. The practical limits of narrowing are illustrated in the pressure diameter curve obtained in the presence of K$^+$ (127 mM) PSS (lower curve) when the smooth muscle cells are maximally contracted. Thus, the myo-

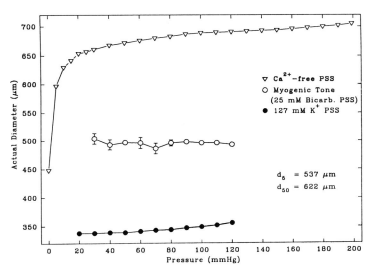

Fig. 1. The relationship between intravascular pressure and diameter of a human pial artery in which stretch-induced myogenic tone was allowed to develop in bicarbonate (25 mM) PSS, in the presence of K$^+$ (127 mM) PSS that caused maximum increase in smooth muscle tone and in Ca^{2+}-free PSS containing 1 mM EGTA when active muscle tone could not develop. The latter curve reflects passive wall properties. At 50 mmHg, the diameter of the artery after all muscle tone was abolished was 672 μm. The level of myogenic tone represents a 26.0% decrease in vessel lumen size. The segment was obtained from a frontal pial artery of a 69-yr-old male whose history included obesity, hypertension, and who was undergoing a craniotomy for a tumor. This result was obtained 48 h after surgery. Vessels from this patient maintained a similar level of myogenic tone 24 h after surgery.

genic tone level of this vessel is approx 50% of the maximum obtainable constriction. We do not know what percent of maximal smooth muscle tone shortening is actually represented by this measurement. The upper pressure–diameter curves obtained when all vascular smooth muscle tone is abolished represents the passive pressure/diameter relationship for the segment. Both the upper and lower relationships show a modest increase in diameter with increasing pressure above 100–120 mmHg. The active diameter achieved by the small pial arteries usually remains remarkably constant.

Not all human pial artery preparations behaved in this manner. Figure 2 is an example of a pial artery segment that did not maintain its maximum level of constriction in the face of increasing pressure. At 120–130 mmHg, the maximum depolarization-induced contraction had fallen off and was equal to that of the myogenic response, i.e., the stretch-induced contraction was equivalent to tissue maximum. It is significant that despite the fall-off in the maximum maintained contraction, the diameter achieved by the myogenic response maintains arterial diameter constant even with intraluminal pressures that exceed 100 mmHg. This implies that in this vessel, the stretch-induced activity involves an increasing proportion of the contractile capacity of the smooth muscle cells as pressure is raised. It suggests that the sensing and also the coupling of this to contraction remain relatively intact. If the end point of the myogenic response is to maintain a constant cell length, not a proportionate increase in obtainable tone, then this result is consistent with this hypothesis. To maintain cell length in the face of increasing intramural pressure involves increasing wall force as pressure rises. It suggests that the deficiency in the myogenic response in some segments with increased pressure is a defect in the force maintaining apparatus, rather than the stretch sensing and its coupling mechanism.

We have not yet studied a sufficient number of vessels to know what trends there are, if any, in the level of myogenic tone and the pressure range over which it is maintained, in relation, for example, to vessel diameter, age, or some vascular pathology. Results to date suggest that the myogenic response of the human pial arteries is similar at least qualitatively to that seen in laboratory animals.

Flow-Induced Responses of Human Pial Arteries

The technique of mounting small vessels as ring segments in vitro for measurement of isometric wall tension[6,7] and the infusion of PSS into their lumen has been previously described.[8] Briefly, two adjacent 2-mm long arterial or venous segments are mounted in separate myographs, maintained in vitro at 37°C, equilibrated with 95% O_2–5% CO_2, and stretched to their optimum length for agonist-induced contraction. Physiological saline bath solution was

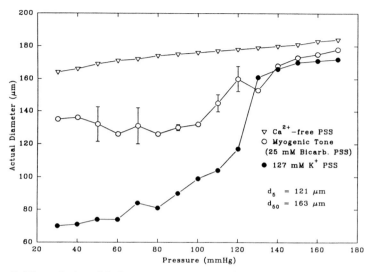

Fig. 2. The relationship between intravascular pressure and diameter of a human pial artery in which stretch-induced myogenic tone was allowed to develop in bicarbonate (25 m*M*) PSS, in the presence of K⁺ (127 m*M*) PSS that caused maximum increase in smooth muscle tone, and in Ca²⁺-free PSS containing 1 m*M* EGTA, which inhibits active muscle tone development. The latter curve reflects passive wall properties. At 50 mmHg, the diameter of the artery after all muscle tone was abolished was 169 µm. The actual diameter associated with stretch-induced myogenic tone was maintained from 30 to 100 mmHg, at a level that represents a 21.9% decrease in vessel lumen size. The segment was obtained from a pial artery of a 56-yr-old male who suffered from a recurrent bilateral frontal meningioma.

infused into the artery lumen through a glass micropipet whose tip was placed just within the open end of the vessel, using a Harvard syringe infusion pump 22 at rates between 0.5 and 3 µL/min for varying time periods. Drugs were added directly to the tissue bath.

Bath temperature was changed by adjusting the thermostatic control on the Laude RM6 refrigerated pump that circulated fluid through the jacketed tissue bath. At the end of each experiment, the contractile response to 127 m*M* KCl plus $10^{-6}M$ vasopressin was recorded at 1 and 37°C. This is taken as the contraction maximum.

Responses to intraluminal infusion of PSS were very variable. Since the size and the direction of the change in tone with flow are very dependent on the level of wall tone and these vessels often show spontaneous maintained, but also unpredictably changing levels of wall tone, the response is difficult to study and quantify. The time-course and pattern of response show considerable variability and are not always quantitatively reproducible even in the same preparation. This probably reflects long-term changes in the excitable state of the blood vessel wall that are not understood. Despite these difficulties and bearing in mind the changes observed in animal tissues as a guide, we can begin to interpret some of the patterns of the flow responses in the human pial arteries.

Both contraction (force increase) and relaxation (force decrease) changes were observed (Fig. 3). Flow contraction was more commonly seen at lower levels of wall force, both spontaneous and agonist-induced. The half-time for contraction is 64.6 ± 19.5 ($n = 19$) s. Flow dilation, the most frequently elicited response, is observed with higher levels of wall force. The half-time for this response is 124.4 ± 17 ($n = 23$) s. Both responses have been observed to reach an equilibrium that is maintained for the duration of the infusion.

A commonly seen variant response is one in which an initial response—contractile—to flow reverses, leveling out below the preflow tone level, which is maintained until the infusion is stopped. Wall tone then usually reverts to its preflow value (Fig. 3). It is tempting to speculate that as proposed for animal vessels, intraluminal flow induces simultaneously both flow contraction and flow dilation of the human pial arteries.[9] Since the latency for flow contraction is shorter than that for dilation, an increase in tone is first observed. Then the consequence of the more slowly developing dilator response is seen. The final effect is the algebraic sum of the two opposite responses. In animal studies, there is much evidence to support the idea that both the contraction and dilation response are activated simultaneously.[10] In addition to the change in the direction of the flow response seen as the preflow level of wall force is increased, there are other observations to support this point of view, specifically:

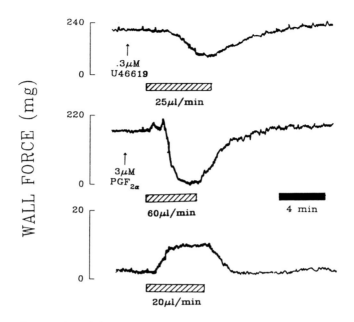

Fig. 3. Examples of changes in isometric wall force of human pial arteries during intraluminal infusion of physiological saline solution. Period of infusion as shown by the hatched bars. **(A)** Pial artery internal lumen diameter 266 μm from 55-yr-old male. Infusion at 25 μL/min caused a 17% inhibition of spontaneously developed wall force. **(B)** Pial artery internal lumen diameter 550 μm from 69-yr-old male. Infusion at 60 μL/min caused complete inhibition of tone induced by $PGF_{2\alpha}$ ($3 \times 10^{-6}M$). Note that the initial contractile response changes within approx 2 min to dilation. **(C)** Pial artery internal lumen diameter 570 μm from a 73-yr-old female without preflow tone. Infusion at 20 μL/min caused a contraction that was 10% of tissue maximum.

1. The effect of nominal zero calcium conditions blocked flow dilation, but not flow contraction.[10]
2. In some vessels where flow dilation is entirely endothelium-dependent, pharmacological block of NO synthase or inhibition of cyclic GMP reversed the effect of flow (Xiao and Bevan, unpublished data).
3. Flow contraction and flow dilation are associated with membrane depolarization and hyperpolarization, respectively.[11]

    A variety of patterns of electrophysiological change can be interpreted as the interaction of these two membrane potential responses.

4. The change in the force record in response to flow is often very complex, but can usually be interpreted as the interaction between two opposite mechanisms with different time-courses.

Our experimental series is too few in number and from too diverse a patient population to permit generalization about the way in which the flow response varies in relation to different patient characteristics.

In a number of experiments on human pial artery segments, we observed reversal of the flow response from contraction to dilation, as the level of wall tone was increased. Flow contraction was usually studied by flowing on baseline or when the vessel did not show significant myogenic tone; in this series, flow dilation was seen at all levels of wall tone between 20 and 100% of tissue maximum. When a regression line was fitted to the peaks of the flow responses, both contraction and relaxation—for each experiment—the level at which this line intercepted zero response was $13.3 \pm 15.2\%$ ($n = 8$) of the maximum tissue force development. We assume this to be an approximation of the flow null or balance point for flow. Although it is not easy to extrapolate from isometric studies in vitro to those that pertain in the body, the data are consistent with the levels of basal intrinsic tone seen in vivo in small resistance vessels.[12]

Synopsis of Animal Studies on Small Artery Myogenic Tone, Flow Contraction, and Dilation

The diagrams in Fig. 4 illustrate the summary from a recent review[13] of some of the cellular mechanisms responsible for stretch-induced tone and the bimodal tone response to intramural flow (for details and references, *see* ref. 13).

Stretch-Induced Tone

A stretch/pressure constriction sensor (Sm) is located in the smooth muscle and endothelial cells. Entry of Ca^{2+} occurs via channels activated directly by stretch and possibly concomitantly by activation of voltage-dependent channels. Stretch/pressure contraction is Ca^{2+}-dependent and is mediated by protein kinase C

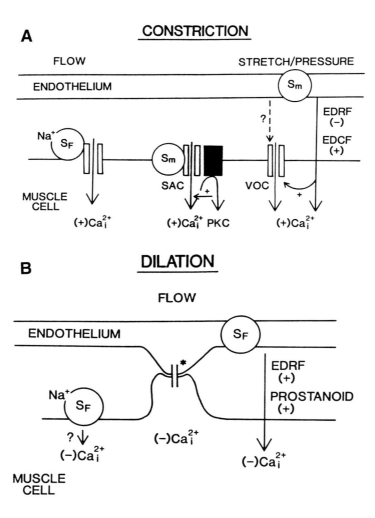

Fig. 4. Diagrammatic representation of mechanisms of pressure, flow-induced vasoconstriction, and flow-induced vasodilation. **(A)** Proposed mechanism of flow and stretch/pressure constriction of blood vessels. Changes in flow influence sensors (Sf) located on vascular smooth muscle cells or adjacent matrix. Alterations in the extracellular concentrations of sodium (Na^+) affect the constrictor response to flow. Stretch/pressure sensors (Sm) are located in the smooth muscle and endothelial cells. Entry of Ca^{2+} occurs via channels activated directly by stretch and by activation of voltage-dependent channels. Stretch/pressure contraction is Ca^{2+}-dependent

(PKC). Inhibition of release of endothelial-derived relaxing factor (EDRF) and the release of an endothelial-derived constricting factor (EDCF) may contribute to the increase in tone in some vessels.

Flow-Induced Changes in Tone

Changes in flow influence sensors (Sf) located on vascular endothelial cells or, if these are removed, on the subjacent extracellular matrix and/or smooth muscle cells. Alterations in the extracellular concentrations of sodium (Na^+) affect the flow sensors and, thus, both the constrictor and dilator responses to flow. Flow contraction is associated with an uptake of calcium.[14] Flow dilation may be related to the release of endothelial-derived relaxing factor (EDRF), and in some blood vessels, prostanoids and also possibly by a muscle-derived endogenous dilator factor.[15]

Flow Sensor

The mechanism that has been proposed for a flow sensor is not included in Fig. 4. Flow over the outer and inner surface of an endothelium-denuded blood vessel results in comparable changes in muscle tone, suggesting the involvement of elements in the flow sensing that exist throughout the thickness of the blood vessel wall.[16] Functional experiments implicating an important role for sodium and flow in shear stress-induced change in tone and biochemical studies showing that shear can result in changes in Na^+ binding to a specific polyanionic site together with other observations have led to a hypothesis that the flow sensor may be the cation binding complex of a proteoglycan. These viscoelastic, anionic, hydrated biopolyelectrolytes under external strain, such as shear, may change

---

and is mediated by protein kinase C (PKC), inhibition of endothelium-derived relaxing factor (EDRF), and release of endothelium-derived constricting factor (EDCF). **(B)** Proposed mechanism of flow dilation of blood vessels. Sensors (Sf) located on the endothelial cells or vascular smooth muscle cells decrease the intracellular concentration of calcium (Ca^{2+}) by releasing endothelium-derived relaxing factors (EDRF) and also muscle-derived relaxing factor.[13] Alternatively or in addition, flow dilation may be associated with hyperpolarization. Flow dilation that occurs both in the presence and absence of the endothelium is sensitive to changes in extracellular Na^+.

from a randomly coiled to a longitudinally oriented state. Our hypothesis is that proteoglycan sulfate is present as a random coil under "no-flow" conditions and as a less furled filamentous structure with increasing flow, and that this change in shape is associated with an increase in binding sites for Na^+.[17,18] The Na^+ ion itself may be related to flow signal transduction; a change in the transmembrane Na^+ gradient has been proposed,[13] but the detailed mechanism involved is unclear. When flow is reduced, intramolecular, elastic recoil forces result in the assumption of the original molecular form and an interruption of the signal.

Role of Perivascular Nerves in the Regulation of Cerebral Blood Flow

In vivo studies of the brain circulation suggest that the most important consequence of activity of the cerebrovascular innervation is to extend the limit of autoregulation.[19,20] If this is correct, then activity of the nerves to the brain vessels is only important when arterial pressure is high or low. Such a conclusion is consistent with observations that stimulation of the sympathetic nervous system has little influence on cerebral blood flow[21,22] when blood pressure is within normal levels.

If function can be inferred from the anatomical arrangement of the distribution of perivascular nerves to the cerebral bed, they would be expected to exert an overall, generalized influence on the main arterial distribution system, and this effect would most likely be small. Differences between the density of innervation of anterior and posterior cerebral arteries have been described, but these relate to the arteries supplying major divisions of the brain, and not to the smaller branches. There is very good reason to view both the constrictor and dilator systems as part of more widespread neural outflows that exert control over much of the vasculature of the head. Within the pial artery network, local adjustments to flow must occur presumably through a local action. The most likely mechanisms for pial arteries not subject to direct metabolic influence from brain tissue and minimally influenced by nerves are those evoked through changes in local intravascular pressure and flow.

Role of Pressure and Flow
in the Regulation of Cerebral Blood Flow

In a myograph-mounted arterial preparation, the level of the flow and membrane potential determines the direction of the flow response of animal pial arteries. When more negative than –58 mV, contraction ensues, and when less negative, dilation.[11] The reported vascular smooth muscle cell membrane potential range in vitro is –60 to –75 mV.[23] In vivo data, although scarce, suggest that membrane potentials are 10–25 mV less negative than in vitro. On the basis of these figures, it might be predicted that in vivo, flow dilation would be the commonly observed response—as almost invariably seems to be the case.[12]

Tone in the resistance vasculature is because of multiple mechanisms. Myogenic tone (stretch) contributes significantly and (it is speculated) is associated with calcium entry through stretch-dependent potential sensitive-channels.[13] Harder et al.[24] subjected the middle cerebral artery of the cat to increasing pressure over the range 40–120 mmHg. E_m decreased from –53.06 ± 2.7 to –22.6 ± 1.4 mV. At the equivalent of physiological pressures (80 mmHg), the mean membrane potential in this artery was of the order of –35 to –40 mV. Brayden and Wellman[25] found a membrane potential of –63 mV in unstretched feline cerebral arteries of 400 μm OD. At 50 mmHg, the membrane potential averaged –48 mV.

Some of the human pial arteries we examined developed myogenic tone that effectively maintained diameter up to intraluminal pressures exceeding 100 mmHg. In others, the ability of the artery to maintain this tone fell off at lower pressures. We can only presume that the first group represents the normal "healthy" response, and the latter some departure from this, either because of patient disease or some technical experimental problem. Unfortunately, membrane potential changes of these human vessels are unknown.

In the human pial arteries, several types of observations favor the conclusion that flow can cause both contraction and dilation. This is evidenced by the biphasic response—flow contraction preceding flow dilation—and the reversal of the flow effect when wall tone is increased. Thus, there is good reason to consider that the flow-related set or balance point seen in animals also occurs in humans. Our observations in animals can be interpreted as suggesting that flow buffers the influence of other factors that affect vascular tone, modifying their effect toward an intermediate tone level—the balance or set point. After an increase in central arterial pressure, for example, it would be expected that most of the smaller arteries would constrict because of the myogenic response. Since this would result in vascular smooth muscle cell depolarization, flow contraction would be diminished and flow dilation augmented. There would be a tendency for the effect of the myogenic response on flow to be restored. However, if the extent of depolarization owing to the myogenic response was small, either flow might decrease or not change. These conclusions, however, contrast with other proposals that emphasize the competitive interaction between myogenic contraction and flow dilation,[26] and the primary role of flow in communication and coordination of small vessel function.[27,28]

In summary, the myogenic response represents a mechanism that protects the microcirculation from excessive changes in pressure, both increases and decreases; this response occurs independently of local tissue needs. The blood-flow-induced changes in tone provide a further dimension to the regulation of local flow. They modify other regulating effects in relation to tissue need. This occurs because the effect of shear stress seems to be exerted through a local mechanism in the blood vessel wall.

Acknowledgments

Arteries were kindly supplied by F. D. Barranco, Neurological Surgeons, P. C., Phoenix, AZ and E. Vijayakumaran, Department of Pediatrics, University of Vermont. This work was supported by the Ray and Ildah Totman Medical Research Fund.

References

[1] Bevan, J. A. and Bevan, R. D. (1993) *NIPS* **8,** 149–153.
[2] Duckworth, J. W., Wellman, G. C., Walters, C. L. and Bevan, J. A. (1989) *Circ. Res.* **65,** 316–324.
[3] Zamir, M. (1977) *J. Gen. Physiol.* **69,** 449–461.

[4] Mayrowitz, H. N. and Roy, J. (1983) *Am. J. Physiol.* **245,** H1031–1038.

[5] Halpern, W., Osol, G., and Coy, G. S. (1984) *Ann. Biomed. Eng.* **12,** 463–479.

[6] Bevan, J. A. and Osher, J. V. (1972) *Agents and Actions* **2,** 257–260.

[7] Mulvany, M. J. and Halpern, W. (1976) *Nature (Lond.)* **260,** 617–619.

[8] Bevan, J. A., Joyce, E. H., and Wellman, G. C. (1988) *Circ. Res.* **63,** 980–985.

[9] Bevan, J. A. and Joyce, E. H. (1990) *Am. J. Physiol.* **258** (*Heart Circ. Physiol.* **27**), H663–H668.

[10] Bevan, J. A. (1994) *Flow Dependent Regulation of Vascular Function in Health and Disease* (Kaley, G., Rubanyi, G., and Bevan, J. A., eds.), Oxford University Press, New York, in press.

[11] Bevan, J. A. and Wellman, G. C. (1993) *Circ. Res.* **73,** 1188–1192.

[12] Bevan, J. A. (1991) *The Resistance Vasculature* (Bevan, J. A., Halpern, W., and Mulvany, M. J., eds.), Humana, Totowa, NJ, pp. 169–191.

[13] Bevan, J. A. and Laher, I. (1991) *FASEB J.* **5,** 2267–2273.

[14] Henrion, D., Laher, I., and Bevan, J. A. (1992) *Circ. Res.* **71,** 339–345.

[15] Gaw, A. G. and Bevan, J. A. (1991) *Resistance Arteries: Structure and Function* (Mulvany, M. J., Aalkjaer, C., Heagerty, A. M., Nyborg, N. C., and Strandgaard, S., eds.), Elsevier Science, The Netherlands, pp. 20–23.

[16] Bevan, J. A. and Siegel, G. (1991) *Blood Vessels* **28,** 552–556.

[17] Siegel, G., Walter, A., Ruckborn, K., Buddecke, E., Schmidt, A., Gustavsson, H., and Lindman, B. (1991) *Polymer J.* **23,** 697–708.

[18] Siegel, G., Walter, A., Schnalke, F., Schmidt, A., Buddecke, E., Loirand, G., and Stock, G. (1991) *Z. Kardiol.* **80(Suppl. 7),** 9–24.

[19] Harper, A. M. (1975) *Cerebral Vascular Diseases* (Whisnant, J. P. and Sandok, B. A., eds.), Grune and Stratton, New York, pp. 27–35.

[20] Hernandez, M. J., Raichle, M. E., and Stone, H. L. (1977) *Neurogenic Control of the Brain Circulation* (Owman, C. and Edvinsson, L., eds.), Pergamon, New York, pp. 377–386.

[21] Gross, P. M., Heistad, D. D., Strait, M. R., Marcus, M. L., and Brody, M. J. (1979) *Circ. Res.* **44,** 288–294.

[22] MacKenzie, E. T., McGeorge, A. P., Graham, D. I., Fitch, W., Edvinsson, L., and Harper, A. M. (1979) *Pfluegers Arch.* **378,** 189–195.

[23] Hirst, G. D. S. and Edwards, F. R. (1989) *Physiol. Rev.* **69,** 546–595.

[24] Harder, D. R., Sanchez-Ferrer, C., Kauser, K., Stekiel, W. J., and Rubanyi, G. M. (1989) *Circ. Res.* **65,** 193–198.

[25] Brayden, J. E. and Wellman, G. C. (1989) *J. Cereb. Blood Flow Metabol.* **9,** 256–263.

[26] Kuo, L., Chilian, W. M., and Davis, M. J. (1991) *Am. J. Physiol.* **261** (*Heart Circ. Physiol.* **30**), H1706–H1715.

[27] Duling, B. R. (1991) *Resistance Arteries, Structure and Function* (Mulvany, M. J., Aalkjaer, C., Heagerty, A. M., Nyborg, N. C. B., and Strandgaard, S., eds.), Elsevier Science, Amsterdam, pp. 3–9.

[28] Segal, S. S. (1992) *NIPS* **7,** 152–156.

Chapter 15

Mechanisms of Hypoxic
and Hypercapnic Cerebral Vasodilatation

William J. Pearce

Introduction

The purpose of this chapter is to give an overview of current thinking regarding the mechanisms of hypoxic and hypercapnic cerebral vasodilatation. Given the great breadth of this topic, the chapter will focus primarily on the general hypotheses proposed to explain these effects, which fall into three main groups. The first and oldest of these is the tissue effect group, which includes hypotheses dealing with a primary effect on the neural and glial tissues of the brain with secondary effects on cerebral vessels. The second collection of ideas is the direct vascular group, which includes proposals involving a direct effect of hypoxia or hypercapnia on cerebrovascular smooth muscle. Finally, the endothelial effect group includes ideas describing a direct effect of hypoxia or hypercapnia on cerebrovascular endothelium, with secondary effects on the underlying smooth muscle (*see* Figs. 1 and 2).

Hypoxic Cerebral Vasodilatation
Extravascular Factors
Potassium Hypothesis/H^+ Hypothesis

Among the tissue effect hypotheses is an idea, first proposed in the mid 1960s, that hypoxia promotes the release of hydrogen ion, perhaps in the form of lactic acid, which then diffuses to the

From *The Human Brain Circulation*, R. D. Bevan and J. A. Bevan, eds.
©1994 Humana Press

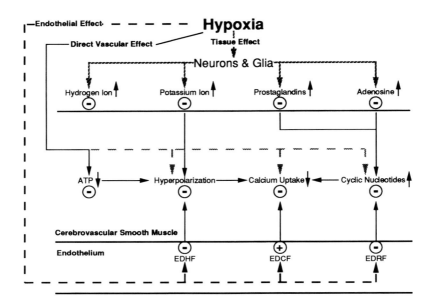

Fig. 1. Mechanisms of hypoxic cerebral vasodilatation. In response to hypoxia, neurons and glia release widely varying quantities of hydrogen ion, potassium ion, prostaglandins, and adenosine, all of which promote vasodilatation through secondary actions on cerebrovascular smooth muscle. Through direct actions on vascular endothelium, hypoxia promotes the release of hyperpolarizing (EDHF), contracting (EDCF), and relaxing (EDRF) factors. Within vascular smooth muscle cells, hypoxia reduces ATP levels enough to promote hyperpolarization and reduce calcium uptake, which led to vasorelaxation. The effects of both tissue and endothelial factors released by hypoxia also appear to be mediated, at least in part, through changes in hyperpolarization and calcium uptake, and may also involve changes in vascular cyclic nucleotide levels. Throughout this diagram, the circled minus signs indicate a net vasodilator influence, and the circled plus signs, a net vasoconstrictor influence.

perivascular surface to promote vasodilatation.[1] Similarly, potassium ion was also proposed as a perivascular signal of tissue hypoxia. This perivascular pH and potassium hypothesis persisted until the late 1970s, when ion-selective electrodes were used to make the first direct measurements of pH and potassium during hypoxic vasodilatation. The consistent finding of these measurements was

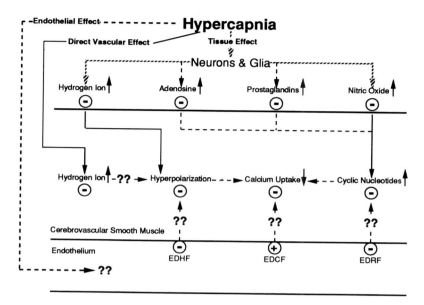

Fig. 2. Mechanisms of hypercapnic cerebral vasodilatation. As for hypoxia, hypercapnia can also potentially act directly on at least three different tissue types within the brain to promote vasodilatation. In response to hypercapnia, neurons and glia appear to release hydrogen ion and possibly also nitric oxide. Hypercapnic release of parenchymal prostaglandins appears to be species-specific. A role for tissue adenosine in hypercapnic cerebral vasodilatation has been reported, but remains controversial. As indicated by the question marks, the effects of hypercapnia on the release of endothelial vasoactive factors remain largely unexplored. Perhaps the most important effect of hypercapnia is on the intracellular pH of vascular smooth muscle cells, although effects on membrane potential and cyclic nucleotide levels have also been reported. Clearly, much less is known of the mechanisms mediating the cerebral vasodilatation owing to hypercapnia than that owing to hypoxia. For abbreviations, *see* the legend for Fig. 1.

that "changes in perivascular potassium and hydrogen ion concentrations are too slow and too small to fully explain hypoxic cerebral vasodilatation."[2–4] Although these measurements were first criticized because the electrodes used were thought to be too inaccurate, or to have too slow a response time to define the pH or potassium time-courses precisely during hypoxia, subsequent measurements using more modern methods have confirmed these early observations.[5] Clearly, changes in perivascular hydrogen and potassium ion contribute to hypoxic vasodilatation, but this contribution is probably significant only under conditions of prolonged severe hypoxia.

Prostaglandin Hypothesis

Another member of the tissue effects family of ideas is the prostaglandin hypothesis, which proposes that hypoxia promotes the release of vasodilator prostaglandins. First originated from work in coronary arteries by Kalsner and others in the mid 1970s,[6] this idea was explored in the rat cerebral circulation in the late 1970s by Sakabe and Siesjo, who found that indomethacin had little effect on hypoxic responses.[7] Similarly, Kontos et al. found that indomethacin had little effect on cat pial artery responses to hypoxia.[8] However, McCalden et al. reported in 1984 that hypoxia increased cerebral prostacyclin syntheses in the baboon brain, and that both this increase and the attendant vasodilatation were attenuated by indomethacin.[9] Working in newborn piglets, Leffler and Busija reported in 1985 that indomethacin could block the pial vasodilatation produced by asphyxia.[10] Bian and Toda[11] and Inoue et al.[12] have also recently suggested that prostacyclin contributes to hypoxic vasodilatation in the dog. Given this range of findings, there is now some consensus that prostaglandins may be involved in hypoxic cerebral vasodilatation, but that the extent of this involvement is highly species, and perhaps age, specific. Given the sensitivity of the baboon[9] and human[13–15] cerebral circulations to indomethacin, a role for prostaglandin synthesis in hypoxic cerebral vasodilatation in humans seems possible, although direct evidence in support of this view has yet to be obtained.

Adenosine Hypothesis

Perhaps the least controversial of the tissue-effect family of ideas is the adenosine hypothesis, which attributes hypoxic vasodilatation to increases in perivascular adenosine concentration. First originated by Berne and colleagues based on work in the coronary and skeletal muscle circulations,[16] this idea gained relevance to the cerebral circulation when Winn et al. demonstrated definitively in rats that "adenosine concentrations in brain are increased during hypoxia."[17]

The adenosine hypothesis, however, cannot completely explain hypoxic cerebral vasodilatation. As shown in rabbits, a maximal dose of theophylline can block only about half of the cerebral response to hypoxia (*see* Fig. 3). Although theophylline is not the cleanest or most selective antagonist of the A2 adenosine receptor, other studies have yielded similar results, thus reinforcing the notion that adenosine is an important, but not the only, mediator of hypoxic cerebral vasodilatation.[18]

Direct Vascular Effects of Hypoxia

Given that changes in perivascular hydrogen and potassium ion are important primarily during severe or prolonged hypoxia, prostaglandins play a variable species-dependent role, and adenosine can explain only about half of the response to acute moderate hypoxia, other mechanisms must be involved in the cerebrovascular responses to hypoxia. Principal among these are the direct vascular effects of hypoxia.

Early Hypotheses

Early in the search for mechanisms of hypoxic vasodilatation, Pittman and Duling proposed that hypoxia may simply precipitate the depletion of vascular ATP, which in turn would limit contraction.[19] Despite a series of elegant arguments and indirect data in support of this hypothesis, direct measurements of vascular ATP reveal that, although ATP concentrations do fall between 20 and 30%, hypoxic relaxation is well developed long before vascular ATP levels become limiting for either actomyosin ATPase or myosin light-chain kinase.[20-22] Although it remains possible that decreases in ATP during hypoxia may be compartmentalized within the vascular cell, the early version of the ATP-limitation hypothesis has now been largely abandoned.[23] Similarly, a proposal by Coburn et al. that a specific intracellular oxygen receptor mediates hypoxic relaxation[24] has also been generally abandoned.[25] This oxygen-receptor idea was based on the ability of cyanide to inhibit hypoxic relaxation.[26,27] However, cyanide also interferes with multiple intracellular mechanisms within smooth muscle. Most

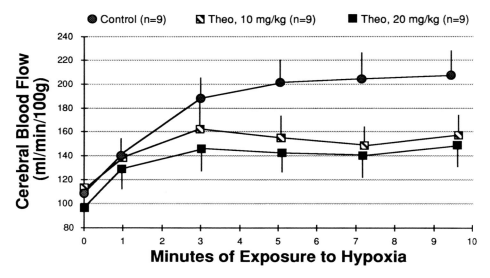

Fig. 3. Effects of theophylline on hypoxic cerebral vasodilatation. Cerebral blood flow was measured by the helium wash-out method[44] in lightly anesthetized rabbits after 0, 1, 3, 5, 7, and 9 min of hypoxia, produced by reducing the inspired oxygen content to 8%. Arterial oxygen tensions dropped to ≈35 torr within 2 min of lowering the inspired oxygen and remained stable thereafter. Theophylline at either 10 or 20 mg/kg administered iv 15 min prior to hypoxia, completely blocked the vasodilator response to 100 µg/kg iv adenosine, but only blocked approx 50% of the vasodilatation response to hypoxia. The vertical error bars indicate standard errors for the number of animals indicated in parentheses.

importantly, other laboratories have been unable to reproduce a selective effect of cyanide on the direct relaxant effects of hypoxia on vascular smooth muscle.[28]

Hyperpolarization Hypothesis

A more modern explanation of hypoxic relaxation is provided by the membrane hyperpolarization hypothesis, which proposes that hypoxia acts to hyperpolarize the vascular smooth muscle membrane. Based on indirect observations of the effects of ouabain and sodium-free Krebs on hypoxic relaxation of rabbit aorta, Detar and Bohr first proposed this hypothesis in the late 1960s.[29] Detar later refined and more explicitly stated the hyperpolarization hypothesis in 1980, but the evidence in support of the hypothesis was still entirely indirect.[30] The first direct evidence in support of the hyperpolarization hypothesis was provided by Grote et al. in the late 1980s.[31] These studies demonstrated, in isolated dog carotid artery, that a decrease in oxygen tension produced a simultaneous hyperpolarization and vasorelaxation. Unfortunately, however, this effect began at pO_2 values near 150 torr and was complete at pO_2 values above 50 torr. Thus, the maximum effect occurred over a pO_2 range not typically associated with hypoxic vasodilatation, in vivo. Thus, these data were not universally taken as direct support for the hyperpolarization hypothesis.

In the late 1980s, another idea related to hyperpolarization was gaining rapid acceptance, and that was related to ATP-sensitive potassium channels.[32-34] As we now know, these channels increase their conductance to potassium when intracellular ATP concentrations fall and, thus, act to hyperpolarize the smooth muscle membrane.[35] More importantly, the K_m for ATP of these channels[34,36] is up to an order of magnitude higher than that for actomyosin ATPase or myosin light-chain kinase,[37,38] which predicts that if ATP levels fall at all, then ATP-sensitive potassium channels should be among the first cellular components to respond.

To test this idea in cerebral arteries, we have recently examined the effects of glibenclamide, a specific blocker of the ATP-sensitive potassium channel, on hypoxic cerebral vasodilatation in rabbit cerebral arteries. We found that doses of glibenclamide, which block the responses to cromakalim, a specific activator of ATP-sensitive potassium channels, also blocked hypoxic relaxation in isolated rabbit carotid arteries and attenuated the response in cerebral arteries in a size-dependent manner.[39] Because of the indirect nature of our measurements, however, we could not determine if the size dependency of this effect was the result of either a decreased density of ATP-sensitive potassium channels in the smaller arteries or a smaller decrease in ATP owing to the thinner wall and thus a smaller oxygen gradient in the smaller vessels.

Direct evidence that ATP-sensitive channels are important in the cerebrovascular responses to hypoxia has recently been provided by Bonnet et al.[40] Using cell-attached patch-clamp techniques, these experiments demonstrate that hypoxia increases K^+ channel activity in cat cerebral arterial muscle cells. Because these increases were largely inhibited by selective concentrations of glibenclamide, it appears that this increased activity is mediated by ATP-sensitive potassium channels.

Calcium Hypothesis

As suggested by a wide variety of electrophysiological studies, membrane hyperpolarization leads to vasorelaxation by inhibiting the calcium conductance of voltage-operated membrane calcium channels.[35] Consistent with such a mechanism, it was proposed in the early 1980s by Ebeigbe, long before the existence of ATP-sensitive potassium channels was established, that "a decrease in calcium uptake may be a mechanism for hypoxic relaxation."[41] Because Ebeigbe's hypothesis was based entirely on work with rabbit aorta, my laboratory decided to test this hypothesis in rabbit cerebral arteries. Using direct measurements of calcium uptake, we found that hypoxia had little effect on unactivated arteries, but significantly depressed calcium uptake in arteries activated with either potassium or serotonin.[42] Interestingly, the magnitude of this inhibitory effect of hypoxia appeared greater in potassium depolarized than in serotonin-contracted arteries. Because increased potassium conductance owing to ATP-sensitive channels would have little influence under potassium depolarized conditions, these data suggest that hypoxia may also affect calcium uptake through pathways independent of hyperpolarization produced by ATP-sensitive potassium channels. The identity of these additional pathways, however, remains uncertain.

Endothelium Hypothesis

In addition to the established effects of hypoxia on vascular ATP, membrane potential, and calcium uptake, hypoxia also has other effects in isolated arteries. For example, recent data from Coburn et al.[43] suggest that hypoxia may attenuate receptor-induced mobilization of inositol trisphosphate and, thus, reduce contractile capacity. More importantly, hypoxia also appears to increase vascular cyclic nucleotide levels, both in response to increased parenchymal synthesis of cyclic-nucleotide-dependent relaxants, but also through the release of endothelial factors.[44,45]

Based on work in dog coronary arteries, Busse et al. proposed in 1983 that the "endothelium plays a crucial role in the dilator response to hypoxia."[46] As suggested by these initial studies, hypoxia was proposed to release both prostacyclin and endo-thelium-derived relaxing factor. To explore this hypothesis in the cerebral circulation, my laboratory mounted intact and denuded segments of rabbit basilar, internal carotid, and common carotid arteries in vitro, contracted them with potassium or serotonin, and then exposed them to hypoxia.[45] In the potassium-contracted arteries, removal of the endothelium attenuated hypoxic relaxation approx 50% in the basilar and 20% in the internal carotid, but poten-tiated relaxation in the common carotid, suggesting the hypoxic release of a contracting factor in this artery. In the serotonin-con-tracted arteries, the hypoxic release of a contracting factor became even more evident, and again, this effect was artery dependent. Together these data suggest that hypoxia releases both relaxing and contracting factors from rabbit cerebral endothelium, and that this release is weighted more toward relaxing factors in the more distal cerebral arteries and more toward contracting factors in the more proximal vessels.

Given our data suggesting the hypoxic release of endothelial factors in isolated cerebral arteries, we measured cGMP levels and found they were increased by hypoxia in the large cerebral arteries of the rabbit.[44] However, when we administered methylene blue in vivo, at a dose sufficient to block the cerebral vasodilatation pro-duced by a bolus of nitroglycerin, we found that the cerebral blood flow response to hypoxia, measured by helium clearance in lightly anesthetized rabbits, was unchanged. This finding suggests that the endothelial effects of hypoxia are probably different in the large cerebral arteries we study in vitro and the small cerebral arteries, which determine cerebral blood flow, in vivo. It also remains pos-sible that endothelium-derived hyperpolarizing factor may be released during hypoxia as suggested by Grote and Siegel based on their work in canine carotid.[47] Such an effect in the small cere-bral arteries would be independent of methylene blue, as we have observed, and would also be consistent with hyperpolarizing effects of hypoxia in small middle cerebral arteries, as reported by Bonnet et al.[40] Whether this latter hyperpolarization is the result of release of EDHF or a direct vascular effect is currently under investigation.

Hypercapnic Cerebral Vasodilatation

Just as described for hypoxic mechanisms, the mechanisms of hypercapnic cerebral vasodilatation can be divided into three main families: the tissue effects, the direct vascular effects, and the endothelial effects. As indicated in Fig. 2, however, the mechanisms of hypercapnic cerebral vasodilatation have been less intensively investigated than those for hypoxia.

Extravascular Factors

Neural Hypothesis

One of the oldest ideas concerning hypercapnic cerebral vaso-dilatation was put forth by Molnar and Shalit in the late 1960s[48–50] who based the inhibitory effect of either brain stem transections or selective lesions, attributed the response to the action of intracere-bral vasodilator pathways. Unfortunately, however, these studies have not been easily corroborated, and many observations to the contrary have been reported. In particular, Kontos et al. found that local bicarbonate superfusion could eliminate hypercapnic vasodi-latation in cat pial arteries, and concluded that "the action of CO_2 is entirely local."[51] In their studies of the seventh cranial nerve, Hoff et al. concluded that hypercapnic responses "were unaltered by either unilateral or bilateral section of the nerves."[52] In light of these and other similar data, the neural hypothesis of hypercapnic vaso-dilatation has been largely abandoned and still awaits definitive experimental support.

Extracellular pH Hypothesis

More widely accepted is the extracellular pH hypothesis of hypercapnic vasodilatation, but as for the hypoxic version of this hypothesis, changes in extracellular pH measured by microelec-trodes are consistently too slow and too small to explain hyper-capnic vasodilatation.[2–4] In light of such data, Azin has proposed that "changes in the intracellular pH are of the greatest importance in the action of CO_2 whereas changes in the extracellular pH have but a modulating effect."[53] Extensive studies by Toda's group further corroborate this view.[54]

Prostaglandin Hypothesis

Another group of parenchymal products proposed to mediate hypercapnic vasodilatation are the prostaglandins. Based on work in baboons, Pickard et al. concluded early on that "indomethacin, a prostaglandin synthesis inhibitor, blocks the cerebrovascular response to hypercapnia."[55] Based on work in rats, Siesjo's group, quoted here from Dahlgren et al.,[56] agreed and suggested that "metabolites of arachidonic acid mediate the CBF response to increased CO_2 tension." Not everyone agreed, however, including Kontos, who found in cat pial arteries that cyclo-oxygenase inhibitors did not affect responses to arterial hypercapnia.[8] Similarly, Hoffman et al. found in goats that prostaglandins "have no role in increasing CBF during hypercapnia."[57] Thus, once again, it appears that the role of prostaglandins is highly species-specific. Given that indomethacin appears to attenuate the response in baboons, it seems reasonable to expect a similar effect in the human cerebral circulation, although studies of this effect in humans remain controversial.

Nitric Oxide Hypothesis

A more recent hypothesis concerning the mechanism of hypercapnic cerebral vasodilatation suggests that nitric oxide may mediate this response. Based on the ability of arginine analogs to inhibit hypercapnic cerebral vasodilatation in rats, Iadecola has recently concluded that the "effects of CO_2 on the cerebral circulation are mediated by arginine derived EDRF/NO."[58] Similarly, Dale Pelligrino's group have come to the same conclusion based on work in rats.[59] However, once again, not everyone agrees. Adachi et al. have also reported this year that, in rats, "inhalation of 10% CO_2 for 15 seconds induced an increase in cortical blood flow that was not affected by L-nitro-arginine."[60] Certainly, species differences are not a major factor among these contradictory findings, so other factors must be involved. Paramount among these are the high and variable concentrations of arginine analogs used in these studies; arginine is a critical enzyme involved in transamination, the urea cycle, and polyamine synthesis, as well as nitric oxide synthesis, and it is logical to expect that such high doses probably have multiple and wide ranging effects. The early results of Iadecola's and Pelligrino's groups are fascinating, but much more careful work is needed before their hypothesis can be fully accepted.

Direct Vascular Effects of Hypercapnia

At the direct vascular level, very little is known of the effects of hypercapnia. Harder's group has shown that extracellular acidification can lead to hyperpolarization,[61] but as mentioned previously, the physiological significance of this effect remains in question. More importantly, the relationship among decreases in intracellular pH, hyperpolarization, calcium uptake, and cyclic nucleotides also remain in question. It does appear quite likely, however, that decreases in intracellular pH precipitate vasodilatation. As shown in preliminary studies from our laboratory using rabbit middle cerebral arteries,[62] switching from 5 to 10% CO_2 causes both a vasodilatation and an acidification of the tissue baths. However, when the baths are titrated back to normal pH with bicarbonate, much of the original vasodilatation remains, thus strongly implicating depression of intracellular pH as a mechanism of hypercapnic cerebral vasodilatation. It is important to note, however, that the participation of the endothelium in this effect remains completely unexplored. No studies yet published have examined the effects of hypercapnia on the release of either EDRF, EDCF, or EDHF.

Summary

In cerebral tissue, the mechanisms that link tissue oxygen and CO_2 balance with tissue perfusion can be grouped into three categories:

1. Direct tissue effects with secondary vascular effects.
2. Direct vascular effects.
3. Direct endothelial effects with secondary vascular effects.

For oxygen, hypoxia acts directly on cerebral tissue to promote the release of adenosine, and in some cases, prostanoids, which contribute significantly to cerebral vasodilatation. Hypoxia also acts directly on cerebrovascular smooth muscle to produce hyperpolarization and reduce calcium uptake, both of which enhance vasodilatation. Hypoxia also appears to promote the release of both relaxing and contracting factors from the endothelium, the combined effect of which can either promote or attenuate vasodilatation, depending on the artery and species under study. For hypercapnia, the mechanisms linking it to hyperemia are less well studied than for hypoxia. Hypercapnia appears to act directly on cerebral tissue to promote the release of prostanoids and possibly nitric oxide, but these effects do not appear to be universal and remain controversial. More importantly, hypercapnia depresses intracellular pH, which produces cerebral vasodilatation through mechanisms that at present are unclear. In addition, hypercapnia may also modulate the release of vasoactive factors from the vascular endothelium, but such effects have thus far received relatively little scientific scrutiny and remain as promising topics for future investigation.

References

[1] Lassen, N. A. (1968) *Scand. J. Clin. Lab. Invest.* **22**, 247–251.

[2] Urbanics, R., Leniger, F. E., and Lubbers, D. W. (1977) *Adv. Exp. Med. Biol.* **94**, 611–616.

[3] Silver, I. A. (1978) *Ciba Found. Symp.* **56**, 49–67.

[4] Astrup, J., Heuser, D., Lassen, N. A., Nilsson, B., Norberg, K., and Siesjo, B. K. (1978) *Ciba Found. Symp.* **56**, 313–337.

[5] Allen, K., Busza, A. L., Crockard, H. A., and Gadian, D. G. (1992) *NMR Biomed.* **5**, 48–52.

[6] Kalsner, S. (1978) *Prostaglandins Med.* **1**, 231–239.

[7] Sakabe, T. and Siesjo, B. K. (1979) *Acta Physiol. Scand.* **107**, 283–284.

[8] Kontos, H. A., Wei, E. P., Ellis, E. F., Dietrich, W. D., and Povlishock, J. T. (1981) *Fed. Proc.* **40**, 2326–2330.

[9] McCalden, T. A., Nath, R. G., and Thiele, K. (1984) *Life Sci.* **34**, 1801–1807.

[10] Leffler, C. W. and Busija, D. W. (1985) *Circ. Res.* **57**, 689–694.

[11] Bian, K. and Toda, N. (1988) *J. Cereb. Blood Flow Metab.* **8**, 808–815.

[12] Inoue, S., Kinoshita, M., and Toda, N. (1988) *Eur. J. Pharmacol.* **148**, 69–77.

[13] Kraaier, V., Van, H. A. C., Wieneke, G. H., Van der Worp, H. B., and Bar, P. R. (1992) *Electroencephalogr. Clin. Neurophysiol.* **82**, 208–212.

[14] Edwards, A. D., Wyatt, J. S., Richardson, C., Potter, A., Cope, M., Delpy, D. T., and Reynolds, E. O. (1990) *Lancet* **335**, 1491–1495.

15 Seideman, P. and von Arbin, M. (1991) *Br. J. Clin. Pharmacol.* **31,** 429–432.

16 Berne, R. M., Rubio, R., Dobson, J. G. J., and Curnish, R. R. (1971) *Circ. Res.* **28 (Suppl. 1),** 115–121.

17 Winn, H. R., Rubio, G. R., and Berne, R. M. (1981) *J. Cereb. Blood Flow Metab.* **1,** 239–244.

18 Pinard, E., Puiroud, S., and Seylaz, J. (1989) *Brain Res.* **481,** 124–130.

19 Pittman, R. N. and Duling, B. R. (1973) *Microvasc. Res.* **6,** 202–211.

20 Namm, D. H. and Zueker, J. L. (1973) *Circ. Res.* **32,** 464–470.

21 Fisher, M. J. and Dillon, P. F. (1988) *NMR Biomed.* **1,** 121–126.

22 Ishida, Y. and Paul, R. J. (1990) *J. Physiol. Lond.* **424,** 41–56.

23 Ekmehag, B. L. and Hellstrand, P. (1988) *Acta Physiol. Scand.* **133,** 525–533.

24 Coburn, R. F., Grubb, B., and Aronson, R. D. (1979) *Circ. Res.* **44,** 368–378.

25 Scott, D. P. and Coburn, R. F. (1989) *Am. J. Physiol.* **257,** H597–H602.

26 Ekmehag, B. L. (1989) *Acta Physiol. Scand.* **137,** 41–51.

27 Ekmehag, B. L. and Hellstrand, P. (1989) *Acta Physiol. Scand.* **136,** 367–376.

28 Mathew, R., Burke-Wolin, T., Gewitz, M. H., and Wolin, M. S. (1991) *J. Appl. Physiol.* **71,** 30–36.

29 Detar, R. and Bohr, D. F. (1968) *Am. J. Physiol.* **214,** 241–244.

30 Detar, R. (1980) *Am. J. Physiol.* **238,** H761–H769.

31 Grote, J., Siegel, G., Zimmer, K., and Adler, A. (1988) *Adv. Exp. Med. Biol.* **222,** 481–487.

32 Benham, C. D. (1989) *J. Physiol. Lond.* **419,** 689–701.

33 Ohya, Y. and Sperelakis, N. (1989) *Pflugers Arch.* **414,** 257–264.

34 Standen, N. B., Quayle, J. M., Davies, N. W., Brayden, J. E., Huang, Y., and Nelson, M. T. (1989) *Science* **245,** 177–180.

35 Nelson, M. T., Patlak, J. B., Worley, J. F., and Standen, N. B. (1990) *Am. J. Physiol.* **259,** C3–C18.

36 Ashcroft, F. M. (1988) *Annu. Rev. Neurosci.* **11,** 97–118.

37 Serventi, I. M. and Coffee, C. J. (1986) *Arch. Biochem. Biophys.* **245,** 379–388.

38 Sohma, H. and Morita, F. (1987) *J. Biochem. Tokyo* **101,** 497–502.

39 Pearce, W. J., Brayden, J. E., Hull, A. D., and Long, D. M. (1991) *J. Cereb. Blood Flow Metab.* **11 (Suppl. 2),** S24.

40 Bonnet, P., Gebremedhin, D., Rush, N. J., and Harder, D. R. (1991) *Z. Kardiol.* **80 (Suppl. 7),** 25–27.

41 Ebeigbe, A. B. (1982) *Experientia* **38,** 935–937.

42 Pearce, W. J., Ashwal, S., Long, D. M., and Cuevas, J. (1992) *Am. J. Physiol.* **262,** H106–H113.

43 Coburn, R. F., Baron, C., and Papadopoulos, M. T. (1988) *Am. J. Physiol.* **255,** H1476–H1483.

44 Pearce, W. J., Reynier, R. A., Lee, J., Aubineau, P., Ignarro, L., and Seylaz, J. (1990) *J. Pharmacol. Exp. Ther.* **254,** 616–625.

45 Pearce, W. J., Ashwal, S., and Cuevas, J. (1989) *Am. J. Physiol.* **257,** H824–H833.

[46] Busse, R., Pohl, U., Kellner, C., and Klemm, U. (1983) *Pflugers Arch.* **397,** 78–80.

[47] Grote, J., Siegel, G., Adler, A., and Zimmer, K. (1989) *Prog. Clin. Biol. Res.* **301,** 199–203.

[48] Shalit, M. N., Reinmuth, O. M., Shimojyo, S., and Scheinberg, P. (1967) *Arch Neurol.* **17,** 342–353.

[49] Shalit, M. N., Shimojyo, S., Reinmuth, O. M., Lockhart, W. S. J., and Scheinberg, P. (1968) *Prog. Brain Res.* **30,** 103–106.

[50] Molnar, L. (1968) *Scand. J. Clin. Lab. Invest.* **22 (Suppl. 102),** 6–8.

[51] Kontos, H. A., Wei, E. P., Raper, A. J., and Patterson, J. L. J. (1977) *Stroke* **8,** 227–229.

[52] Hoff, J. T., MacKenzie, E. T., and Harper, A. M. (1977) *Circ. Res.* **40,** 258–262.

[53] Azin, A. L. (1981) *Biull. Eksp. Biol. Med.* **91,** 387–388.

[54] Toda, N., Hatano, Y., and Mori, K. (1989) *Am. J. Physiol.* **257,** H141–H146.

[55] Pickard, J., Tamura, A., Stewart, M., McGeorge, A., and Fitch, W. (1980) *Brain Res.* **197,** 425–431.

[56] Dahlgren, N., Nilsson, B., Sakabe, T., and Siesjo, B. K. (1981) *Acta Physiol. Scand.* **111,** 475–485.

[57] Hoffman, W. E., Albrecht, R. F., Pelligrino, D., and Miletich, D. J. (1982) *Prostaglandins* **23,** 897–905.

[58] Iadecola, C. (1992) *Proc. Natl. Acad. Sci. USA* **89,** 3913–3916.

[59] Pelligrino, D. A., Koenig, H., and Sharp, A. (1992) *FASEB J.* **6,** A1462.

[60] Adachi, T., Inanami, O., and Sato, A. (1992) *Neurosci. Lett.* **139,** 201–204.

[61] Bonnet, P., Rusch, N. J., and Harder, D. R. (1991) *Pflugers Arch.* **418,** 292–296.

[62] Aubineau, P., Pearce, W., Cuevas, J., and Issertial, O. (1989) *J. Cereb. Blood Flow Metab.* **9 (Suppl. 1),** S507.

Chapter 16

Regulation of Pituitary Circulation

Daniel F. Hanley, David A. Wilson, and Richard J. Traystman

Introduction

The pituitary gland has neural and endocrine tissues that form its working structure. Both portions of the gland serve a vital role in an organism's response to stress by secreting multiple peptide hormones. It is a so-called neural-hemal organ: that is a portion of the central nervous system acting as a vascular portal by which the brain communicates trophic and regulatory signals to the body. In the case of the mammalian pituitary, there are a diverse set of functions under regulation: thyroid, adrenal, growth, sex, lactation, skin coloration, renal, and uterine. These functions can be divided by the site of secretory activity with the first six being served by the endodermal-derived anterior portion of the gland and the last two being served by the neuro-ectodermal-derived posterior pituitary. The posterior pituitary is the terminal field of axons derived from the magnocellular hypothalamic neurons that synthesize and release vasopressin and oxytocin. Thus, there are two distinct regions of this gland that share a common vascular territory. It is the goal of this chapter to describe the anatomic and physiologic principles of the circulatory control mechanisms by which the glandular activities of the pituitary take place.

From *The Human Brain Circulation*, R. D. Bevan and J. A. Bevan, eds.
©1994 Humana Press

Arterial Anatomy

Initially, anatomic descriptions of the pituitary vasculature have focused on the portal venous system and its novel neurovascular relationship to the (adenohypophysis) anterior pituitary.[1,2] The anatomy of small (100–300 µ) resistance arteries of the neurohypophysis has recently been defined.[3] The superior hypophyseal artery was initially thought to provide blood to the median eminence and pars distalis, whereas a separate inferior hypophyseal supply to the neural lobe was postulated.[1] Video angiography studies, however, demonstrated the importance of the inferior hypophyseal route as a major source of neural lobe, infundibular process, and median eminence blood flow.[4] Our studies demonstrated one or two inferior hypophyseal branches from each carotid pass medially along the floor of the cavernous sinus until they reach the clivus, where they turn rostral and eventually reach the infundibular process. A significant, bilateral, intracranial arterial supply to the neurohypophysis also occurs from the Circle of Willis, where the superior hypophyseal arteries supply the median eminence as one to three branches of the initial portion of both right and left posterior communicating arteries. These two sets of vessels represent the only circulatory route to the anterior lobe, which has no direct arterial inflow with the possible exception of adenomas, which appear to develop a separate arterial supply.[5]

Vascular Control Mechanisms

Neurohypophyseal blood flow regulation is unique when contrasted to other cerebral regions.[6–8] The absolute level of flow is about ten times greater than resting cerebral flow, and the patterns of flow responses are different for the pituitary when compared to adjacent cerebral tissue. Finally, flow is different in the different regions of the gland. These characteristics may relate to the constraints of a portal circulation including the absence of a blood–brain barrier, the functionally restricted nature of neurohypophyseal axon terminals, or the metabolic differences between neurosecretion and cortical neuronal activities. Although the precise nature of pituitary flow regulation remains uncertain, it is clear both anatomically and physiologically that the neurohypophysis is the site of significant resistance to flow and, thus, the apparent regulatory center for the gland's circulation. Significant progress in our understanding of mechanisms of neurohypophyseal regulation of pituitary circulatory events has occurred in the last decade.

Page et al. provided a nontraumatic, validated measure of neurohypophyseal flow that clearly demonstrated a marked elevation of resting flow levels.[8] The response of the neurohypophysis to alterations of arterial blood gases suggested the possibility of heterogenous physiologic mechanisms of circulatory regulation. Page demonstrated the absence of a CO_2 response in neurohypophyseal tissue when a significant increase of cerebral flow was occurring concurrently.[8] We confirmed this finding in a second species and demonstrated that the response to hypoxia was present in the neurohypophysis.[6] Subsequent studies demonstrated the chemoreceptor dependence of this hypoxic response.[7] Comparison of hypoxic hypoxia stimulation to carbon monoxide hypoxia stimulation suggested that neurohypophyseal vasodilation was dependent on P_aO_2, but not delivery of O_2. This finding was confirmed by denervation studies, which demonstrated the need for either aortic or carotid chemoreceptor stimulation to produce an increase of neurohypophyseal blood flow (Fig. 1). Parallel studies demonstrated the independence of this vasodilation on the blood pressure changes produced by hypoxia. Concurrent assessment of plasma AVP levels demonstrated an increase of hormone levels with hypoxia. This did not occur after denervation. Thus, in the neurally intact system, vasodilation and hypoxia were concurrent events. Because vasodilation did not occur under hypoxic conditions after denervation, this brain region appeared to be insensitive to local oxygen delivery changes for the same levels of P_aO_2 where other cerebral tissues demonstrate sensitivity.

Autoregulation of cerebral blood flow is defined as the stability of flow over a wide range of perfusion pressures. For most cerebral regions, this range is 60–150 mmHg. However, the neurohypophyseal response to a decrease in perfusion pressure is more complex, since baroreceptor stimulation occurs with small drops in either cardiac pressures or arterial pressures. We demonstrated

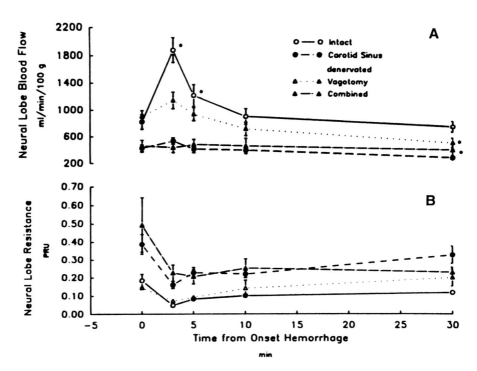

Fig. 1. The neurohypophyseal response to 10 min of hypoxic hypoxia. Either intact carotid sinus nerves or aortic arch nerves are necessary for the response.

a transient increase in blood flow with a decreasing perfusion pressure (Fig. 2). This transient increase was sustained for several minutes, and the flow gradually returned to baseline.[9] A concurrent increase in Plasma AVP occurred with the transient vasodilation. The aortic and carotid baroreceptors are important to the transient vasodilation that occurs with hypotension. This dilation is significantly blunted with denervation of either type of baroreceptor. However, both reflex pathways must be blocked in order to impair the AVP neurosecretory response to hypotension. Thus, it appears there is an association of vasodilation with neurosecretion for both hypoxia and hypotension with neural pathways mediating the vasodilation, but vasodilation is not a necessary condition for neurosecretion.

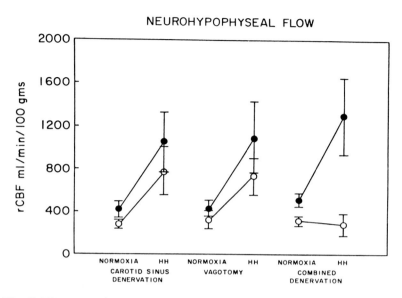

Fig. 2. The neurohypophyseal response to hemorrhagic hypotension. Note that there is a transient drop in resistance with the initial period of hypotension, but blood flow returns to control after 10 min.

Vasodilating Mechanisms

Cholinergic

Evidence supporting a vasomotor role for cholinergic nerves in the neural lobe is both direct and indirect. Ach, applied topically to the hypothalamic nuclei, causes AVP release.[10] It has no effect on the isolated neural lobe, however.[11] Sooriyamoorthy and Livingston[12] showed that neural lobe blood volume significantly increases in response to saline treatment (drinking water replacement with 2% saline for 120 h), hemorrhage, $CaCl_2$ injection, and right vagal nerve stimulation. Atropine (0.5 mg/kg, sc) raised control neural lobe blood volume and attenuated the neural lobe response to these stimuli. Intravenous methacholine was accompanied by vasodilation and was blocked by atropine. These authors did not quantify changes in hypothalamic–hypophyseal function in these experiments. Thus, it is not possible to differentiate neurosecretory-linked blood volume changes from direct effects of muscarinic receptor stimulation at the blood vessel level.

Vasoactive Intestinal Polypeptide

VIP has been demonstrated to increase neurohypophyseal blood flow in two separate studies.[13,14] Both show a large increase of flow, but do not define the site of action of this substance. Neurohypophyseal resistance arteries have demonstrated a dose-dependent dilation to VIP.[13] This occurred for both extracranial and intracranial origins of hypophyseal vessels. The ED_{50}s for relaxation of proximal inferior, distal inferior, and superior hypophyseal vessels were $10^{-8.26}$, $10^{-8.18}$, and $10^{-8.58}M$, respectively. The effect of innervation on resistance artery tone has been investigated with transmural nerve stimulation. Both the inferior and superior hypophyseal arteries demonstrated a frequency-dependent nonadrenergic, noncholinergic vasodilation to TNS. Although the presence of physiologically active VIP nerves on neurohypophyseal resistance vessels strengthens the likelihood of a selective VIP dilator system, the possibility remains that VIP-induced hypotension and not direct vasodilation is the cause of this phenomenon.

Other Dilators

Dopamine has not been demonstrated to produce an increase of median eminence blood flow.[15] Effects of β-adrenergic, prostaglandins, adenosine, substance P, and CGRP have not been described on neurohypophyseal flow. Similarly, the possible effects of Somatostatin and Corticotrophin releasing factor on median eminence flow remain to be investigated.

Vasoconstricting Mechanisms

Adrenergic Constriction

A role for the sympathetic nervous system in decreasing neurohypophyseal blood flow has been suggested by several lines of evidence. Pharmacologic studies using the α_2-adrenergic agents phenylephrine and phenoxybenzamine have demonstrated significant vasoconstrictor effects in the neurohypophysis.[16] Bilateral stimulation of the superior cervical ganglion also produces a decrease of neurohypophyseal blood flow, but the flow does not return to its control condition after stimulation. The blunted blood flow response to hypercapnia appears to be partially related to a strong α-adrenergic vasoconstrictor effect during CO_2 breathing.[17] The site or sites of action of these agents and nerves are not completely understood. Afferent arteries and the neurohypophyseal parenchyma are potential sympathetic vasoconstrictor sites. We have investigated the afferent arteries. The inferior neurohypophyseal artery is responsive to norepinephrine, but not the superior hypophyseal artery.[13] The ED_{50}s for the proximal and distal portions of the inferior hypophyseal arteries are $10^{-5.73}$ and $10^{-5.61}M$, respectively. These vessels demonstrate a constrictor response to transmural nerve stimulation. This response was about 10–20% of the maximal constriction produced by potassium. However, it only occurred in about 50% of artery segments studied. These effects are consistent with the presence of NE in the neurohypophysis and on large afferent arteries supplying the region. The physiologic role for adrenergic nerves is less clear. One hypothesis would be that vasoconstriction improves delivery of neurosecretory material to the general circulation. This is possible if transient decreases in neurohypophyseal flow alter Frank-Starling forces and promote AVP diffusion from the interstitial space to the intravascular space. Alternatively, tonic sympathetic vasoconstrictor influences on large afferent arteries could provide important control mechanisms for modulating local neurohypophyseal vasodilation.

Enkephalin

We have demonstrated a significant decrease in NHBF with both LEU- and MET-Enkephalin (Enk) analogs. This decrease is naloxone-reversible, suggesting an opiate-receptor-mediated process.[18] The mechanism of this vasoconstriction is not certain, since isolated pituitary vessels have not been studied and many brain sites for neurally mediated opiate inhibition have been demonstrated at the neurohypophyseal, magnocellular, and brainstem levels. Our study suggests NHBF and AVP release may both be decreased by local enkephalinamide. The effects of magnocellular or nonmagnocellular enkephalins on neurohypophyseal vessels could be directly mediated via precapillary arterioles or secondarily through an action on axon terminals or glial cells. Evidence exists for all three possibilities, since NHBF,[18] glial cell morphology,[19] and AVP release[20] all appear to undergo local regulation.

Other Vasoconstrictors

The possibility of additional vasoconstrictor substances regulating neurohypophyseal blood flow exists. Possible factors include prostaglandins, ATP, neuropeptide Y, serotonin, or histamine. Angiotensin has been used to elevate systemic blood pressure and test the steady-state response to elevated blood pressure. In this situation it did not alter neurohypophyseal blood flow.[8] Further investigation will be required, since there may be significant effects of blood pressure elevation on neurohypophyseal blood flow and neurosecretion.

Physiologic Implications of Alterations in Blood Flow

Neurohypophyseal flow is unique among brain regions. Flow seems to increase and decrease with activation of the sensory limb of many different magnocellular reflexes. The neural anatomy of secretion is well understood. The physiologic functions are few and well represented by discrete populations of axon terminals. There is no blood–brain barrier. It seems an ideal model to study the relationship of brain activity to regional flow regulation. Initially we proposed there might exist a simple relationship among neurohypophyseal blood flow, neurohypophyseal metabolism, and neurosecretion. All evidence to date suggests that normal central nervous system metabolic regulatory mechanisms do not apply to the neurohypophysis. This system appears to have an excess of oxygen in relation to traditional metabolic needs. There are several potential explanations for this finding:

1. Increased perfusion is required to maintain the normal function of the portal circulation.
2. Elevated flow is important to the wash-out of an unidentified neuronal inhibitory waste product.
3. Complex neurosecretory processes require rapid manipulations of local blood flow as required in stress responses and circadian rhythms.

A better understanding of the regulation of neurohypophyseal flow will come from a precise knowledge of the factors that account for a low resting resistance to blood flow and that can account for the blood flow responses to neural activation.

References

[1] Daniel, P. M. and Pritchard, M. M. L. (1975) *Acta Endocrinol* **80(Suppl. 201),** 1–205.

[2] Green, J. D. and Harris, G. W. (1947) *J. Endocrinology* **5,** 136–146.

[3] Hanley, D. F., Wilson, D. A., Conway, M. A., Traystman, R. J., Bevan, J. A., and Brayden, J. E. (1992) *Amer. J. Physiol.* **263,** H1605–H1615.

[4] Page, R. B. (1983) *Endocrinology* **112,** 157–165.

[5] Gorczyca, W. and Hardy, J. (1988) *Neurosurgery* **22,** 1–6.

[6] Hanley, D. F., Wilson, D. A., and Traystman, R. J. (1986) *Am. J. Physiol.* **250,** H7–H19.

[7] Hanley, D. F., Wilson, D. A., Feldman, M. A., and Traystman, R. J. (1988) *Am. J. Physiol.* **254,** H742–H750.

[8] Page, R. B., Funsch, J. J., Brennan, R. W., and Hernandez, M. J. (1981) *Am. J. Physiol.* **241** (*Regulatory Integrative Comp. Physiol.* **10**), R36–R43.

[9] Vella, L. M., Hanley, D. F., Wilson, D. A., and Traystman, R. J. (1989) *Am. J. Physiol.* **257,** H1498–H1506.

[10] Daniel, A. R. and Lederis, K. (1967) *J. Physiol. (Lond.)* **190,** 171–187.

[11] Douglas, W. W. and Poisner, A. M. (1964) *J. Physiol. (Lond.)* **172,** 1–18.

[12] Sooriyamoorthy, T. and Livingston, A. (1972) *J. Endocrinology* **54,** 407–415.

[13] Wilson, D. A., O'Neill, J. T., Said, S. I., and Traystman, R. J. (1981) *Circ. Res.* **48,** 138–148.

[14] Hanley, D. F., Struble, R., Wilson, C., Kirsch, J., Wilson, D., and Traystman, R. J. (1987) *J. CBF Metab.* **7(Suppl. 1),** S318.

[15] Page, R. B., Gropper, M., Woodard, E., Townsend, J., Davis, S., and Bryan, R. M. (1990) *Am. J. Physiol.* **258,** R1242–1249.

[16] Wilson, D. A., Hanley, D. F., Rogers, M. C., and Traystman, R. J. (1983) *J. Cereb. Blood Flow Metab.* **3(Suppl.),** 166,167.

[17] Bryan, R. B., Meyers, C. L., and Page, R. B. (1988) *Am. J. Physiol.* **255,** R295–R302.

[18] Kirsch, J. R., Hanley, D. F., Wilson, D. A., and Traystman, R. J. (1988) *J. Cereb. Blood Flow Metab.* **8,** 385–394.

[19] Van Leeuwen, F. W. and DeVries, B. J. (1983) *Prog. Brain Res.* **60,** 343–351.

[20] Iversen, L. I., Iversen, S. D., and Bloom, F. E. (1980) *Nature* **284,** 350–351.

Chapter 17

Aspects
of the Choroid Plexus–
Cerebrospinal Fluid System

Christer Nilsson and Christer Owman

Introduction

The choroid plexus is located in each of the four cerebral ventricles, secreting the cerebrospinal fluid (CSF), which acts as a mechanical support and protection for the brain. Since these have been considered the main functions of the choroid plexus and CSF, there has been considerable interest in the regulation of CSF production in relation to clinical disorders, such as increased intracranial pressure. Studies in this field have been hampered by the limitations of available methods for measuring CSF production, which have been highly invasive and mostly limited to experimental animals. The recent introduction of magnetic resonance imaging (MRI) for noninvasive measurement of CSF production in human volunteers[1,2] has made it possible to investigate both physiological and pharmacological regulation of human CSF production directly.

In addition to the purely mechanical protection of the brain by the CSF, evidence accumulated during the past decade suggests a more specific interaction in the environment between the choroid plexus and the brain by the bidirectional transport of substances via the CSF. The high levels of receptors for 5-HT, atrial natriuretic

From *The Human Brain Circulation*, R. D. Bevan and J. A. Bevan, eds.
©1994 Humana Press

peptide (ANP), and vasopressin (AVP) in the choroid plexus epithelium,[3] indicates that chemical messengers released from nerve terminals in the nervous tissue into the CSF can activate cellular responses in the choroid plexus, e.g., during brain volume regulation.[4] On the other hand, the choroid plexus synthesizes and secretes several types of proteins into the CSF, such as the thyroid hormone transport protein transthyretin (TTR; formerly called prealbumin),[5] and a peptide growth factor named insulin-like growth factor-II (IGF-II).[6] These proteins could act as neuroendocrine messengers for communication between the peripheral tissues and compartments, and the brain.[3]

In this chapter, we will highlight these aspects of choroid plexus and CSF function, and present some of our own recent data related to this topic. Although most research on the choroid plexus has been performed on experimental animals because of the inaccessibility of this structure deep in the brain, the situation in humans will be emphasized wherever possible.

Choroid Plexus Structure

The choroid plexus is a villous structure located in all four cerebral ventricles, consisting of a cuboidal epithelium overlying a highly vascularized connective tissue stroma. In contrast to the intraparenchymal endothelium of the brain, choroid plexus endothelial cells are fenestrated, permitting free passage of macromolecules and hydrophilic substances from blood to the interstitial tissue. The epithelial cells, on the other hand, are connected with tight junctions, thereby forming the blood–CSF barrier (B-CSF-B). The epithelial cells have well-developed apical microvilli and locally oriented mitochondria, as well as abundant rough endoplasmic reticulum, characteristic of transporting epithelia and protein synthesis, respectively.

The Blood–CSF Barrier

The B-CSF-B can be considered a very specialized part of the blood–brain barrier (BBB), forming an interface regulating the transport of hydrophilic substances and macromolecules between blood and CSF. The presence of the B-CSF-B explains the low protein content of the CSF. The main function of the B-CSF-B is to maintain a stable concentration of ions and nutrients comparable to that of the brain extracellular fluid. In addition, the B-CSF-B provides an enzymatic barrier, with the capacity of uptake and degradation of organic acids, bases, and peptides, including many neuro-transmitters and their metabolites.[7-9] Although in most cases the B-CSF-B acts only as a supplement to the transport and barrier functions of the BBB, some micronutrient carrier mechanisms and peptidases appear to be present only in the choroid plexus and not in the cerebral endothelium,[10,11] indicating that the choroid plexus serves as the main gateway for transport or degradation of these substances in the brain.

Secretion of CSF

The composition of the CSF clearly shows that it cannot be a passively formed ultrafiltrate of plasma, but rather a fluid modi-fied by active secretion.[12] The secretory morphology of the choroid plexus, the localization of Na^+/K^+-ATPase to the apical part of the plexus epithelium,[13] and the analysis of freshly secreted fluid from the tissue,[14] strongly suggest that the choroid plexus secretes CSF. Current estimates of the proportion of CSF originating in the chor-oid plexus range from 60–90%,[12,15] the remainder probably being formed by extracellular fluid formed by the brain endothelial cells and draining into the ventricles.[12]

Choroid Plexus Blood Flow

The blood supply to the choroid plexus in mammals, including humans, derives mainly from the anterior and posterior choroidal arteries, originating from the internal carotid and posterior cere-bral arteries, respectively.[16] Vascular casts of the rat choroid plexus, examined by scanning electron microscopy, have revealed an exceedingly complex vascular pattern of both arterioles and sinusoids/capillaries,[17] the functions of which are still unknown. The turnover rate of CSF is high in mammals, around 0.5% of the total volume/min or 4–5 times the total vol/d.[12] Accordingly, the choroid plexus is provided with a very rich blood supply, several times higher than the cerebral cortical blood flow.[18] This has led to the suggestion that CSF production by the choroid plexus is determined by the blood flow.[19] Recent studies in our laboratory have demonstrated that the neuropeptide vasoactive intestinal polypeptide (VIP) decreases CSF production in the rat during intraventricular perfusion, although the choroid plexus blood flow is increased, probably because of the well-known vasodilatory action of VIP[20] (Fig. 1). Similarly, azetazolamide, a carbonic anhydrase inhibitor, inhibits CSF production by 55% after iv injection, at the same time increasing choroid plexus blood flow by 100%.[21,22] These results clearly demonstrate that the CSF production is not a simple reflection of changes in choroid plexus blood flow, although the rate of blood perfusion might still set a maximum limit to the rate of CSF secretion.[19] Studies in dogs using radioactive microspheres have shown that several different vasoactive stimuli, e.g., AVP, angiotensin II, and endothelin, regulate choroid plexus blood flow when given intravenously, whereas cerebral blood flow remains unchanged. This is probably because of the fenestrated nature of the choroid plexus capillaries, allowing blood-borne substances to reach the vascular smooth muscle. The physiological relevance of these observations is not known yet, although a role for blood-borne AVP in regulation of intracranial pressure has been suggested.

Regulation of CSF Production

The choroid plexus epithelium might be a target for neuroendocrine mediators that regulate CSF production.[3] For example, ANP and AVP have high levels of receptors on choroid plexus epithelial cells and have been shown to influence CSF production in the rabbit,[23,24] as is discussed further below. However, since the methods used are highly invasive, utilize anesthetized experimental animals, and could be influenced by several different factors affecting cerebral hydrodynamics, the physiological relevance of these studies remains to be determined.

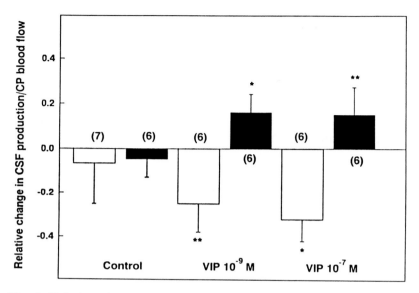

Fig. 1. Relative changes in cerebrospinal fluid (CSF) production (open bars) and choroid plexus blood flow (filled bars; measured by laser-doppler flowmetry) during the second perfusion period of a ventriculcisternal perfusion experiment, compared to the initial, control perfusion period, with or without (control) intraventricular administration of VIP. The figures within parentheses are the numbers of experiments in each group. All values are means ± SD. Statistically significant differences, as measured by Student's *t*-test for paired observations, are shown as *$p < 0.05$, **$p < 0.01$. Reproduced from ref. 20 with permission.

Direct measurements of human CSF production have been performed using ventriculo-lumbar perfusions in neurosurgical patients.[25,26] Studies of the physiological regulation of human CSF production in healthy individuals have been restricted to indirect methods, such as measurements of CSF pressure after lumbar puncture or estimates of CSF volume.[27,28] With the development of CSF flow measurements by magnetic resonance phase imaging,[1,29] which measures the net flow of CSF through the cerebral aqueduct in healthy human volunteers, a powerful new tool is available for studies of human CSF production and its regulation. We have used this method to elucidate the possibility of circadian variations in human CSF production.[2]

A prominent circadian rhythm was found, with CSF production values being two to three times higher around 200 h compared to 1800 h (Fig. 2). The concept of circadian variation in human CSF production is supported by continuous measurements of ventricular fluid pressure in hydrocephalic children, which show increases in pressure during nighttime in patients with acute hydrocephalus.[30] Further studies have confirmed these results and also demonstrated that the nocturnal rise in CSF production is curtailed by treatment with the β_1-adrenoceptor antagonist, Atenolol® (submitted). This indicates that sympathetic nerves might regulate human CSF production in a circadian manner, either directly at the choroid plexus epithelium or indirectly via the secretion of melatonin by the pineal gland.[31,32] Previous investigations have shown that choroid plexus epithelial cells in the rabbit contain β_1-adrenoceptors,[33] through which the sympathetic nerves appear to inhibit CSF production tonically,[34] in contrast to the situation in the human, where, instead, the sympathetic nerves might stimulate CSF production.

Secretion of Plasma Proteins by the Choroid Plexus

Through the work of Schreiber and collaborators, it has become well established that the choroid plexus synthesizes and secretes a number of different plasma proteins.[35] Such proteins known to be synthesized by the choroid plexus are summarized in Table 1. This feature of choroid plexus function seems to be very well preserved phylogenetically, as noted for the thyroid hormone transport protein, TTR,[37] and the protease inhibitor, cystatin C.[39] The presence of high levels of TTR mRNA in the choroid plexus has been noted also in humans.[44,45] Although the CSF has a low protein content because of the existence of the B-CSF-B, the CSF/plasma concentration ratio differs for several proteins in a manner that cannot be explained on the basis of molecular size.[46] These proteins (e.g., TTR, ceruloplasmin, transferrin, and cystatin C) should accumulate in the CSF either because of a specific transport mechanism or intracerebral synthesis, rather than by passive leakage of protein through

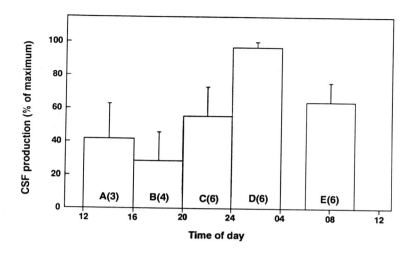

Fig. 2. CSF production rate relative to each individual's maximum production in five different time intervals during the day–night cycle, calculated from CSF flow velocities in the cerebral aqueduct in six healthy volunteers aged 25–32 yr. Each bar represents average CSF production (%maximum) in each time interval ± SE. Numbers within parentheses in each bar represent the number of measurements in each time interval (*n*). Reproduced from ref. 2 with permission.

Table 1
Secretory Proteins in the Choroid Plexus Epithelium[a]

Protein	Species	Refs.
Transthyretin	Mammals, birds, reptiles	36,37
Cystatin C	Mammals, birds	38,39
Transferrin	Rat, mouse	40
Ceruloplasmin	Rat	41
α_2-Macroglobulin	Rat	42
β_2-Microglobulin	Rat	38
β-A4-amyloid precursor protein	Sheep	39
Insulin-like growth factor II	Rat, pig, sheep	3,6,43

[a]The proteins, the species that they have been described in, and the respective references are summarized in the table. For further details, *see text.*

the B-CSF-B from the blood. This problem can now be explained by the high rate of synthesis and secretion of these proteins by the choroid plexus, and has been proven unequivocally by the findings that choroid plexus TTR is secreted into the CSF and not to the blood, and that newly synthesized TTR in the CSF derives predominantly from an intracerebral source,[5] namely the choroid plexus, as shown in rat, sheep, and humans.[36,47,48] The function of TTR in the CSF is not yet known, although some experimental data suggest a role in intracerebral transport or distribution of thyroxine.[3,5]

IGF-II is another peptide/protein that, in the adult rat brain, appears to be almost exclusively expressed in the choroid plexus and meninges.[49] We and others have recently demonstrated that both IGF-II mRNA and mRNA for the IGF-II transport protein, IGF binding protein-2 (IGFBP-2), are expressed at high levels in the rat and pig choroid plexus.[43,49,50] Both mRNA and the mature peptide are synthesized by sheep choroid plexus epithelial cells in primary culture.[54] IGF-II and IGFBP-2, but not IGF-I, are found in human CSF,[52] and receptors for IGF-II are present in many areas of the brain.[53] Although the widespread cerebral expression of IGF-II in the fetus points to a paracrine, mitogenic action, the role of choroid plexus IGF-II in the adult is not yet clear. However, it is possible that IGF-II acts as a growth factor for the adult brain as well, perhaps stimulating glial cell proliferation.

The Choroid Plexus as a Target for Neuroendocrine Signaling

In classical endocrine signaling, hormones are released from their site of origin and travel with the blood to their target tissue. Also the CSF seems to be a pathway for transport of hormones from their site of synthesis to their target cells.[3,54] Theoretically, a hormone can pass from blood to CSF via the choroid plexus or brain regions lacking a BBB, and reach the brain or part of it by bulk flow and diffusion in the brain extracellular fluid.[55] This appears to be the case for prolactin: This hormone has been suggested to be transported from blood to CSF via the choroid plexus,[56] which is enriched in prolactin binding sites.[57] The function of such a transport system could be a negative feedback loop to inhibit prolactin secretion either at the level of the dopaminergic cell bodies in the hypothalamus or their nerve terminals in the median eminence.[56] Alternatively, substances synthesized in a brain region can diffuse into the CSF to reach another part of the brain by bulk flow.[3,54] The various suggested roles of the choroid plexus in neuroendocrine signalling have been summarized in Fig. 3.

Advances in receptor autoradiography, immunohistochemistry, and *in situ* hybridization have revealed a great number of receptor types for different neuronal and endocrine messengers, some of which are listed in Table 2. It is therefore conceivable that one of the target tissues in the brain for neuroendocrine signaling is the choroid plexus. This is most clearly shown for 5-HT. The choroid plexus contains large amounts of the 5-HT_{1C} receptor subtype, with levels 10 times higher than other brain regions.[58,62] The 5-HT_{1C} receptor appears to be localized to the apical, CSF-facing membrane of the choroid plexus epithelial cells.[63] Chemical denervation of the 5-HT innervation of the brain by centrally injected 5,7-dihydroxytryptamine induces a marked receptor supersensitivity in the choroid plexus.[64] The 5-HT reaching the choroid plexus appears to be released into the CSF from supraependymal nerve fibers lining the ventricle walls.[65,66] We have proposed a model where 5-HT released from the supraependymal nerve fibers diffuses into the CSF and is taken by bulk flow to the CSF side of the choroid plexus epithelium; here it interacts with the apically located 5-HT_{1C} receptors, thereby stimulating synthesis of the inositoltriphosphate second-messenger system.[67]

Although the function of 5-HT in the CSF remains unclear, evidence has accumulated that ANP and AVP might be involved in brain ion and volume homeostasis.[4] There is a high density of receptors for both these peptides in the choroid plexus.[59,60] Although the origin of the ANP and AVP that reacts with the choroid plexus has not been determined, it seems likely that centrally released peptides could be the primary source.[4,68,69] ANP has been shown to stimulate cyclic GMP production in the choroid plexus[70] and decreases CSF production in rabbits.[23] Inhibition of CSF produc-

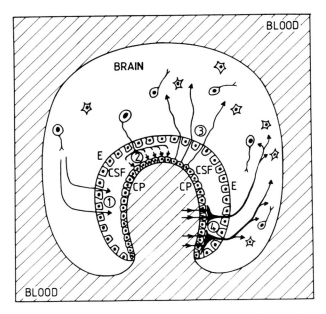

Fig. 3. Schematic drawing of neuroendocrine signaling pathways involving the choroid plexus–CSF system. Neurotransmitters released within the
brain parenchyma can diffuse or flow between the cells of the ependyma
(E) into the CSF and there be transported to apically located receptors on
the choroid plexus epithelium (CP) (1). The CP might here participate as
part of a general functional response involving several parts of the brain.
Two substances that might be released in such a fashion are AVP and ANP.
In the case of 5-HT, the releasing nerve fibers have been identified. These
are dense, supraependymal, serotonergic nerve fiber plexuses located in
several parts of the ventricle walls. Several lines of evidence suggest that
these nerve fibers release 5-HT into the CSF from where it reaches the CP
epithelium (2). Apart from acting as a target for centrally released transmitters (1,2), the CP also produces insulin-like growth factor II (*see* Choroid
Plexus Structure) (3) and transport proteins for peripheral hormones (4).
These substances have been suggested to mediate endocrine signals to brain
neurons and glia via CSF bulk flow and diffusion within the brain parenchyma (3,4). Reproduced from ref. 3, with permission.

tion might occur through inhibition of amiloride-sensitive Na$^+$
transport, as demonstrated in cerebral capillaries.[71] Furthermore,
ANP injected intraventricularly during hypoosmolar fluid load-
ing in rats leads to sodium loss and water accumulation in the

Table 2
Some Neuroendocrine Mediators
with High Receptor Densities
in the Choroid Plexus Epithelium[a]

Ligand	Function	Refs.
Noradrenalin	+cAMP	33
5-HT	+PI-hydrolysis	58
ANP	+cGMP	59
AVP	+PI-hydrolysis	60
IGF-I	+tyrosine kinase	61
Prolactin	Transcytosis	57

[a]The demonstrated (in the case of prolactin, suggested) cellular function of the respective receptor for each ligand is given in the middle column: stimulation (+) of cyclic AMP (cAMP), cyclic GMP (cGMP), PI (phosphatidyl inositol) hydrolysis, and tyrosine kinase. It is believed that prolactin is transported by transcytosis through the choroid plexus epithelial cells from blood to CSF. For further details, see text.

brain,[72] indicating that ANP has a general role in brain fluid homeostasis. Normal CSF levels of ANP[73] are far below the association constant reported for the ANP receptor in the choroid plexus, precluding activation during physiological conditions. However, ANP receptor density is increased in kaolin-induced, but lowered in congenital hydrocephalus,[74] and ANP levels are higher in patients with elevated intracranial pressure.[75]

For a full discussion of AVP in human CSF, see the review by Sörensen (1986).[76] In general, AVP appears to increase the ion content of the brain, whereas ANP has the opposite effect.[4] Increases in CSF osmolality are followed by raised AVP levels in the CSF.[77] This could be a compensatory response, since AVP enhances capillary permeability and brain water content,[78,79] and might mediate bulk flow of water and electrolytes from the CSF into the brain.[4] In fact, AVP and ANP seem to mediate opposite effects on many different systems in the body. Furthermore, since ANP as well as brain natriuretic peptide both inhibit AVP secretion, they could also interact with each other in the regulation of brain ion and volume homeostasis.

The studies reviewed above suggest that the choroid plexus–CSF system could constitute an important pathway for neuroendocrine signaling in the brain, as summarized in Fig. 3. However, clear-cut evidence for such a role is still largely lacking.[3]

Acknowledgments

Parts of the material presented in this chapter were supported by grants from the Medical Faculty of Lund University and the Swedish Medical Research Council (Grant No. 14X-5680).

References

[1] Thomsen, C., Ståhlberg, F., Stubgaard, M., and Nordell, B. (1990) *Radiology* **77,** 659–665.

[2] Nilsson, C., Ståhlberg, F., Herning, M., Henriksen, O., and Owman, C. (1992) *Am. J. Physiol.* **262,** R20–R24.

[3] Nilsson, C., Lindvall-Axelsson, M., and Owman, C. (1992) *Brain Res. Rev.* **17,** 109–138.

[4] Cserr, H. F. and Patlak, C. S. (1991), in *Advances in Comparative and Environmental Physiology,* vol. 9 (Gilles, R., Hoffmann, E. K., and Bolis, L., eds.), Springer, Berlin/Heidelberg, pp. 61–80.

[5] Schreiber, G., Aldred, A. R., Jaworowski, A., Nilsson, C., Achen, M. G., and Segal, M. B. (1990) *Am. J. Physiol.* **258,** R338–R345.

[6] Hynes, M. A., Brooks, P. J., van Wyk, J. J., and Lund, P. K. (1988) *Mol. Endocrinol.* **2,** 47–54.

[7] Bourne, A. and Kenny, A. J. (1990) *Biochem. J.* **271,** 381–385.

[8] Forn, J. (1972) *Biochem. Pharmacol.* **21,** 619–624.

[9] Tochino, Y. and Schanker, L. S. (1965) *Biochem. Pharmacol.* **14,** 1557–1566.

[10] Spector, R. (1989) *J. Neurochem.* **53,** 1667–1674.

[11] Solhonne, B., Gros, C., Pollard, H., and Schwartz, J.-C. (1987) *Neuroscience* **22,** 225–232.

[12] Davson, H., Welch, K., and Segal, M. B. (1987) *The Physiology and Pathophysiology of the Cerebrospinal Fluid,* Churchill Livingstone, Edinburgh.

[13] Ernst, S. A., Palacios, J. R., and Siegel, G. J. (1986) *J. Histochem. Cytochem.* **34,** 189–195.

[14] Ames, A., III, Sakanoue, M., and Endo, S. (1964) *J. Neurophysiol.* **27,** 672–681.

[15] Pollay, M., Hisey, B., Reynolds, E., Tomkins, P., Stevens, F. A., and Smith, R. (1985) *Neurosurgery* **17,** 768–772.

[16] Netsky, M. G. and Shuangshoti, S. (1975) in *The Choroid Plexus in Health and Disease* (Netsky, M. G. and Shuangshoti, S., eds.), John Wright and Sons, Bristol, pp. 151–161.

[17] Hodde, K. C. (1981) *Cephalic Vascular Patterns in the Rat,* Thesis Rodopi, Amsterdam, pp. 52–54.

[18] Faraci, F. M., Mayhan, W. G., Williams, J. K., and Heistad, D. D. (1988) *Am. J. Physiol.* **254,** H286–H291.

[19] Cserr, H. F. (1975) in *The Choroid Plexus in Health and Disease* (Netsky, M. G. and Shuangshoti, S., eds.), John Wright and Sons, Bristol, pp. 175–195.

[20] Nilsson, C., Lindvall-Axelsson, M., and Owman, C. (1991) *J. Cereb. Blood Flow Metab.* **11,** 861–867.

[21] Faraci, F. M., Mayhan, W. G., and Heistad, D. D. (1990) *J. Pharmacol. Exp. Ther.* **254,** 23–27.

[22] Faraci, F. M. and Heistad, D. D. (1991) *Hypertension* **17,** 917–922.

[23] Steardo, L. and Nathanson, J. A. (1987) *Science* **235,** 470–473.

[24] Faraci, F. M., Mayhan, W. G., and Heistad, D. D. (1990) *Am. J. Physiol.* **27,** R94–R98.

[25] Rubin, R. C., Henderson, E. S., Ommaya, A. K., Walker, M. D., and Rall, D. P. (1966) *J. Neurosurgery* **25,** 430–436.

[26] Cutler, R. W. P., Page, L., Galicich, J., and Watters, G. V. (1968) *Brain* **91,** 707–720.

[27] Grant, R., Condon, B., Lawrence, A., Hadley, D. M., Patterson, J., Bone, I., and Teasdale, G. M. (1988) *J. Comput. Assist. Tomogr.* **12,** 36–39.

[28] May, C., Kaye, J. A., Atack, J. R., Schapiro, M. B., Friedland, R. P., and Rapoport, S. I. (1990) *Neurology* **40,** 500–503.

[29] Ståhlberg, F., Mogelvang, J., Thomsen, C., Nordell, B., Stubgaard, M., Ericsson, A., Sperber, G., Greitz, D., Larsson, H., Henriksen, O., and Persson, B. (1989) *Magn. Reson. Imaging* **7,** 655–667.

[30] Hayden, P. W., Shurtleff, D. B., and Foltz, E. L. (1970) *Arch. Neurol.* **23,** 147–154.

[31] Decker, J. F. and Quay, W. B. (1982) *J. Neural. Transm.* **55,** 53–67.

[32] Reiter, R. J. (1991) *Endocrine Rev.* **12,** 151–180.

[33] Lindvall-Axelsson, M., Gustafson, Å., Hedner, P., and Owman, C. (1985) *Neurosci. Lett.* **54,** 153–157.

[34] Lindvall, M., Edvinsson, L., and Owman, C. (1978) *Science* **201,** 176–178.

[35] Schreiber, G. and Aldred, A. R. (1990) in *Pathophysiology of the Blood–Brain Barrier* (Johanson, B., Owman, C., and Widner, H., eds.), Elsevier, Amsterdam, pp. 89–103.

[36] Dickson, P. W., Howlett, G. J., and Schreiber, G. (1985) *J. Biol. Chem.* **260,** 8214–8219.

[37] Harms, P. J., Tu, G.-F., Richardson, S. J., Aldred, A. R., Jaworowski, A., and Schreiber, G. (1991) *Comp. Biochem. Physiol.* **99B,** 239–249.

[38] Cole, T., Dickson, P. W., Esnard, F., Averill, S., Risbridger, G. P., Gauthier, F., and Schreiber, G. (1989) *Eur. J. Biochem.* **186,** 35–42.

[39] Tu, G.-F., Cole, T., Southwell, B. R., and Schreiber, G. (1990) *Dev. Brain Res.* **55,** 203–208.

[40] Aldred, A. R., Dickson, P. W., Marley, P. D., and Schreiber, G. (1987) *J. Biol. Chem.* **262,** 5293–5297.

[41] Aldred, A. R., Grimes, A., Schreiber, G., and Mercer, J. F. B. (1987) *J. Biol. Chem.* **262,** 2875–2878.

[42] Thomas, T., Schreiber, G., and Jaworowski, A. (1989) *Dev. Biol.* **134,** 38–47.

[43] Nilsson, C., Blay, P., Nielsen, F. C., and Gammeltoft, S. (1992) *J. Neurochem.* **58,** 923–930.

[44] Dickson, P. W. and Schreiber, G. (1986) *Neurosci. Lett.* **66,** 311–315.

[45] Jacobsson, B., Collins, V. P., Grimelius, L., Pettersson, T., Sandstedt, B., and Carlström, A. (1989) *J. Histochem. Cytochem.* **37,** 31–37.

[46] Felgenhauer, K. (1974) *Klin. Wochenschr.* **52,** 1158–1164.

[47] Stauder, A. J., Dickson, P. W., Aldred, A. R., Schreiber, G., Mendelsohn, F. A. O., and Hudson, P. (1986) *J. Histochem. Cytochem.* **34,** 949–952.

[48] Hamberger, A., Nyström, B., Silvenius, H., and Wikkelsö, C. (1990) *Neurochem. Res.* **15,** 307–312.

[49] Stylianopoulou, F., Herbert, J., Soares, M. B., and Efstratiadis, A. (1988) *Proc. Natl. Acad. Sci. USA* **85,** 141–145.

[50] Tseng, L. Y. H., Brown, A. L., Yang, Y. W. H., Romanus, J. A., Orlowski, C. C., Taylor, T., and Rechler, M. M. (1989) *Mol. Endocrinol.* **3,** 1559–1568.

[51] Holm, N. R., Hansen, L. B. H., Nilsson, C., and Gammeltoft, S. (1993) *Mol. Brain Res.* (in press).

[52] Haselbacher, G. and Humbel, R. (1982) *Endocrinology* **110,** 1822–1824.

[53] Lesniak, M. A., Hill, J. M., Kiess, W., Rojeski, M., Pert, C. B., and Roth, J. (1988) *Endocrinology* **123,** 2089–2099.

[54] Wood, J. G. (1982) *Neurosurgery* **11,** 293–305.

[55] Johanson, C. E. (1993) in *Pharmaceutical Biotechnology, vol 5: Biological Barriers to Protein Delivery* (Audus, K. L. and Raub, T. J., eds.), Plenum, New York, pp. 467–486.

[56] Nicholson, G., Greeley, G. H., Humm, J., Youngblood, W. W., and Kizer, J. S. (1980) *Brain Res.* **190,** 447–457.

[57] Posner, B. I., van Houten, M., Patel, B., and Walsh, R. J. (1983) *Exp. Brain Res.* **49,** 300–306.

[58] Yagaloff, K. A. and Hartig, P. R. (1985) *Neuroscience* **15,** 3178–3183.

[59] Mantyh, C. R., Kruger, L., Brecha, N. C., and Mantyh, P. W. (1987) *Brain Res.* **412,** 329–342.

[60] Gerstberger, R. and Fahrenholz, F. (1989) *Eur. J. Pharmacol.* **167,** 105–116.

[61] Davidson, D. A., Bohannon, N. J., Corp, E. S., Lattemann, D. P., Woods, S. C., Porte, D., Jr., Dorsa, D. M., and Baskin, D. G. (1990) *J. Histochem. Cytochem.* **38,** 1289–1294.

[62] Pazos, A., Probst, A., and Palacios, J. M. (1987) *Neuroscience* **21,** 97–122.

[63] Giordano, J. and Hartig, P. R. (1987) *Neuroscience* **22,** 223P.

64 Conn, P. J., Janowsky, A., and Sanders-Bush, E. (1987) *Brain Res.* **400,** 396–398.

65 Chan-Palay, V. (1976) *Brain Res.* **102,** 103–130.

66 Ternaux, J. P., Boireau, A., Bourgoin, S., Hamon, M., Hery, F., and Glowinski, J. (1976) *Brain Res.* **101,** 533–548.

67 Nilsson, C., Lindvall-Axelsson, M., and Owman, C. (1991) in *Volume Transmission in the Brain* (Fuxe, K. and Agnati, L., eds.), Raven, New York, pp. 307–315.

68 Standaert, D. G., Needleman, P., and Saper, C. B. (1986) *J. Comp. Neurol.* **253,** 315–341.

69 Raichle, M. E. and Grubb, R. L., Jr. (1978) *Brain Res.* **143,** 191–194.

70 Tsutsumi, K., Niwa, M., Kawano, T., Ibaragi, M., Ozaki, M., and Mori, K. (1987) *Neurosci Lett.* **79,** 174–178.

71 Ibaragi, M., Niwa, M., and Osaki, M. (1989) *J. Neurochem.* **53,** 1802–1806.

72 Dóczi, T., Joó, F., Szerdahelyi, P., and Bodosi, M. (1987) *Neurosurgery* **21,** 454–458.

73 Marumo, F., Masuda, T., and Ando, K. (1987) *Biochem. Biophys. Res. Commun.* **143,** 813–818.

74 Mori, K., Tsutsumi, K., Kurihara, M., Kawaguchi, T., and Niwa, M. (1990) *Child's Nerv. Syst.* **6,** 190–193.

75 Dóczi, T., Joó, F., Vecsernyés, M., and Bodosi, M. (1988) *Neurosurgery* **23,** 16–19.

76 Sörensen, P. S. (1986) *Acta Neurol. Scand.* **74,** 81–102.

77 Morris, M., Barnard, R. R., Jr., and Sain, L. E. (1984) *Neuroendocrinology* **39,** 377–383.

78 Dóczi, T., Szerdahelyi, P., Gulya, K., and Kiss, J. (1982) *Neurosurgery* **11,** 402–407.

79 Rosenberg, G. A., Kyner, W. T., Fenstermacher, J. D., and Patlak, C. S. (1986) *Am. J. Physiol.* **251,** F485–F489.

Chapter 18

Collateral Pial Arteries

Peter Coyle

Collateral Pial Arteries in Humans

Where Are the Anastomoses?

More than 300 years ago, Willis characterized the arterial ring at the base of the brain and began debate concerning whether the circle functions primarily as a flow equalizer or as an anastomosis.[1,2] In the Circle of Willis, the single anterior communicating artery joins each side of the bilateral anterior cerebral circulation supplied by the internal carotid artery. The paired posterior communicating artery joins each anterior circulation with the posterior circulation receiving supply from the vertebral arteries. Communicating arteries are present in most brains.[3] Colored media injected into cerebral arteries demonstrate that distal pial surface branches of the three major cerebral arteries are not end arteries.[4-9] Rather, end branches of the middle (MCA) cerebral artery anastomose with end branches of the anterior (ACA) or posterior (PCA) cerebral artery on the pial surface of the brain. Such distal end-to-end anastomoses define anatomical border zones between the major cerebral arteries and are located where branch angles of opposing vessels reverse direction.[8] Also, anastomoses join side branches of adjacent small arteries and arterioles arising from the same major cerebral artery in many species, including primates,[10] and in humans, an absence of microcircle anastomoses seems unlikely. End-to-end anastomotic patterns exist between major pial arteries

From *The Human Brain Circulation*, R. D. Bevan and J. A. Bevan, eds.
©1994 Humana Press

of the cerebellum.[6-8] Arterial-venous anastomoses are not normally observed on the pial surface of the brain.[8,11] In summary, pial surface arterial anastomotic segments are located in the Circle of Willis, in border zones separating major arteries of the brain, and probably within defined vascular territories.

Significance of the Anastomoses

Anastomoses are connecting passageways allowing alternate blood supply to circulations, territories, and local tissue regions. Normally, the major cerebral circulations receive autonomous ipsilateral supply with only minimal mixing of different input streams in the Circle of Willis in humans[12] and other mammals.[13] With reduction of flow in one or more major afferent vessels to the Circle of Willis, communicating arteries permit flow allotments to more than one major circulation (Fig. 1). The allotment depends on many factors, including the differential blood pressure across the segment, size, and flow reserve of the communicating arteries that can also be compromised by disease.[14] Blood flow is proportional to the fourth power of the luminal radius of the anastomotic segment. Mean luminal diameters of communicating arteries determined from 35 autopsied brains, presumably human, were: anterior 1.00 mm, left posterior 0.85 mm, right posterior 0.88 mm, but size variability was not stated.[15] Asymmetry in size occurs in the Circle of Willis more often than not,[16] and asymmetry in luminal size of the communicating arteries suggests that no single standard size exists. Because carotid artery or vertebral artery occlusion may occur slowly without any neurological sign, asymmetry in the circle could reflect unrecognized collateral blood flow and adaptive remodeling of vessels. After occlusion of a major cerebral or cerebellar artery in humans, wider distal end-to-end anastomoses appear to correlate with more tissue protection,[6-8] suggesting that greater collateral blood flow protects more of the arterial territory at risk of infarction. Mechanisms controlling luminal size of the distal anastomoses are unknown. Microcircle anastomoses[10] likely contribute to local autoregulation of blood flow when local metabolic demands require more or less blood supply. Thus, Circle of Willis anastomoses channel blood into major cerebral circulations,

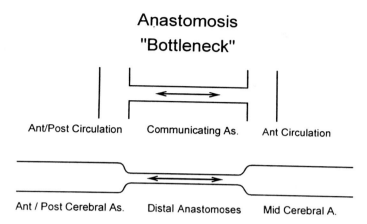

Fig. 1. Scheme of collateral pathways. Anterior communicating artery is the anastomotic segment in the Circle of Willis that joins the bilateral anterior (Ant) circulation. Posterior (Post) circulation is linked to the anterior circulation through the paired posterior communicating arteries (As). Distal anastomoses join distal branches of the anterior and posterior cerebral arteries with distal branches of the middle (Mid) cerebral artery (A). Note luminal width of the anastomosis is narrower than the connecting supply or delivery segment, thus producing a "bottleneck" with higher resistance to blood flow in the pathway.

distal anastomoses of major cerebral arteries convey blood into major arterial territories, and microcircle anastomoses route blood to local tissue fields.

Some Determinants of Collateral Circulation

Prior to developed collateral flow, the anastomotic segment, the intermediate component of the collateral pathway, is normally of narrower luminal width with greater resistance to blood flow than the connecting supply or delivery artery (Fig. 1). Most anastomoses are arranged in parallel, thus making the total anastomotic resistance to blood flow less than the resistance of any given one.[17] Compared to a serial arrangement, the parallel pattern provides greater safety if a segment becomes occluded, because alternate routes remain functional even though vascular conductance is reduced. A gradient in blood pressure forces blood to flow through the anastomotic segment into the downstream vessel where blood pressure is lower.[14] The drop in driving pressure across the anastomotic segment is inversely related to the luminal width and directly related to the length.[17] Narrow anastomoses with little dilator capacity present greater vascular resistance to blood flow and, thus, produce a larger drop in the driving pressure than do wider anastomoses. Below the critical blood pressure level required for autoregulation, collateral blood flow becomes pressure-dependent,[18] and flow decreases with distance into the tissue area at risk of infarction.[19,20] Thus, the anastomosis is a necessary component of the collateral pathway, and its luminal width, location, parallel pattern, and blood pressure are important parameters that determine the approximate position and field size protected by collateral circulation. When protection from injury is lost because of inadequate blood flow, secondary events resulting from the lesion probably determine final infarct size.

Ultrasound Studies and Other Investigations in Humans

Noninvasive human blood flow studies utilizing transcranial Doppler ultrasonography detect velocity and direction of blood flow around the Circle of Willis.[21,22] Ultrasonography is used to evaluate collateral blood flow in individual vessels. Compression of a common carotid artery reverses flow through the ipsilateral anterior cerebral artery, thus indicating flow through the anterior communicating artery.[21] Compression of the vertebral arteries below the mastoid process produces flow through the posterior communicating arteries and reversal of flow in the basilar artery. An index of cerebral circulatory resistance (R) is obtained[23] by subtracting the diastolic velocity (D) of the common carotid artery from the maximal velocity (A) and dividing the difference by the maximal velocity, $R = (A - D)/A$. R increases with progressive internal carotid artery occlusion because diastolic velocity falls to zero.[23] Thus, noninvasive ultrasound detects flow direction in the communicating arteries, and velocity amplitude during the cardiac cycle can provide information about the downstream vascular resistance, which increases with arterial blockage.[22,23]

In 1961, Reivich et al. demonstrated with serial arteriography reversed blood flow in the left vertebral artery in two patients with cerebral ischemia.[24] Atherosclerotic narrowing or occlusion of the subclavian artery proximal to the vertebral artery reduces blood pressure distal to the stenosis below that at the vertebral–basilar junction, thus reversing the pressure gradient and blood flow in the vertebral artery. Ultrasound directional studies provide evidence that reversed flow in the vertebral artery comes via the Circle of Willis and from the other vertebral artery before supplying an upper extremity.[22] Arm compression, which increases vascular resistance, decreases diastolic velocity in the ipsilateral internal carotid artery providing more evidence of flow via the internal carotid artery.[22] In some patients with so-called subclavian steal syndrome, perhaps a misnomer,[25] arm exercise prevents adequate blood flow to the brain to the extent that motor-sensory functions are impaired.[26] Thus, anastomoses of the arterial Circle of Willis are capable of providing collateral blood supply not only to the brain but also to somatic regions with detrimental expense to the brain if pressure gradients between the arterial circle and brain tissue are reduced.[25]

Vander Eecken reported in more detail than any prior publication the location, number, and width of anastomoses joining distal branches of the major cerebral arteries.[8] Unlike prior studies that attempted to identify functional border zones by location of injected colored media, Vander Eecken correctly positioned major vascular territories anatomically by location of the distal anastomoses. Anatomical border zones were located on the lateral pial surface near the vertex, in the inferior lateral temporal region, on the basal aspect over the orbit, and medially above the splenium. Anastomoses ranged in luminal width from 200–760 μ, contained an elastic lamina, and histologically were like other arteries of similar size. Average diameter of 131 anastomoses from 12 cerebral hemispheres was 312 μ. Luminal width was observed not to vary with age. No quantitative data were given to differentiate larger end-to-end anastomoses from the generally narrower candelabra type.

Illustrations and photographs demonstrated that major cerebral artery occlusions produced cortical infarcts located within areas at risk of infarction defined by anastomotic borders.[7,8] Large regions of tissue were shown to exist between centrally located grossly infarcted softened areas and the peripherally positioned anastomoses. Protective supply from a noncollateral source seems unlikely, because cortical vessels do not interdigitate or overlap, intracortical precapillary and capillary anastomoses of penetrating radial arteries have very limited laterally directed perfusion fields, and no source for supply to the cortex exists deep to the cortex. Thus, without protection from collateral blood flow through pial surface distal anastomoses, such small infarcts after major arterial occlusions are otherwise difficult to explain.

Mathematical models were designed to study hemodynamic features of anastomotic communicating arteries in the arterial Circle of Willis under conditions of luminal width asymmetry, changes in vertebral artery resistance, and ratios of efferent vessel peripheral resistances.[27] A change in luminal width of a communicating artery was shown to have effect on flow in the afferent vessels and flow within the arterial Circle of Willis. Flow reductions resulting from increased vertebral artery resistance were compensated for by the system to maintain efferent fluxes constant.[27]

Anastomoses also bridge distal rami of the middle meningeal artery with the MCA near the vertex, but little is known of the number, size, or possible functional significance of these junctional segments that join internal and external carotid arterial beds.[28] For other sources of collateral supply to the human brain, the reader is referred to the summary study by Gillilan.[9]

Collateral Pial Arteries in Nonhumans

Development of Collateral Circulation

By 15 s of temporary occlusion of a common carotid artery, blood flow measured by laser Doppler flowmetry in the ipsilateral territory of the MCA falls to a minimum level, and then collateral flow escapes to baseline level in normotensive Wistar rats (NW). In contrast, in spontaneously hypertensive stroke-prone rats (SHRSP), blood flow falls to the minimum level and collateral flow is 48% below baseline level at 15 s of occlusion ($p < 0.05$). Release of the occlusion immediately unloads the anastomoses, and flow through normal channels is restored to normal or higher levels within seconds in both strains. Thus, in SHRSP collateral blood flow through the anastomoses is impaired at initiation time, possibly because of narrower, stiffer anastomoses in the Circle of Willis or a reduced rate of relaxation of vascular smooth muscle. At 5 min of MCA occlusion above the rhinal fissure, collateral blood flow to the cortical territory of the occluded artery is less in SHRSP (13 ± 3 mL/min/100 g) than NW (23 ± 4 mL/min/100 g, $p < 0.05$).[29] One month after MCA occlusion, blood flow and blood flow reserve are restored to virtually normal levels in NW protected from infarction,[30] but a large atrophic infarct precludes flow measurement in SHRSP. Distal anastomoses are appreciably narrower in luminal width in SHRSP ($32 \pm 2 \mu$, mean $\pm$ SEM) than in normotensive rats ($55 \pm 3 \mu$),[31] as are communicating arteries in the Circle of Willis, but numbers of anastomoses do not differ appreciably in the two strains. Thus, at occlusion time, narrow anastomoses with high resistance to flow reduce driving pressure and conduct less collateral blood, which results in a larger infarct after MCA occlusion in SHRSP compared to protected normotensive rats[32] or to SHRSP receiving antihypertensive treatment.[33]

Vessel Remodeling
in Response to Chronic Occlusion

Changes in neural activity, hemodynamic shear stress, and drag might be stimuli-initiating dilatory vascular events, but little is known of the events in the anastomoses. Increased blood flow through an anastomotic segment produces functional and structural changes in the vessel wall. Permanent occlusion of the common carotid artery in young normotensive rats produces a wider, thicker, longer posterior communicating artery ipsilateral to the occlusion. The wider, thicker, longer basilar artery in rabbits after chronic carotid occlusion is the result of hyperplasia, not hypertrophy.[34] In basilar artery ring segments, contractile response to potassium chloride is more potent and, after precontraction by $10^{-6}M$ serotonin, relaxation to acetylcholine is more sensitive in ligated rabbits.[34] Permanent occlusion of the MCA in 10-d-old normotensive rats produces distal ACA-MCA anastomoses 90–110 d later that are wider, but shorter (less tortuous) than control anastomoses,[35] whereas anastomoses remodeled from 36 to 56 d of age are 24–29% longer than controls.[35] Increased tritiated thymidine update in pia-arachnoid containing distal anastomoses, but not in underlying cortex or contralateral controls, suggests proliferating cells remodel existing distal anastomotic segments into longer, wider, thicker-walled vessels mostly occurring within several days of the occlusion.[36] Oldendorf suggested that disinhibition of growth may occur with increased blood flow causing local wash-out of a growth-inhibiting factor.[37] Basic fibroblast growth factor might stimulate vessel growth as in coronary arterial collaterals,[38] but we find no evidence of synthesis of additional new blood vessels, only modification of vessels existing at occlusion time. The purpose of increasing the anastomotic segment length in juvenile rats, but not in very young rats, is unknown. Thus, increased blood flow through anastomotic segments produces adaptive structural change to the Circle of Willis and distal anastomoses existing at occlusion time, but no new vessels are added.

Summary

On the pial surface of the human cerebrum, communicating arteries in the Circle of Willis are anastomotic segments with potential to channel incoming blood to the anterior or posterior circulation. In border zones of major cerebral and cerebellar arteries, distal anastomoses are positioned to communicate alternate supply into a major arterial territory. Within major pial arterial territories in human, as in other species, microcircle anastomoses probably regulate alternate vascular supply to local cortical tissue fields. Compensatory blood flows through the anastomosis when a pressure gradient exists across the segment. A pressure gradient occurs when the usual supply pathway is compromised by flow blockage or progressively narrowing disease. Systemic blood pressure, luminal width and location of the anastomosis, site of blockage, and blood pressure downstream to the anastomosis are important variables that determine whether compensatory flow is partially or totally protective of tissue in the area at risk of infarction.

Measurement of blood flow in hypertensive rats before, during, and after temporary common carotid artery occlusion suggests that the earliest initiation of collateral blood flow is impaired in the anastomoses. Impaired initiation of collateral blood flow, less blood flow, and less reserve blood flow suggest narrower anastomoses predispose to large infarcts in hypertensive rats compared to normotensive rats. After common carotid artery or MCA occlusion, anastomotic segments increase in size beyond that explained by vasodilation. Anastomotic segments existing at occlusion time are remodeled into wider luminal, thicker, longer segments by addition of new cells. Much remains to be learned about mechanisms controlling anastomotic segments with potential for alternate sources of blood and protection against infarction.

Acknowledgment

Support for this study was provided by National Institutes of Health Grant HL 18575.

References

[1] Symonds, C. (1955) *Brit. Med. J.* **1**, 119–124.

[2] Rogers, L. (1947) *Brain* **70**, 171–178.

[3] Fawcett, E. and Blachford, J. V. (1906) *J. Anat. Physiol.* **40**, 63–70.

[4] Duret, H. (1874) *Arch. Physiol. Norm. Pathol.* **1**, 60–91, 316–353.

[5] Beevor, C. E. (1908) *Brain* **30**, 402–425.

[6] Vander Eecken, H. M., Fisher, M., and Adams, R. D. (1952) *J. Neuropath. Exper. Neurol.* **11**, 91–94.

[7] Vander Eecken, H. M. and Adams, R. D. (1953) *J. Neuropath. Exp. Neurol.* **12**, 132–157.

[8] Vander Eecken, H. M. (1959) *The Anastomoses Between the Leptomeningeal Arteries of the Brain.* C. Thomas, Springfield, IL, pp. 1–160.

[9] Gillilan, L. A. (1974) *Neurology* **24**, 941–948.

[10] Mchedlishvili, G. and Kuridze, N. (1984) *J. Cereb. Blood Flow Metabol.* **4**, 391–396.

[11] Duvernoy, H. M., Delon, S., and Vannson, J. L. (1981) *Brain Res.* **7**, 519–579.

[12] Shenkin, H. A., Harmel, M. H., and Kety, S. S. (1948) *Arch. Neurol. Psychiat.* **60**, 240–252.

[13] McDonald, D. A. and Potter, J. M. (1951) *J. Physiol.* **114**, 356–371.

[14] Fields, W. S., Bruetman, M. E., and Weibel, J. (1965) *Monograph in Surg. Sci.* **2,** 183–259.

[15] Murray, K. D. (1964) *J. Neurosurg.* **21,** 26–34.

[16] Riggs, H. E. and Rupp, C. (1963) *Arch. Neurol.* **8,** 8–14.

[17] Berne, R. M. and Levy, M. N. (1977) *Cardiovascular Physiology,* 3rd ed., CV Mosby, St. Louis, MO, pp. 53–74.

[18] Muhonen, M. G., Sawin, P. D., Loftus, C. M., and Heistad, D. D. (1992) *Stroke* **23,** 988–994.

[19] Loftus, C. M., Greene, G. M., Detwiler, K. N., Baumbach, G. L., and Heistad, D. D. (1990) *Am. J. Physiol.* **259,** H560–H566.

[20] Liu, X. L., Branston, N. M., Kawauchi, M., and Symon, L. (1992) *Stroke* **23,** 40–44.

[21] Arnolds, B. J. and von Reutern, G.-M. (1986) *Ultrasound in Med. Biol.* **12,** 115–123.

[22] Klingelhofer, J., Conrad, B., Benecke, R., and Frank, B. (1988) *Stroke* **19,** 1036–1042.

[23] Pourcelot, L. (1976) *Present and Future of Diagnostic Ultrasound* (Donald, I. and Levi, S., eds.), Kooyker, Rotterdam, pp. 141–147.

[24] Reivich, M., Holling, H. E., Brooke, R., and Tolle, J. F. (1961) *New Engl. J. Med.* **265,** 878–885.

[25] Fronek, A. (1992) *J. Vascular Surg.* **15,** 938–940.

[26] Greenfield, N. N. (1982) *Heart Lung* **11,** 327–331.

[27] Hillen, B., Hoogstraten, H. W., and Post, L. (1986) *J. Biomechanics* **19,** 187–194.

[28] Batson, O. V. (1944) *Fed. Proc.* **3,** 139–144.

[29] Coyle, P. and Heistad, D. D. (1986) *Hypertension* **8 (Suppl II),** II-67–II-71.

[30] Coyle, P. and Heistad, D. D. (1987) *Stroke* **18,** 407–411.

[31] Coyle, P. (1987) *Anat. Rec.* **218,** 40–44.

[32] Coyle, P. and Jokelainen, P. T. (1983) *Stroke* **14,** 605–611.

[33] Fugii, K., Weno, B., Baumbach, G. L., and Heistad, D. D. (1992) *Hypertension* **19,** 713–720.

[34] Lehman, R. M., Owens, G. K., Kassell, N. F., and Hongo, K. (1991) *Stroke* **22,** 499–504.

[35] Coyle, P. (1984) *Anat. Rec.* **210,** 357–364.

[36] Myers, S. F. and Coyle, P. (1987) *Anat. Rec.* **218,** 162–165.

[37] Oldendorf, W. H. (1989) *J. Neuropath. Exp. Neurol.* **48,** 534–547.

[38] Yanagisawa-Miwa, A., Uchida, Y., Nakamura, F., Tomaru, T., Kido, H., Kamijo, T., Sugimoto, T., Kaji, K., Utsuyama, M., Kurashima, C., and Ito, H. (1992) *Science* **257,** 1401–1403.

Chapter 19

The Intracerebral Circulation

Wolfgang Kuschinsky

Capillary Morphology and Brain Function

Of the whole substance of the brain, a fraction of about 1% is occupied by intracerebral vessels. Most of this fraction consists of capillaries. Because of their small diameter and large number per volume of brain tissue, this small fraction is sufficient to provide a large surface area between the blood and the tissue allowing for diffusion of metabolites and waste products.

Craigie[1] speculated that the capillary network in the brain "corresponds to its varying metabolic activity." Meanwhile, evidence has accumulated that supports such a concept. The network structure of cerebral capillaries and the local variations of their density have been shown in three-dimensional casts using scanning electron microscopy.[2] A positive correlation has been established between the local density of perfused capillaries, and both local cerebral glucose utilization and local cerebral blood flow,[3] as shown in Figs. 1 and 2. A similar kind of relationship has also been verified to exist between the density of morphologically stained capillaries, and both local blood flow and the maximal transport capacity of the glucose transport system at the same location.[4] It even exists within different parts of a single brain structure, for example, the inferior colliculus of the rat, a structure that displays a heterogeneous pattern of blood flow and glucose utilization.[5] Regional differences in blood-to-brain glucose uptake were paralleled by differences in leucine transport.[6] Although relationships

From *The Human Brain Circulation*, R. D. Bevan and J. A. Bevan, eds.
©1994 Humana Press

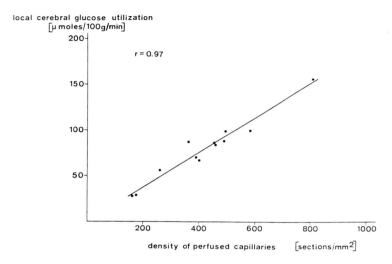

Fig. 1. Correlation between density of perfused capillaries and local cerebral glucose utilization. Each point represents values obtained for one brain structure. Densities of perfused capillaries and local cerebral glucose utilization were measured in different groups of conscious rats. From Klein et al.,[3] with permission.

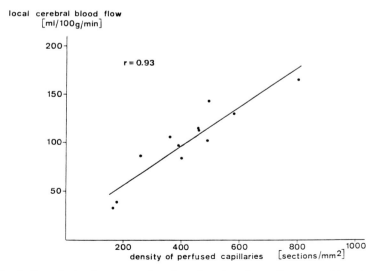

Fig. 2. Correlation between density of perfused capillaries and local cerebral blood flow. For details, *see* legend to Fig. 1. From Klein et al.,[3] with permission.

between capillary density and either glucose utilization or blood flow appear to hold for the large majority of gray and white matter brain structures, there are exceptions to the rule with respect to structures that lack the common blood–brain barrier. The neural lobe of the pituitary displays extremely high values of local blood flow and capillary density, although its metabolic rate would not require such high flow.[7] In conjunction with its high permeability,[7] this enables the neural lobe of the pituitary to secrete pituitary hormones effectively into the circulating blood. Mismatches among capillary density, glucose utilization, and permeability have also been verified for structures of the dorsal vagal complex[8,9] and of the subfornical organ and area postrema.[8]

The relationship between local cerebral glucose utilization and local capillary density has been confirmed by Borowsky and Collins.[10] These authors analyzed, in addition, the local patterns of a typical oxidative enzyme, cytochrome oxidase, and of a typical glycolytic enzyme, lactate dehydrogenase. The relationships between these enzymes and capillary density were not impressive. Both enzymes showed lower activity in white matter (with its low capillary density) than in gray matter (with its higher capillary density). A better correlation may be expected to exist between the volume density of mitochondria and capillary density, although not yet verified for the brain. Such a relationship has been convincingly demonstrated in skeletal muscle.[11,12] Although the relationship between the density of capillaries and that of mitochondria in skeletal muscle suggests a better performance with higher capillary densities, this could not be verified as a general rule, as discussed by Hudlicka et al.[13] This shows that we do not understand all components of the interaction between oxygen consumption and capillarity.

The Question of a Perfusion Fraction

The dynamics of capillary perfusion in the brain are a highly controversial issue. The answer to the question of whether all capillaries are perfused at any time-point appears to be critically dependent on the method used. Two methods have mainly been employed and need to be discussed: (1) analysis of brain sections obtained after injection of intravascular markers, and (2) direct observation of the exposed brain surface.

Analysis of Brain Sections

This method implies the intravascular injection of a perfusion marker under in vivo conditions and the analysis of the distribution of this marker in the capillaries after a defined circulation time. The perfusion marker and the capillary morphology are observed in brain sections using light or fluorescent microscopy. Compared to the method of direct observation of the exposed brain surface, this method has the advantage that the intravascular marker can be given to the intact, even conscious, animal. In addition, all brain structures can be investigated. The disadvantage of this method lies in the fact that dynamic changes of capillary perfusion, which do occur from one second to the next, cannot be detected with the desirable accuracy. Although the basic approach of this method as used by different groups looks rather similar at first glance, small methodological differences have yielded conflicting results, which have led to contradictory conclusions. The experimental approach is the iv injection of an intravascular perfusion marker and the analysis of the brain tissue taken after a short circulation time of a few seconds. Concerning the amount of capillaries filled within this short time period, Weiss claims to have observed a perfusion of about half of all capillaries,[14–19] whereas Kuschinsky maintains a complete perfusion of all capillaries.[20–22] Comparable methods have been used by Collins et al.[23] and Kikano et al.[24] Collins et al.[23] found 84% of all capillaries to be filled within 15 s. However, only one brain structure, the stratum griseum superficiale, was investigated. Kikano et al.[24] have reported a 70–80% filling in three brain structures.

Methodology of Analysis of Brain Sections

The critical dependence of the results obtained on the method used is apparent. It is therefore mandatory to discuss the methodological approaches. Both light and fluorescent microscopical methods have been applied for the detection of perfused and morphologically existing capillaries. Light microscopical methods, e.g., the alkaline phosphatase method, are widely used in many organs for the quantification of stereological parameters, such as capillary length per volume or capillary surface per volume.[25,26] In contrast, fluorescent microscopical methods (antibody methods for morphology, intravascular markers for perfusion) are not well suited for such a quantification, since the intensity of the fluorescent light depends, in part, on the intensity of the light source. The advantage of fluorescent microscopical methods, however, lies in the high sensitivity, which allows one to detect even capillary sections that are too small to be visible with light microscopy. It is, therefore, not surprising that the morphological densities of capillaries found by fluorescent microscopy[21,22] are higher than those reported by Weiss for light microscopy.[16] Such densities (Na = number of microvessels/mm^2 of brain section) can be detected appropriately with the fluorescent microscopical method, since they do not necessitate the introduction of other stereological parameters. Therefore, Na appears to be the only stereological parameter that can be determined quantitatively using fluorescent microscopy, and even with higher accuracy than using light microscopy. Apart from the principal limitations of light microscopy in the analysis of cerebral capillaries because of its low sensitivity, there are some special problems with the alkaline phosphatase method used by Weiss and his group[14–19] and others.[23,24,27–29] It is well known that the alkaline phosphatase method, as an enzymatic method, is critically dependent on the analytical details.[30] Especially the venous part of the capillary bed is poorly stained.[31–34] This may enhance the underestimation of the capillary density, which is likely with light microscopical methods.

Apart from the choice of light or fluorescent microscopy, the technique of processing the brain slices is a critical point. To avoid a diffusional loss of the intravascular marker, it is necessary to freeze the brain immediately at the end of the experiment and to keep the brain frozen during cutting. To preserve the intravascular marker, the frozen slices are exposed to cold alcohol or acetone immediately after cutting.[3,20–22] This kind of fixation does not interfere with the staining of either intravascular or morphological capillary fluorescent marker. In contrast, Weiss and his group had to avoid fixation of the tissue, since the alkaline phosphatase method could otherwise not be applied. Air-drying was performed instead, which is deleterious to the intravascular marker. By a process of condensation and evaporation at the cold surface of the brain slice, the intravascular marker is dissipated and spreads over the section. This explains why Weiss and his group found only part of the capillaries being perfused. Apparently, some of the intravascular marker (fluoresceinisothiocyanate = FITC, coupled to dextran) had been scattered to such an extent that it could not be detected any longer, as discussed by Göbel et al.[21] The objection of Weiss to the fixation method is that it "causes changes in the FITC label which may cause clumping or movement to noncapillary areas."[16] This has meanwhile been invalidated. Theilen and Kuschinsky[22] showed that fixation did not induce any of the addressed artifacts or a shrinkage of the tissue.

Altogether, fluorescent microscopical methods in combination with tissue fixation are highly sensitive and, therefore, best suited for the detection of perfused capillaries and of capillary morphology. Fixation of the tissue by alcohol or acetone is superior to air drying because it preserves the intravascular marker at its original location in the capillary. This kind of fixation does not induce artifacts. Fluorescent microscopical methods combined with tissue fixation have shown that all capillaries are perfused in the brain of the conscious rat at any time-point.

Direct Observation of the Exposed Brain Surface

Most of the studies using direct observation of the brain surface for the detection of capillary perfusion have not addressed explicitly the question of a complete or partial perfusion of brain capillaries. As will be discussed later, such studies have mainly detected the flow of erythrocytes and not that of plasma. In general, erythrocyte velocities measured in capillaries that are close to the brain surface have been found to be around 1 mm/s,[35–38] which is similar to velocities found in capillaries of other organs. A wide range of velocities has been reported with even a few occasional short periods (less than a second) of complete stop of erythrocyte flow. This fact is well known to anyone who has watched the microcirculation on the brain surface. Since erythrocytes that did not move for longer time periods could not be observed, such studies have not given any indication of the existence of nonperfused capillaries. However, they cannot completely rule out such a possibility, since nonperfused capillaries could contain stagnant plasma without erythrocytes.

The Question of Recruitment

The controversial view concerning the existence of nonperfused capillaries under normal conditions determines which opinions exist about cycling of capillaries and capillary recruitment. Capillary cycling is defined as the opening and closing of capillaries without concomitant changes in the average blood flow in the same area, whereas recruitment means the opening of previously closed capillaries with an enhanced blood flow. It should be pointed out that, in the literature, the term recruitment has also been used to describe increased capillary diffusion capacity in case of capillary perfusion heterogeneity when extra capillaries seemed to be recruited by increasing the flow rate in the slowly perfused capillaries. It is evident that capillary cycling and recruitment are rejected as mechanisms of physiological regulation by those investigators who claim a perfusion of all capillaries is the normal state. Consequently, an increase in the density of perfused capillaries could not be found by the group of Kuschinsky during hypercapnia in any brain structure investigated, although cerebral blood flow was doubled[20] (Fig. 3). Conversely, Weiss and his group have claimed that it takes about 6 min to fill most of the capillaries, which would mean time periods of complete capillary closing that last for minutes.[16]

Recent studies using confocal laser scanning microscopy to observe capillaries within the outer 250 μm of brain cortex have given no indication of capillary recruitment. On and off periods were observed for erythrocyte, but not for plasma flow.[39] Bolwig et al.[40] and Hertz and Paulson[41] found, on the basis of tracer kinetic studies, evidence of capillary recruitment with increased capillary surface area in response to increases in blood flow. As pointed out by these authors, these findings can well be ascribed to a decrease

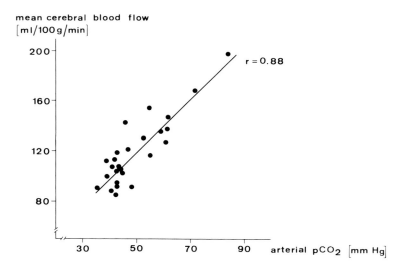

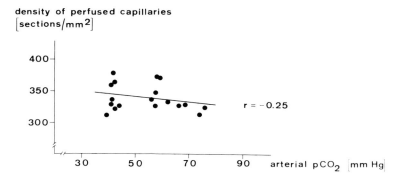

Fig. 3. Dependence of mean cerebral blood flow and mean density of perfused capillaries on the arterial pCO_2. For both cerebral blood flow and density of perfused capillaries, mean values have been calculated from the sum of all local values measured in each structure. Whereas a significant correlation was found between arterial pCO_2 and cerebral blood flow, no correlation could be observed between the arterial pCO_2 and the density of perfused capillaries. The data show the lack of capillary recruitment during hypercapnic hyperemia in the brain. From Göbel et al.,[20] with permission.

in the capillary perfusion heterogeneity in high-flow areas. Altogether, these data show that the concept of capillary cycling and recruitment in the brain has not been convincingly supported by direct experimental evidence and should therefore be abandoned. The classical and the present concept of capillary perfusion with plasma are shown in Fig. 4.

The Role of Erythrocyte Flow

As outlined previously, the capillary circulation of the brain has been analyzed in many studies by direct in vivo observation of the brain surface. Such studies are normally performed during anesthesia and are restricted to the surface of the brain. Since the number of capillaries found on the brain surface is limited, this approach has been used rarely.[35,42] Layers of 50–100 μm below the surface are accessible by transillumination and dark-field microscopy.[36,38] A more invasive technique uses insertion of a micro-transilluminator into the brain tissue.[37,43] All these techniques have measured the flow of erythrocytes. The results were interpreted to represent capillary blood flow. As a more recent technique, confocal laser scanning microscopy has been applied to cortical layers (up to 250 μm depth) in vivo.[39,44–46] Plasmatic flow could be separated from erythrocyte flow in single capillaries. A continuous plasmatic flow was observed, whereas erythrocyte flow was discontinuous and sometimes absent in single capillaries.[39] These results show that the erythrocyte flow, if it exists, can be taken as a qualitative, although not quantitative, marker of capillary flow. With a higher blood flow, the linear velocity of capillary blood increases, which means a higher number of erythrocytes passing through the capillaries during a given time period.

Analysis of Capillary Perfusion Using PET

Gjedde et al.[47] have made efforts to calculate the density of perfused capillaries from hemodynamic variables in humans. They determined the unidirectional clearance of glucose from positron emission tomography studies in stroke patients. Assumptions were

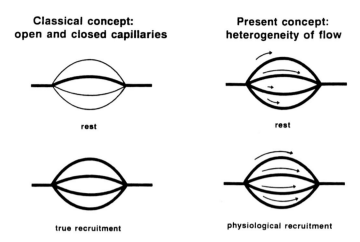

Fig. 4. Schematical outline of previous (left) and present (right) concepts of capillary perfusion in the brain. Thin lines represent nonperfused capillaries; wide lines mean perfused capillaries. The lengths of the arrows on the right side indicate flow velocities.

made of capillary morphology and transport kinetics. These authors came to the conclusion that the postischemic amelioration of cerebral blood flow is not paralleled by an increase in the number of perfused (glucose transporting) capillaries. Although any piece of information that can be obtained from humans is of high interest, the indirect approach, which is unavoidable in patient studies, makes this conclusion rather doubtful.

Acknowledgment

This work was supported by the Deutsche Forschungsgemeinschaft.

References

[1] Craigie, E. H. (1945) *Biol. Rev.* **20**, 133–146.
[2] Yoshida, Y. and Ikuta, F. (1984) *J. Cereb. Blood Flow Metab.* **4**, 290–296.
[3] Klein, B., Kuschinsky, W., Schröck, H., and Vetterlein, F. (1986) *Am. J. Physiol.* **251**, H1333–1340.
[4] Gjedde, A. and Diemer, N. H. (1985) *J. Cereb. Blood Flow Metab.* **5**, 282–289.

[5] Gross, P. M., Sposito, N. M., Pettersen, S. E., Panton, D. G., and Fenstermacher, J. D. (1987) *J. Cereb. Blood Flow Metab.* **7**, 154–160.

[6] LaManna, J. C. and Harik, S. I. (1986) *J. Cereb. Blood Flow Metab.* **6**, 717–723.

[7] Gross, P. M., Sposito, N. M., Pettersen, S. E., and Fenstermacher, J. D. (1986) *Neuroendocrinology* **44**, 401–407.

[8] Gross, P. M. (1991) *Can. J. Physiol. Pharmacol.* **69**, 1010–1025.

[9] Shaver, S. W., Pang, J. J., Wall, K. M., Sposito, N. M., and Gross, P. M. (1991) *J. Comp. Neurol.* **306**, 73–82.

[10] Borowsky, I. W. and Collins, R. C. (1989) *J. Comp. Neuro.* **288**, 401–413.

[11] Conley, K. E., Kayar, S. R., Rösler, K., Hoppeler, H., Weibel, E. R., and Taylor, C. R. (1987) *Respir. Physiol.* **69**, 47–64.

[12] Hoppeler, H., Hudlicka, O., and Uhlmann, E. (1987) *J. Physiol.* **385**, 661–675.

[13] Hudlicka, O., Egginton, S., and Brown, M. D. (1988) *News Physiol. Sci.* **3**, 134–138.

[14] Anwar, M., Buchweitz-Milton, E., and Weiss, H. R. (1988) *Circ. Res.* **63**, 27–34.

[15] Buchweitz-Milton, E. and Weiss, H. R. (1988) *Am. J. Physiol.* **255**, H623–628.

[16] Weiss, H. R. (1988) *Microvasc. Res.* **36**, 172–180.

[17] Frankel, H., Dribben, J., Kissen, I., Gerlock, T., and Weiss, H. R. (1989) *Microcirc. Endoth. Lymphatics* **5**, 319–415.

[18] Kissen, I. and Weiss, H. R. (1991) *Life Sci.* **48**, 1351–1363.

[19] Weiss, H. R., Buchweitz, E., Murtha, T. J., and Auletta, M. (1982) *Circ. Res.* **51**, 494–503.

[20] Göbel, U., Klein, B., Schröck, H., and Kuschinsky, W. (1989) *J. Cereb. Blood Flow Metab.* **9**, 491–499.

[21] Göbel, U., Theilen, H., and Kuschinsky, W. (1990) *Circ. Res.* **66**, 271–281.

[22] Theilen, H. and Kuschinsky, W. (1992) *J. Cereb. Blood Flow Metab.*, in press.

[23] Collins, R. C., Wagman, I. L., Lymer, L., and Matter, J. M. (1987) *J. Cereb. Blood Flow Metab.* **7(Suppl. 1)**, S336.

[24] Kikano, G. E., LaManna, J. C., and Harik, S. I. (1989) *Stroke* **20**, 1027–1031.

[25] Hoppeler, H. and Kayar, S. R. (1988) *News Physiol. Sci.* **3**, 113–116.

[26] Weibel, E. R. and Elias, H. (1967) *Quantitative Methods in Morphology* (Weibel, E. R. and Elias, H., eds.), Springer, Berlin, pp. 89–98.

[27] Iadecola, C., Arneric, S. P., and Reis, D. J. (1989) *Brain Res.* **501**, 188–193.

[28] Meier-Ruge, W. and Schulz-Dazzi, U. (1987) *Life Sci.* **40**, 943–949.

[29] Jucker, M. and Meier-Ruge, W. (1989) *Microvasc. Res.* **37**, 298-307.

[30] Doty, S. B. (1980) *J. Histochem. Cytochem.* **28**, 66–68.

[31] Appell, H. J. and Hammersen, F. (1977) *Kölner Beiträge zur Sportwissenschaft. Jahrbuch der Deutschen Sporthochschule Köln*, Hans Richarz, St. Augustin, pp. 97–113.

[32] Grim, M. and Carlson, B. M. (1990) *J. Histochem. Cytochem.* **38**, 1907–1912.
[33] Osterkamp-Baust, U. and Hammersen, F. (1981) *Biblthca. Anat.* **20**, 126–129.
[34] Romanul, F. C. A. and Bannister, R. G. (1962) *J. Cell. Biol.* **15**, 73–84.
[35] Ma, Y. P., Koo, A., Kwan, H. C., and Cheng, K. K. (1974) *Microvasc. Res.* **8**, 1–13.
[36] Ivanow, K. P., Kalinina, M. K., and Levkovich, Y. I. (1981) *Microvasc. Res.* **22**, 143–155.
[37] Pawlik, G., Rackl, A., and Bing, R. J. (1981) *Brain Res.* **208**, 35–58.
[38] Kislyakov, Y. Y., Levkovitch, Y. I., Shuymilova, T. E., and Vershinina, E. A. (1987) *Int. J. Microirc. Clin. Exp.* **6, 1**, 3–13.
[39] Villringer, A., Dirnagl, U., Gebhardt, R., and Einhäupl, K. M. (1991) *J. Cereb. Blood Flow Metab.* **Suppl. 2**, S441.
[40] Bolwig, T. G., Hertz, M. M., Paulson, O. B., Spotoft, H., and Rafaelsen, O. J. (1977) *Eur. J. Clin. Invest.* **7**, 87–93.
[41] Hertz, M. M. and Paulson, O. B. (1982) *Microvasc. Res.* **24**, 364–376.
[42] Rosenblum, W. I. and Zweifach, B. W. (1963) *Arch. Neurol.* **9**, 414–423.
[43] Yamakawa, T., Yamaguchi, S., Niimi, H., and Sugiyama, I. (1987) *Circulatory Shock* **22**, 323–332.
[44] Dirnagl, U., Villringer, A., Gebhardt, R., Haberl, R. L., Schmiedek, P., and Einhäupl, K. M. (1991) *J. Cereb. Blood Flow Metab.* **11**, 353–360.
[45] Villringer, A., Dirnagl, U., Them, A., Schürer, L., Krombach, F., and Einhäupl, K. M. (1991) *Microvas. Res.* **42**, 305–315.
[46] Villringer, A., Haberl, R. L., Dirnagl, U., Anneser, F., Verst, M., and Einhäupl, K. M. (1989) *Brain Res.* **504**, 159–160.
[47] Gjedde, A., Kuwabara, H., and Hakim, A. M. (1990) *J. Cereb. Blood Flow Metab.* **10**, 317–326.

Chapter 20

Cerebral Circulation
of the Fetus and Newborn

David W. Busija

Introduction

Similar to the adult, the fetal and neonatal cerebral circulations are regulated by four primary factors: metabolic stimuli, perfusion pressure, chemical stimuli, and neural stimuli. However, the relative importance of these factors in regulation of the cerebral circulation in many instances appears to vary with age or developmental stage. The underlying basis for differential responsiveness has to do with considerations such as basal arterial blood gases and arterial blood pressure, completeness of neural development, basal level of brain metabolism, physical features of blood vessels, and characteristics of the blood–brain barrier (BBB). I will review recent studies concerning the roles played by chemical, autoregulatory, metabolic, and neural factors in the regulation of cerebral resistance vessels. Further, since neonatal animals are often exposed to several pathophysiological conditions, I will discuss cerebrovascular responses to asphyxia/reventilation, seizures, and hemorrhagic hypotension in neonates.

Chemical Stimuli

Chemical stimuli include arterial blood gases and circulating vasoactive substances, such as catecholamines, vasopressin, oxytocin, and angiotensin II, as well as cerebrospinal fluid (CSF) gases

From *The Human Brain Circulation*, R. D. Bevan and J. A. Bevan, eds.
©1994 Humana Press

and neurotransmitters. Several features of the cerebral circulation in immature animals could make cerebrovascular responsiveness different from that of adults. For example, fetal arterial blood gases are very different from those of neonates and adults. Arterial PO_2 is very low in the fetus, and PCO_2 is moderately elevated. At the time of birth, arterial blood gases change toward adult values relatively quickly.[1] It has been shown that prolonged exposure to abnormal blood gases alters subsequent exposure to arterial hypercapnia, probably because of altered buffering capacity of CSF.[2] In addition, cardiovascular reflexes might not be fully developed,[3] so that sympathetic-mediated vasoconstriction does not oppose hypoxic or hypercapnic cerebrovascular dilation as occurs in adult animals.[4,5]

A characteristic feature of the cerebral circulation is the dramatic vasodilation that accompanies increases in arterial blood PCO_2. The immediate stimulus for cerebrovascular dilation appears to be increased brain extracellular fluid $[H^+]$,[6] and at least in piglets, the response appears to involve an essential prostanoid component.[7,8] Lack of effect of decreased arterial blood pH by HCl infusions in piglets indicates the presence of a functional BBB in neonates of this species.[9] Cerebrovascular dilation to arterial hypercapnia is a response that occurs at all ages, but appears to be blunted somewhat in fetuses and neonates compared with adults, even when cerebral blood flow (CBF) values are normalized for metabolic rate.[10] However, even in the fetus, the cerebrovascular dilation to arterial hypercapnia is a relatively strong response.

Similar to arterial hypercapnia, immature fetuses show an attenuated cerebrovascular dilation to arterial hypoxia compared with more mature animals.[11,12] Thus, in more mature animals, such as near-term fetus, neonate, and adults, the increased CBF during hypoxia is sufficient to maintain cerebral oxygen delivery constant.[11] However, in immature fetuses, this response is inadequate, and in contrast to older animals, oxygen extraction from blood by the brain increases.[11] The reason for this blunted cerebrovascular response is unclear. It is thought that adenosine is an important mediator of hypoxic-mediated dilation in the cerebral circulation.[13] However, cerebrovascular dilation to adenosine or adenosine agonists is similar across age groups.[14,15]

Major changes in arterial blood gases occur as a normal consequence of birth, and include increased PO_2 and decreased PCO_2.[1] However, sick neonates may be exposed to additional, severe pertubations of blood gases.[16] During asphyxia/reventilation, neonates are exposed to respiratory acidosis, and the initial response is an increase in CBF.[17] Increases in blood flow are larger in brain stem system areas than in the cerebrum. However, with prolonged asphyxia, arterial blood pressure decreases and CBF falls, with brain stem blood flow being better maintained than that of the cerebrum. Derangements of arterial blood gases also contribute to another pathological condition affecting neonates as well as other age groups. During seizure activity there is a tremendous increase in CBF that is associated with increased brain metabolism, arterial hypertension, and metabolic acidosis. We have shown that when neonatal animals are paralyzed during seizures, increased CBF and acidosis are attenuated because of reduction of muscle activity.[18]

In addition to chemical stimuli in blood, chemical stimuli in the CSF, such as neurotransmitters, also can affect cerebral hemodynamics. Neurotransmitters can reach vasoactive levels in perivascular CSF via synaptic overflow during neuronal activation or pathological conditions.[19] Further, we have shown that the endogenous prostanoid system (prostaglandins, thromboxane) can interact with these neurotransmitters in several different ways to determine the final vascular effect in newborn pigs (Table 1). Our criteria to establish a significant interaction are that topical application of the neurotransmitter is able to increase CSF levels of prostanoids, thereby establishing increased synthesis of prostanoids by cerebral vessels and/or tissues, and that indomethacin pretreatment is able to alter arteriolar responsiveness. Thus, we depend on complementary biochemical and pharmacological data in making our judgment. In almost all cases, if CSF levels of prostanoids increase during application of neurotransmitters, then indomethacin administration alters cerebral arteriolar responses. The only exception that we have found so far is with vasopressin during normal arteriolar tone conditions. Thus, although topical application of vasopressin increased CSF levels of prostanoids, indomethacin preadministration under conditions of normal tone did not reduce or reverse arteriolar dilation. Our results indicate

Table 1
Functional Interactions Between Exogenous Neurotransmitters
and the Endogenous Prostanoid System Relating to Changes in Vascular Tone in Newborn Pigs

Neurotransmitter	Vascular effect[a]	CSF levels of prostanoids	Effect of indomethacin	Reference
Constrictor stimulus				
Dopamine	Constricts	No change	None	Busija and Leffler[47]
Noradrenaline	Constricts	Increases	Potentiates	Busija and Leffler[42]
Vasopressin[b]	Constricts	Increases	Potentiates	Armstead et al.[48]
Dynorphin[b]	Constricts	Increases	Potentiates	Armstead et al.[49]
β-endorphin	Constricts	Increases	Potentiates	Armstead et al.[49]
Acetylcholine	Constricts	Increases	Abolishes	Busija et al.,[50] Armstead, et al.,[51] Wagerle and Busija[52,53]
Dilator stimulus				
Glutamate	Dilates	No change	None	Busija[54]
Aspartate	Dilates	No change	None	Busija[54]
Isoprenaline	Dilates	No change	None	Busija and Leffler[42]
Substance P	Dilates	No change	None	Busija and Chen[32]
Calcitonin gene-related peptide	Dilates	No change	None	Busija and Chen[32]
Vasopressin[b]	Dilates	Increases	None	Armstead et al.[48]
Dynorphin[b]	Dilates	Increases	Attenuates	Armstead et al.[49]
Leu-enkephalin	Dilates	Increases	Attenuates	Armstead et al.[49]
Met-enkephalin	Dilates	Increases	Attenuates	Armstead et al.[49]
Histamine	Dilates	Increases	Attenuates	Mirro et al.[55]
Oxytocin	Dilates	Increases	Allows constriction	Busija et al.[56]

[a]Vascular effect represents direction of change of pial arteriolar diameter after topical application of neurotransmitter.
[b]Vasoactive responses of these substances are tone-dependent (Armstead et al.,[48]); application results in dilation in arterioles under baseline conditions and constriction in arterioles previously dilated with other interventions.

that neurotransmitters can interact with prostanoids in the final determination of pial arteriolar responses in several ways. First, neurotransmitters can act independently of prostanoids, e.g, for dopamine (a constrictor agent) and glutamate, aspartate, isoprenaline, substance P, calcitonin-gene related peptide, and vasopressin (dilator agents). Second, prostanoids mediate dilation, e.g., for Met-enkephalin, Leu-enkephalin, histamine, and dynorphin (normal tone). Third, prostanoids counteract and limit vasoconstriction, e.g., for norepinephrine, β-endorphin, dynorphin (increased tone), and vasopressin (increased tone). Fourth, prostanoids are permissive in allowing responses to occur, e.g., for acetylcholine. Fifth, prostanoids can promote dilation and mask constriction, e.g., oxytocin.

Autoregulatory Stimuli

Another characteristic feature of the cerebral circulation is its ability to maintain total and regional blood flows relatively constant over a wide range of arterial blood pressures. The importance of autoregulation is that it allows blood flow to match metabolic needs in spite of fluctuations in arterial blood pressure by maintaining capillary perfusion pressure at levels to ensure adequate exchange between plasma and tissues. Usually autoregulation is discussed in terms of arterial blood pressure vs blood flow for the sake of convenience, because cerebral venous or CSF pressures are normally low. However, it is more precise to define autoregulation as the relationship between perfusion pressure and CBF. Perfusion pressure is the difference between arterial blood pressure and cerebral venous or CSF pressure, whichever of the latter two is greater. There are several situations that arise in the fetus and neonate when cerebral venous and CSF pressures need to be considered, because with relatively low arterial blood pressure, any increases in these pressures might decrease perfusion pressure below the level needed to maintain CBF. For example, during labor and delivery, external compression can transiently increase intracranial pressure. In addition, for sick babies, situations such as asphyxia, intratracheal suctioning, hydrocephalus, and positive pressure ventilation, can increase cerebral venous and CSF pressures.[16,20]

The autoregulatory curve for neonates is shifted to the left, as a compensation to low arterial blood pressure. Thus, fetal and neonatal animals have been shown to maintain CBF down to values of 35 mmHg,[21–23] and CBF can be maintained for at least 60 min at these low arterial blood pressure levels.[23] However, the upper limit of cerebral autoregulation is shifted to the left also.[24] The shift in the autoregulatory response is opposite that seen in hypertensives, where the autoregulatory curve is shifted to the right.[25] The reason for this shift is the autoregulatory curve in younger animals, but may be the result of such factors as wall thickness of arteries and arterioles and relatively low resistance of the cerebral circulation.[26,27]

Metabolic Stimuli

Brain metabolic rate varies according to age and developmental stage, and in anesthetized animals is lowest in the fetus, higher in adults, and highest in neonates.[10] These differences probably are related to basal activity and level of development. In neonates[28,29] as well as adults,[30] CBF changes correspond to increases and decreases in metabolic rate. Based on indirect evidence, the same relationship apparently exists for the fetus.[11,12]

We have shown that CBF increases dramatically in newborn pigs during seizure activity.[18] However, only part of this increase is probably the result of augmented metabolic rate. When the animals are paralyzed and ventilated, changes in arterial blood pressure and blood gases are minimized, and CBF does not change as much. Further, recovery from seizure activity is faster than in the paralyzed group. Thus, cerebrovascular responses to seizures in unparalyzed neonates are the result of factors both intrinsic and extrinsic to the brain.

Neural Stimuli

Depending on the species studied, or in the case of babies born prematurely, overall neural development may or may not be essentially complete at birth. For example, rodents and rabbits are born blind and helpless, whereas lambs and piglets are born fairly mature. Autonomic innervation of the cerebral circulation, which can have an effect on hemodynamics, may or may not be functional at birth. For example, sympathetic innervation of brain blood vessels is largely absent at birth in rabbits, and is not fully developed to the adult pattern until 3–6 wk after birth.[31] In contrast, in piglets only a couple of days old, substance P and oxytocin/vasopressin–neurophysin innervation are fairly complete (ref. 32; unpublished observations). In addition, neurotransmitters are able to change diameter of pial arterioles, thereby indicating that functional receptors are present. Further, stimulation of preganglionic sympathetic fibers is able to constrict pial arterioles in piglets, indicating that ganglionic and effector components are functional.[33] Lastly, sympathetic nerves are able to have a restraining effect on cerebrovascular dilation during asphyxia and seizures,[34,35] thereby indicating that reflex pathways are functioning. However, results from other laboratories[2] indicate that not all cardiovascular reflexes, such as the baroreceptor reflex, are functional in piglets at this time. We have found that blockade of α-adrenoceptors is not able to affect cerebrovascular responses to hemorrhagic hypotension in newborn pigs.[36]

There is considerable evidence that indicates that there are age-related differences in cerebral resistance vessels to neural stimuli. For example, both in vivo and in vitro, cerebrovascular constrictor responses to norepinephrine or electrical transmural stimulation are greater in fetal and neonatal animals than in adult animals (Fig. 1).[37,38] Further, we have shown that pial arterioles constrict to sympathetic nerve stimulation in piglets,[33] whereas cerebral arteries in older swine do not constrict to transmural electrical stimulation.[39] The mechanisms for this age-related decrease are unclear, but could be the result of such factors as loss of number or affinity of α-adrenoceptors with development,[40] or competing, progressive dominance of counteracting neural[41] or prostanoid[42] mechanisms.

However, changes in cerebrovascular sensitivity to α-adrenoceptor stimuli may not occur with aging in all species. For example, we have shown that electrical or reflex activation of sympathetic nerves reduces CBF in adult rabbits,[43,44] and it has been shown in vitro that rabbit cerebral arteries shown little age-related change in

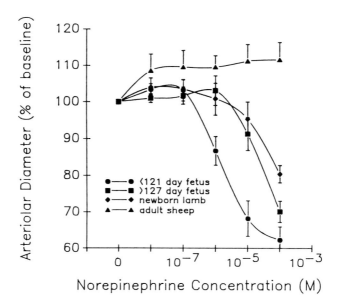

Fig. 1. Responses of sheep pial arteries to norepinephrine in fetus, neonate, and adult. From Wagerle et al.,[38] with permission.

responsiveness to norepinephrine.[45] Reasons for age-related species differences are unclear. Since sympathetic nerves protect the cerebral circulation from hyperemia associated with even modest elevations in arterial blood pressure,[46] this decrease in sympathetic potency with aging could be detrimental to the cerebral vasculature.

Summary

Although the cerebral circulation of the fetus, neonate, and adult responds to chemical, autoregulatory, metabolic, and neural stimuli, there are important although sometimes subtle age-related differences in responsiveness. First, cerebrovascular dilator responses to arterial hypercapnia or hypoxia appear to be attenuated in immature animals. Second, the autoregulatory curve is shifted to the left, such that CBF is maintained at normal levels at arterial pressures that are associated with falling CBF in adults. Third, cerebrovascular responsiveness to α-adrenoceptor stimuli may decrease in most species with development and aging, and thus expose the cerebral circulation to risk during arterial hypertension.

Acknowledgment

This work supported by Grants HL30260 and HL46558 from the National Institutes of Health.

References

[1] Davidson, D. (1987) *J. Appl. Physiol.* **63**, 676–684.

[2] Pourcyrous, M., Leffler, C., Busija, D. W., Mirro, R., Bada, H., and Korones, S. (1991) *FASEB J.* **5**, A374, abstract.

[3] Gootman, P. M. (1986) *Developmental Neurobiology of the Autonomic Nervous System* (Gootman, P. M., ed.), Humana, Clifton, NJ, pp. 279–325.

[4] Busija, D. W. and Heistad, D. D. (1984) *J. Physiol. (Lond.)* **347**, 35–45.

[5] Busija, D. W. (1984) *Am. J. Physiol.* **247**, H446–H451.

[6] Kontos, H. A., Wei, E. P., Raper, A. J., and Patterson, J. L., Jr. (1977) *Stroke* **8**, 226–229.

[7] Leffler, C. W. and Busija, D. W. (1985) *Circ. Res.* **57**, 689–694.

[8] Wagerle, L. C. and Mishra, O. P. (1988) *Circ. Res.* **62**, 1019–1026.

[9] Wagerle, L. C., Kumar, S. P., Belik, J., and Delivoria-Papadopoulos, M. (1988) *J. Appl. Physiol.* **65**, 776–781.

[10] Rosenberg, A. A., Jones, M. D., Jr., Traystman, R. J., Simmons, M. A., and Molteni, R. A. (1982) *Am. J. Physiol.* **242**, H862–H866.

[11] Koehler, R. C., Traystman, R. J., Zeger, S., Rogers, M. C., and Jones, M. D., Jr. (1984) *J. Cereb. Blood Flow Metab.* **4**, 114–122.

[12] Gleason, C. A., Hamm, C., and Jones, M. D., Jr. (1990) *Am. J. Physiol.* **258**, H1064–H1069.

[13] Park, T. S., Van-Wylen, D. G., Rubio, R., and Berne, R. M. (1987) *J. Cereb. Blood Flow Metabol.* **7**, 178–183.

[14] Toda, N. and Hagashi, S. (1979) *J. Pharmacol. Exp. Ther.* **211**, 716–721.

[15] Kurth, C. D. and Wagerle, L. C. Manuscript in preparation.

[16] Fanconi, S. and Duc, G. (1987) *Pediatrics* **79**, 538–542.

[17] Pourcyrous, M., Leffler, C. W., Busija, D. W. (1990) *Am. J. Physiol.* **259**, H662–H667.

[18] Pourcyrous, M., Leffler, C. W., Bada, H. S., Korones, S. B., Stidham, G. L., and Busija, D. W. (1992) *Ped. Res.* **31**, 636–639.

[19] Hagberg, H., Andersson, P., Kjellmer, I., Thiringer, K., and Thordstein, M. (1987) *Neurosci. Lett.* **78**, 311–317.

[20] Mirro, R., Leffler, C. W., Armstead, W., Beasley, D. G., and Busija, D. W. (1988) *Ped. Res.* **24**, 59–62.

21 Ashwal, S., Dale, P. S., and Longo, L. C. (1984) *Ped. Res.* **18**, 1309–1315.
22 Leffler, C. W., Busija, D. W., Beasley, D. G., and Fletcher, A. M. (1986) *Circ. Res.* **59**, 562–567.
23 Pasternak, J. F. and Groothuis, D. R. (1985) *Biol. Neonate* **48**, 100–109.
24 Fletcher, A. M., Leffler, C. W., and Busija, D. W. (1989) *Am. J. Vet. Res.* **50**, 754–757.
25 Strandgaard, S., Olesen, J., Skinhoj, E., and Lassen, N. A. (1973) *Br. J. Med.* **1**, 507–510.
26 Sadoshima, S., Busija, D. W., and Heistad, D. D. (1983) *Am. J. Physiol.* **244**, H406–H412.
27 Pearce, W. J. and Ashwal, S. (1987) *Ped. Res.* **22**, 192–196.
28 Busija, D. W. and Leffler, C. W. (1987) *Am. J. Physiol.* **22**, H869–H873.
29 Busija, D. W., Leffler, C. W., and Pourcyrous, M. (1988) *Am. J. Physiol.* **24**, H343–H346.
30 Sokoloff, L., Reivich, M., Kennedy, D., Des Rosiers, C. S., Patlak, K. D., Pettigrew, K. D., Sakurada, O., and Hinohara, M. (1977) *J. Neurochem.* **28**, 897–916.
31 Lindvall, M. and Owman, C. (1981) *J. Cereb. Blood Flow Metabol.* **1**, 245–266.
32 Busija, D. W. and Chen, J. (1992) *J. Dev. Physiol.* **18**, 67–72.
33 Busija, D. W., Leffler, C. W., and Wagerle, L. C. (1985) *Ped. Res.* **19**, 1210–1214.
34 Goplerud, J. M., Wagerle, L. C., and Delivoria-Papadopoulos, M. (1991) *Am. J. Physiol.* **260**, H1575–H1580.
35 Kurth, C. D., Wagerle, L. C., and Delivoria-Papadopoulos, M. (1988) *Am. J. Physiol.* **255**, H563–H568.
36 Armstead, W. M., Leffler, C. W., Busija, D. W., Beaslely, D. G., and Mirro, R. (1988) *Am. J. Physiol.* **23**, H671–H677.
37 Toda, N. (1991) *Am. J. Physiol.* **260**, H1443–H1448.
38 Wagerle, L. C., Kurth, C. D., and Roth, R. A. (1990) *Am. J. Physiol.* **258**, H1432–H1438.
39 Winquist, R. J., Webb, R. C., and Bohr, D. F. (1982) *Circ. Res.* **51**, 769–776.
40 Yamada, S., Yamamura, H. I., and Roeske, W. R. (1980) *Eur. J. Pharmacol.* **68**, 217–221.
41 Moskowitz, M. A., Wei, E. P., Saito, K., and Kontos, H. A. (1988) *Am. J. Physiol.* **255**, H1–H6.
42 Busija, C. W. and Leffler, C. W. (1987) *Brain Res.* **403**, 243–248.
43 Busija, D. W. (1984) *Am. J. Physiol.* **247**, H446–H451.
44 Busija, D. W. (1985) *Brain Res.* **345**, 341–344.
45 Toda, N. and Hayashi, S. (1979) *J. Pharmacol. Exp. Ther.* **211**, 716–721.
46 Busija, D. W., Heistad, D. D., and Marcus, M. L. (1980) *Circ. Res.* **48**, 62–69.

47 Busija, D. W. and Leffler, C. W. (1989) *J. Cereb. Blood Flow Metabol.* **9,** 264–267.
48 Armstead, W. M., Mirro, R., Busija, D. W., and Leffler, C. W. (1989) *Cir. Res.* **64,** 136–144.
49 Armstead, W. M., Mirror, R., Busija, D. W., and Leffler, C. W. (1990) *J. Pharmacol. Exp. Ther.* **255,** 1083–1089.
50 Busija, D. W., Wagerle, L. C., Pourcyrous, M., and Leffler, C. W. (1988) *Brain Res.* **439,** 122–126.
51 Armstead, W. M., Mirro, R., Busija, D. W., and Leffler, C. W. (1989) *J. Pharmacol. Exp. Ther.* **251,** 1012–1019.
52 Wagerle, L. C. and Busija, D. W. (1989) *J. Pharmacol. Exp. Ther.* **247,** 926–933.
53 Wagerle, L. C. and Busija, D. W. (1990) *Circ. Res.* **66,** 824–831.
54 Busija, D. W. and Leffler, C. W. (1989) *Am. J. Physiol.* **257,** H1200–H1203.
55 Mirro, R., Busija, D. W., Armstead, W. M., and Leffler, C. W. (1988) *Am. J. Physiol.* **23,** H1023–H1026.
56 Busija, D. W., Khreis, I., and Chen, J. (1992) *Am. J. Physiol.* **264,** H1023–H1027.

Chapter 21

Functional Changes in the Aging Cerebrovasculature

James R. Docherty

Introduction

This chapter looks at how aging affects the cerebrovasculature and the control of cerebral blood flow. With the increasing number of elderly people in Western societies, it becomes crucial that we learn more about how the elderly differ in the control of cerebral blood flow, and how alterations in cerebral blood flow may contribute to decline in cognitive function and to neurological disorders.

The Cerebral Circulation

We must first consider the basic physiology of the cerebral circulation. The major feature of the cerebral circulation that makes it different from the systemic circulation is that blood flow is maintained relatively constant by autoregulation over a wide range of systemic pressures. Various factors influence cerebral blood flow: metabolites, CO_2, autacoids from the vascular smooth muscle, platelets or endothelium, as well as, to a lesser extent than in the systemic circulation, neural and hormonal control. Larger cerebral arteries are by and large more influenced than small arterioles by nervous and hormonal factors that act to modulate autoregulation.

We will examine how aging affects these various factors, using as far as possible examples from the limited number of studies of

From *The Human Brain Circulation*, R. D. Bevan and J. A. Bevan, eds.
©1994 Humana Press

cerebral blood vessels. These results will be supplemented by examples of age-related changes in other blood vessels.

Cerebral Blood Flow

Cerebral blood flow is reported to decrease with age both in control subjects[1-3] and in migraine sufferers.[2] Furthermore, the decline in cerebral blood flow is matched by a decline in glucose utilization and O_2 consumption[4] as well as by a decline in brain mass,[5,6] so that it is possible that, at least in healthy subjects, the age-related decline in cerebral blood flow can be explained by a decreased brain mass. This decline may be increased by atherosclerosis. In a study of subjects over 50 yr old, the age-related decline in blood flow correlated with increased resistance or decreased compliance of cerebral arteries, probably because of atherosclerosis.[3] Cerebral blood flow is reported to be higher in females than males, partly as a result of a lower hematocrit, but aging affects cerebral blood flow in males and females similarly.[3,6,7] Studies of regional blood flow show that the age-related decline in cerebral blood flow is not uniform: the decrease in flow is less in the motor cortex than in the parietal.[8] Despite these changes in blood flow,[9] Muller et al. found no significant correlation between diameters of cerebral and carotid arteries with age.

In rats, a decrease[10] or no difference[11] with age was found in cerebral blood flow, and there is a report of decreased blood flow to certain brain regions in the aged rat.[12] In aged rats, the resting diameter of the pial arteries is reduced, and the relative proportions of the distensible elements elastin and smooth muscle are decreased with no change in collagen so that distensibility is reduced.[13] Other structural changes reported with age include thickening of the basement membrane and subtle changes in cerebrovascular capillary permeability in the rat.[14]

Stroke

The incidence of stroke increases markedly with age. Atherosclerosis is related to age, and usually starts in the carotid or cerebral arteries or Circle of Willis, extending later to the small intracerebral vessels. Also, the level of atherosclerosis of small vessels is usually less than that of large vessels.[15] In stroke-prone spontaneously hypertensive rats, there is evidence for an increased sympathetic innervation of cerebral arteries.[16] In the cat, it has been shown that the ability to form a collateral circulation following middle cerebral artery occlusion decreases with age,[17] so that the aged cerebral circulation may be more vulnerable to ischemic injury.

Nervous Control

The cerebral vasculature is innervated predominantly by the sympathetic arm of the autonomic nervous system, with major neurotransmitter noradrenaline (NA). However, other amine neurotransmitters, such as 5-hydroxytryptamine (5-HT), as well as peptides, such as neuropeptideY (NPY), calcitonin gene related peptide (CGRP), vasoactive intestine peptide (VIP), and substance P (SP), may innervate cerebral blood vessels.

Neurotransmission is likely to be affected by changes in nerve activity, density of innervation, presynaptic control of neurotransmission, and neurotransmitter disposition mechanisms, and in addition, by alterations in target organ responsiveness. In rabbit cerebral arteries, there is an age-related decline in 5-HT content,[18] whereas in arteries of the rat Circle of Willis, there is an age-related decrease in the presence of nerves for vasoconstrictor neurotransmitters (NA and 5-HT) and an age-related increase in the presence of nerves for vasodilator neurotransmitters (VIP, CGRP), with no change in the expression of NPY and SP.[19] In contrast, there is an age-related decline in CGRP and SP with no change in NA with age in guinea pig carotid arteries.[20] In rat small pial vessels, there is no change with age in choline acetylase (marker for cholinergic nerves) or in glutamic acid decarboxylase (marker for GABA).[21]

In monkey cerebral arteries, transmural nerve stimulation produces an α-adrenoceptor-mediated contraction in immature animals, but in arteries from older animals a nonadrenergic noncholinergic relaxation predominates, suggesting changes in the relative importance of different nerve types[22] (*see also* section on α-adrenoceptors).

In humans, one of the most consistently reported changes during aging is an increased plasma level of noradrenaline owing to an increased rate of appearance in the plasma or to a decreased plasma clearance, or both, and could be at least partly explained by a decline in the reuptake of NA into nerve terminals,[23] perhaps because of a decreased innervation. However, cerebral blood vessels have a low sensitivity to NA *(see below)* and are unlikely to respond to circulating levels of NA, although a diminished reuptake of NA may make them more sensitive to nerve activation. Furthermore, there is evidence that the prejunctional α_2-adrenoceptor-mediated inhibition of adrenergic neurotransmission declines with age,[23] so that any decreased innervation may be counteracted by this factor and diminished reuptake.

Actions of Autacoids and Metabolites

Cerebral blood vessels are under the influence of hormones, such as adrenaline and angiotensin II, and locally released autacoids, such as prostaglandins and EDRF (endothelium-derived relaxant factor). Autacoids, which have been extensively studied with respect to aging, will be dealt with individually as vasoconstrictors or vasodilators.

Vasoconstrictors

α-Adrenoceptors

Both α_1- and α_2-adrenoceptors mediate contraction of vascular smooth muscle, using different second-messenger systems (phosphoinositol hydrolysis and inhibition of adenylate cyclase, respectively). Cerebral arteries are much less responsive to NA than systemic arteries, so that the maximum contraction to NA in rabbit basilar artery is only 15% of the maximum possible.[24] This is likely to be the result of the presence of only a small number of α-adrenoceptors, so that there are no spare receptors. As a result, small changes in receptor number might be expected to produce large effects on the maximum contraction to NA. In dog[25] and monkey cerebral arteries,[22] during maturation, the maximum contraction to NA is reported to decrease, both in absolute terms and relative to the contraction to KCl, but in rat carotid arteries, there is no change with age in the response to NA.[26] In systemic blood vessels, most studies have failed to find any change with age in contractile responses mediated by α_1-adrenoceptors, perhaps because many spare receptors are present in most of these vessels. Very few studies have looked at the effects of aging on α_2-adrenoceptor function, but in the human saphenous vein, noradrenaline became less potent at producing α_2-mediated contractions with increasing age.[27]

5-Hydroxytryptamine

In the rat basilar artery, there was no change in the contractile response to 5-HT with age,[21] whereas in the rat carotid artery there was an increase in the maximum contraction to 5-HT.[26,28] During maturation, there was no change in the maximum response to 5-HT in the dog cerebral artery, although the potency of 5-HT was significantly decreased,[25] suggesting that there are spare receptors for 5-HT, but not for NA in the immature dog cerebral artery *(see above)*. In systemic vessels, most studies report no age-related change in the contractile potency of 5-HT.[23,27]

Angiotensin

There are several reports of an age-related decline in the renin-angiotensin-aldosterone system in terms of renin and aldosterone levels.[29]

Prostaglandins

In the rat basilar artery, there was a significant reduction in the maximum contractile response to $PGF_{2\alpha}$ with age, despite no change in the responses to KCl, but no change in potency.[21] In rat cerebral arterioles, the contraction to thromboxane A_2 was unchanged by aging.[30]

Vasodilators

CO₂ and Acidity

An increased CO_2 concentration in cerebral arteries causes an increased cerebral blood flow, and the vasodilator response is thought to be the result of the increased brain acidity, so that metabolic acids, such as lactic acid, also increase cerebral blood flow. Cerebral arteries are much less responsive to changes in systemic pH, since the blood–brain barrier hinders the passage of H^+. In one study, age-related differences in cerebral blood flow at rest (decreased blood flow with age) were not maintained under hyperventilation, suggesting that there is an age-related decrease in the response to changes in pCO_2, at least in terms of the decrease in blood flow to a fall in pCO_2.[7] However, Takeda et al.[6] and Ackerstaff et al.[3] found that the decreased cerebral blood flow in the elderly could not be explained by a decreased end-tidal pCO_2. Elderly smokers showed significantly lower regional cerebral blood flow than elderly nonsmokers, and this may be the result of either cerebral arteriosclerosis[31] or to hypocapnia owing to compensatory hyperventilation.[1]

Potassium

Increased K^+ owing to hypoxia or seizures can increase cerebral blood flow, and this effect can be demonstrated on isolated cerebral blood vessels where low pharmacological doses of KCl, which represent physiological hyperkalemia, cause vascular relaxation. In maturation of dog cerebral arteries, there was no change in the relaxation produced by low pharmacological doses of KCl.[25]

β-Adrenoceptors

The vasodilation to isoprenaline decreases during maturation in monkey cerebral[22] and rabbit basilar arteries,[32] but increases during maturation in the dog basilar artery.[25] There are many reports of reduced vasodilator responses to β-adrenoceptor agonists in isolated tissues, particularly arteries, during maturation and aging.[23] The relaxation to isoprenaline also decreases during maturation in the rat aorta.[33]

Atrial Natriuretic Peptide

In rat carotid artery, the maximum relaxation to ANP decreases with no change in potency during maturation,[28] but there is no further decline in aging.[26,28] In humans, the higher plasma levels of atriopeptin found in the elderly may be caused by a decreased clearance, a decreased renal responsiveness to atriopeptin, or increased atrial pressure.

Other Agents

The relaxation to PGI_2 is decreased in maturation in the rat carotid artery,[25] and the relaxation to somatostatin is unchanged by aging in the rat basilar artery.[21]

Calcium Channel Blockers

Calcium channel blockers like nimodipine can retard the decline of motor and cognitive function in aged rats, at least partly by altering microvascular structure,[34] so that this decline may be the result of an imbalance between vasoconstrictor and vasodilator influences in which vasoconstrictor influences dominate.

Endothelium-Dependent Relaxations

The endothelium is the main barrier to the passage of substances from the blood to the tissues, but also functions as an endocrine gland to modulate vascular resistance. Whereas some vasodilators, such as adrenaline and ANP, produce vasodilation by action at receptors on vascular smooth muscle, various physiological (including stretch) and pharmacological stimuli cause release of a substance from the endothelium, endothelium-dependent relaxant factor (EDRF), thought to be nitric oxide (NO),[35] which acts on vascular smooth muscle to activate the enzyme guanylate cyclase and so cause vascular relaxation.

Endothelium-dependent relaxations (EDR) to histamine and acetylcholine (ACh) are reported to be unchanged by aging in the rat basilar artery,[21] whereas EDR to ACh or bradykinin are significantly reduced by aging in rat cerebral arteries, without change in the relaxation to nitroglycerine.[30] During maturation, the relaxation to ACh was unchanged in the dog basilar artery.[25] In systemic arteries, relaxations to ACh are generally reported to be unchanged or decreased in maturation and aging.[23]

In rat cerebral arterioles, the relaxation to ADP was decreased in aging, and the response to 5-HT was changed from a small relaxation to a small contraction.[30] Levels of adenosine are increased in ischemia, but relaxation to adenosine is unchanged by maturation in the dog cerebral artery[25] and by aging in the rat basilar artery.[21]

Since these studies have looked at the effects of aging on vascular relaxations mediated by EDRF in terms of the ability of a substance like histamine to cause vascular relaxation, age-related changes may occur not only in the effects of EDRF, but also in the ability of the substance to release EDRF or in the tissue response to activation of guanylate cyclase. Since EDRF and nitrovasodilators are thought to act through the same mechanism, i.e., activation of guanylate cyclase, the use of nitrovasodilators would help to answer this question, though few studies of cerebral blood vessels have done so. Atherosclerosis and structural changes in the vascular wall may diminish the importance of the endothelium in maintaining regional cerebral blood flow.

Platelet Function

The aggregatory response of platelets to a variety of stimuli, such as adrenaline, NA, ADP, collagen, and arachidonic acid, is reported to be increased or unchanged by aging,[36-39] with no change in the number of α_2-adrenoceptor ligand binding sites with age.[23] 5-HT content of platelets is reported to be decreased in aged male (but not female) rats[40] and in humans,[41] but this decreased content is not the result of diminished uptake, since uptake of 5-HT into platelets is reported to increase with age in humans.[42] Hence, this decreased 5-HT content could be the result of enhanced release, since it has been shown that the release of 5-HT to collagen is increased in platelets from aged rats.[40]

Summary

The age-related decline in cerebral blood flow is linked to a decline in brain mass, but may be influenced by changes in microvascular structure and by atherosclerosis. Alterations in neural, hormonal, and particularly endothelial control may affect regional cerebral blood flow, and the effectiveness of calcium channel blockers in animal models of age-related cognitive deficit may suggest that the balance of control shifts toward vasoconstriction in aging.

Acknowledgments

Work carried out in the author's laboratory was supported by the Royal College of Surgeons in Ireland, the Health Research Board (Ireland), and by the Irish Heart Foundation.

References

1. Yamashita, K., Kobayashi, S., Yamaguchi, S., and Kitani, M. (1988) *Gerontology* **34,** 199–204.
2. Robertson, W. M., Welch, K. M., Levine, S. R., and Schultz, L. R. (1989) *Neurology* **39,** 947–951.
3. Ackerstaff, R. G., Keunen, R. W., van Pelt, W., Montauban van Swijndregt, A. D., and Stijnen, T. (1991) *Neurol. Res.* **12,** 187–191.
4. Kuhl, D. E., Metter, E. J., Riege, W. H., and Phelps, M. E. (1983) *J. Cereb. Blood Flow Metab.* **2,** 163–171.
5. Barron, S. A., Jacobs, L., and Kinkel, W. R. (1976) *Neurology* **26,** 1011–1113.
6. Takeda, S., Matsuzawa, T., and Matsui, H. (1988) *J. Am. Geriatr. Soc.* **36,** 293–297.
7. Vriens, E. M., Kraaier, V., Musbach, M., Wieneke, G. H., and van Huffelen, A. C. (1989) *Ultrasound Med. Biol.* **15,** 1–8.
8. Shaw, T. G., Mortel, K. F., Meyer, J. S., Rogers, R. L., Hardenberg, J., and Cutaia, M. M. (1984) *Neurology* **34,** 855–862.
9. Muller, H. R., Brunholzl, C., Radu, E. W., and Buser, M. (1991) *Neuroradiology* **33,** 212–216.
10. Goldman, H., Berman, R. F., Gershon, S., Murphy, S. L., and Altman, H. J. (1987) *Neurobiol. Aging* **8,** 409–416.
11. Tuma, R. F., Irion, G. L., Vasthare, U. S., and Heinel, L. A. (1985) *Am. J. Physiol.* **249,** H485–H491.
12. Ohata, M., Sundaram, U., Fredericks, W. R., London, E. D., and Rapoport, S. I. (1981) *Brain* **104,** 319–332.
13. Hajdu, M. A., Heistad, D. D., Siems, J. E., and Baumbach, G. L. (1990) *Circ. Res.* **66,** 1747–1754.
14. Goldman, H., Berman, R. F., Gershon, S., Murphy, S. L., Morehead, M., and Altman, H. J. (1991) *Neurobiol. Aging* **13,** 57–62.
15. Reed, D. M., Resch, J. A., Hayashi, T., MacLean, C., and Yano, K. (1988) *Stroke* **19,** 820–825.
16. Kondo, M., Miyazaki, T., Fujiwara, T., Yano, A., and Tabei, R. (1991) *Virchows Arch. B Cell Path.* **61,** 117–122.
17. Yamaguchi, S., Kobayashi, S., Murata, A., Yamashita, K., and Tsunematsu, T. (1988) *Gerontology* **34,** 157–164.
18. Gale, J. D., Alberts, J. C. J., and Cowen, T. A. (1989) *J. Auton. Nerv. Syst.* **28,** 51–60.
19. Mione, M. C., Dhital, K. K., Amenta, F., and Burnstock, G. (1988) *Brain Res.* **460,** 103–113.
20. Dhall, U., Cowen, T., Haven, A. J., and Burnstock, G. (1986) *J. Auton. Nerv. Syst.* **16,** 109–126.
21. Hamel, E., Assumel-Lurden, C., Bouloy, M., and MacKenzie, E. T. (1990) *Neurobiol. Aging* **11,** 631–639.

22 Toda, N. (1991) *Am. J. Physiol.* **260,** H1443–H1448.
23 Docherty, J. R. (1990) *Pharmacol. Rev.* **42,** 103–125.
24 Duckles, S. P. and Bevan, J. A. (1976) *J. Pharmacol. Exp. Ther.* **197,** 371–378.
25 Toda, N., Shimizu, I., Okamura, T., and Miyazaki, M. (1986) *J. Cardiovasc. Pharmacol.* **8,** 681–688.
26 Duckles, S. P. (1987) *J. Pharmacol. Exp. Ther.* **200,** 697–700.
27 Docherty, J. R. (1992) *Br. J. Pharmacol.* **105,** 305P.
28 Emmick, J. T. and Cohen, M. L. (1986) *Clin. Exper. Hypertens.* **A8,** 75–90.
29 James, G., Sealey, J., Mueller, B., Alderman, M., Madhavan, S., and Laragh, J. (1986) *J. Hypertens.* 4 **(Suppl. 5),** S387–S389.
30 Mayhan, W. G., Faraci, F. M., Baumbach, G. L., and Heistad, D. D. (1990) *Am. J. Physiol.* **258,** H1138–H1143.
31 Rogers, R. L., Meyer, J. S., Shaw, T. G., Mortel, K. F., and Thornby, J. (1984) *J. Am. Geriat. Soc.* **32,** 415–420.
32 Toda, N. and Hayashi, S. (1979) *J. Pharmacol. Exp. Ther.* **211,** 716–721.
33 Hyland, L., Warnock, P., and Docherty, J. R. (1987) *Naunyn-Schmiedeberg's Arch. Pharmacol.* **335,** 50–53.
34 de Jonge, G. I., Jansen, A. S. P., Horvath, E., Gispen, W. H., and Luiten, P. G. M. (1991) *Neurobiol. Aging* **13,** 73–81.
35 Furchgott, R. F. (1990) *Acta Physiol. Scand.* **139,** 257–270.
36 Kamal, L. A., Cloix, J. F., Deuynck, M. A., and Meyer, P. (1983) *Eur. J. Pharmacol.* **92,** 167–168.
37 Yokoyama, M., Kusui, A., Sakamoto, S., and Fukazaki, H. (1984) *Thromb. Res.* **34,** 287–295.
38 Davis, P. B. and Silski, C. (1987) *Clin. Sci.* **73,** 507–513.
39 Johnson, M., Ramey, E., and Ramwell, P. W. (1975) *Nature* **253,** 355–357.
40 Yonezawa, Y., Kondo, H., and Nomaguchi, T. A. (1989) *Mech. Aging Dev.* **47,** 65–75.
41 Shuttleworth, R. D. and O'Brien, J. R. (1981) *Blood* **57,** 505–509.
42 Marazziti, D., Falcone, M. F., Rotondo, A., and Castrogiovanni, P. (1989) *Naunyn-Schmiedeberg's Arch. Pharmacol.* **340,** 593–594.

Chapter 22

Species Differences in Pial Functional Characteristics

Noboru Toda

Endogenous vasoactive mediators and autonomic efferent nerves regulate vascular resistance and blood flow in the brain as a whole or in various regions, and participate in the pathogenesis of cerebral circulatory disturbances. There are variations in the response of cerebral arteries from primate and subprimate mammals, and the data obtained from subprimate arteries cannot always be applied to humans. Therefore, information as to similarities and differences in their response is quite important in evaluating the physiological role and involvement in the pathogenesis of the mediators and nerves in healthy individuals and patients. From the experimental data obtained to date, vasoactive mediators can be classified into three groups:

1. Mediators that produce opposite responses in primate and subprimate cerebral arteries, such as dopamine and histamine.
2. Those that produce quantitatively different magnitudes of response, such as norepinephrine, angiotensin II, and prostaglandin (PG) $F_{2\alpha}$.
3. Those that produce similar responses, including serotonin, isoproterenol, and nicotine.

The present chapter will describe responsiveness to norepinephrine, dopamine, histamine, and vasodilator nerve stimulation of isolated cerebral arteries from humans and Japanese monkeys, compared with that of arteries from dogs and cows.

From *The Human Brain Circulation*, R. D. Bevan and J. A. Bevan, eds.
©1994 Humana Press

Norepinephrine

Human, Japanese monkey, and dog cerebral arteries respond to norepinephrine with a concentration-dependent contraction.[1] The magnitude of contraction is markedly greater in the primate arteries than in dog arteries (maximal contraction: 70 and 68% vs 18% relative to contraction caused by 30 mM K^+). The values in baboon cerebral[2] and bovine middle cerebral arteries[3] are 118 and 11%, respectively. Mean EC_{50} values in these arteries are 2.1, 2.7, 4.1, 3.2, and 9.2 × $10^{-7}M$, respectively. The EC_{50} tends to be related inversely to the magnitude of response.

In human, monkey, and bovine arteries, the amine-induced contraction is attenuated by low concentrations (3 × 10^{-10}–$10^{-9}M$) of prazosin, an α_1-adrenoceptor blocker, but not influenced by yohimbine (10^{-8}–$10^{-7}M$), an α_2 blocker.[1,3] Phenylephrine contracts the arteries, whereas clonidine is ineffective. The opposite is true in the case of dog and cat cerebral arteries.[1,4] It appears that the α_1-receptor subtype is involved in the human, monkey, and bovine artery contraction, and the α_2-subtype mediates the contraction of dog and cat arteries.

Dopamine

Dopamine in low concentrations (5 × 10^{-8}–5 × $10^{-6}M$) produces a relaxation in human and monkey cerebral artery strips contracted with $PGF_{2\alpha}$ but contracts the arteries in response to the higher concentrations.[5,6] In the same preparations, norepinephrine elicits only a contraction (Fig. 1). The relaxation caused by dopamine is potentiated, and the contraction is attenuated by treatment with phentolamine or prazosin. The relaxant response is not influenced by endothelium denudation. The relaxation is inhibited by droperidrol, a nonselective dopaminergic receptor antagonist,[7] and SCH23390, a selective DA_1 antagonist,[8] but not by β-adrenoceptor blockers and domperidone, a DA_2 antagonist. The primate cerebral arteries vasodilate in response to dopamine without α-receptor blockade. Intravenous infusion of low doses of dopamine is expected to dilate pial arteries, as do renal and mesenteric vasculatures in patients under treatment with dopamine.

DOG BASILAR ARTERY

HUMAN MIDDLE CEREBRAL ARTERY

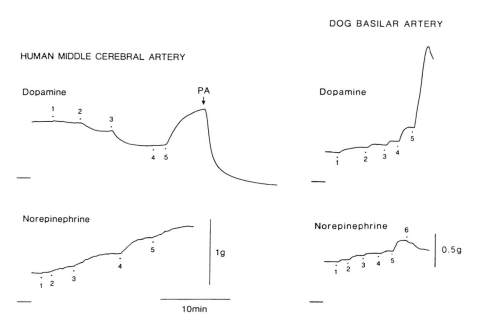

Fig. 1. Responses to dopamine and norepinephrine of a human middle cerebral and a dog basilar artery strip partially contracted with $PGF_{2\alpha}$. Responses to dopamine and norepinephrine were obtained from the same strip. Concentrations of dopamine from 1 to 5 = 5×10^{-8}, 2×10^{-7}, 10^{-6}, 5×10^{-6}, and $2 \times 10^{-5}M$, respectively; concentrations of norepinephrine from 1 to 6 = 5×10^{-9}, 2×10^{-8}, 10^{-7}, 5×10^{-7}, 2×10^{-6}, and $10^{-5}M$, respectively. PA = $10^{-4}M$ papaverine to obtain the maximal relaxation.

In contrast, dog cerebral arteries respond to dopamine with a concentration-related contraction, as seen with norepinephrine (Fig. 1). The maximal contraction caused by dopamine is approximately double the contraction induced by norepinephrine, and the EC_{50} of dopamine is about 100 times the value of norepinephrine. The dopamine-induced contraction is reversed to a small relaxation by treatment with high concentrations of α-antagonists.[9] The relaxation is not influenced by propranolol, but is suppressed by droperidol or SCH23390. Dopamine has an ability to vasodilate cerebral arteries via stimulation of DA_1 receptor located in smooth muscle and to vasoconstrict those by a mediation of α-adrenoceptors. In primate arteries, vasodilation predominates over vasoconstriction, whereas vasoconstriction is predominant in dog arteries.

Histamine

Human cerebral artery strips respond to low concentrations of histamine (up to $10^{-7}M$) with a slight, but significant relaxation, but to the higher concentrations with a dose-dependent contraction (Fig. 2).[10] Endothelium denudation depresses the relaxation and potentiates the contraction. The relaxation is attenuated by cimetidine, an H_2 receptor antagonist, and in addition by chlorpheniramine, an H_1 antagonist. The histamine-induced contraction is also suppressed by the H_1 antagonist (Fig. 2). In monkey basilar and middle cerebral arteries contracted with $PGF_{2\alpha}$, histamine produces only a relaxation, which is partially endothelium-dependent.[10] Cimetidine inhibits the relaxation, and additional treatment with chlorpheniramine or methylene blue, an inhibitor of soluble guanylate cyclase, abolishes the response in endothelium-intact strips. In the strips denuded of the endothelium, cimetidine abolishes the relaxation. Indomethacin does not alter the response to histamine, suggesting that PGI_2 is not involved. In endothelium-intact, cimetidine-treated artery strips, N^G-nitro-L-arginine, a nitric oxide (NO) synthase inhibitor,[11] abolishes the relaxation or reverses it to a contraction. The D-enantiomer of the inhibitor is ineffective. The inhibitory effect is completely reversed by L-, but not D-arginine. These findings may indicate that histamine possesses three actions: phasic relaxation mediated by endothelium-derived relaxing factor or NO released by stimulation of H_1 receptors in the endothelium ("2" in Fig. 3), tonic relaxation caused by activation of H_2 receptors in smooth muscle ("3" in Fig. 3), and contraction mediated by smooth muscle H_1 receptors ("1" in Fig. 3). The endothelium-dependent and independent relaxation is evidently greater in monkey cerebral arteries than in human arteries, whereas the contraction is more marked in human arteries.

Dog cerebral artery strips respond to histamine with only a contraction,[12] which is abolished or reversed to a small relaxation by treatment with chlorpheniramine. The contraction is not influ-

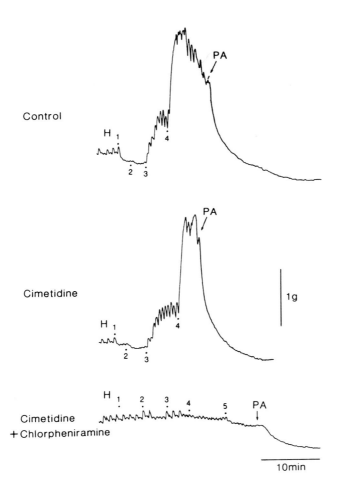

Fig. 2. Modification by cimetidine ($10^{-5}M$) and chlorpheniramine ($10^{-6}M$) of the responses to histamine (H) of a human middle cerebral artery strip partially contracted with $PGF_{2\alpha}$. Concentrations of histamine from 1 to 5 = 2 × 10^{-8}, 10^{-7}, 5 × 10^{-7}, 2 × 10^{-6}, and $10^{-5}M$, respectively. PA = $10^{-4}M$ papaverine to obtain the maximal relaxation. (Reproduced from ref. 10 with permission.)

enced by endothelium denudation or treatment with indomethacin. The relaxation is abolished by cimetidine. Thus, H_1 receptors appear to participate in the contraction, and the H_2 subtype in smooth muscle is involved in the relaxation. As compared with the

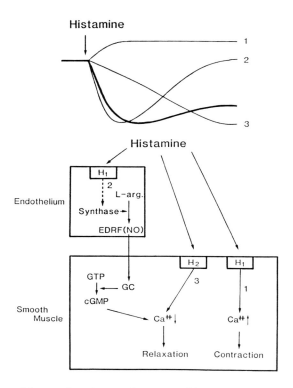

Fig. 3. Possible mechanisms of action of histamine in cerebral arteries from humans, monkeys, and dogs. L-arg. = ʟ-arginine; Synthase = NO synthase; GC = guanylate cyclase. Small squares represent histaminergic H_1 and H_2 receptors. The heavy line in upper tracings denotes the observed response, a sum of the curves 1, 2, and 3.

responses of primate cerebral arteries, those of dog arteries are quite small and inconsistent.

Nonadrenergic, Noncholinergic Nerve Function

Nicotine and transmural electrical stimulation produce a relaxation of a nonadrenergic, noncholinergic nature in dog, cat, rabbit, cow, monkey, and human cerebral arteries.[13–18] The neurally induced relaxation of dog and monkey cerebral arteries is not mediated by substance P, vasoactive intestinal peptide, calcitonin gene related peptide, or atrial natriuretic peptide,[16,19,20] despite the fact that perivascular nerve fibers containing immunoreactivity of a variety of cerebral vasodilator peptides are present.

Treatment with NO synthase inhibitors abolishes the relaxant response to chemical and electrical stimulation of nerves, which is restored by the addition of L-, but not D-arginine (Fig. 4).[21–23] Human cerebral artery strips contracted with $PGF_{2\alpha}$ also respond to the nerve stimulation with relaxations, which are abolished by NO synthase inhibitors, as seen in dog and monkey cerebral arteries. L-arginine antagonizes the inhibitory action. Bovine basilar arteries relax in response to transmural electrical stimulation, but not to nicotine. In the experiments on dog cerebral arteries without the endothelium, we determined the increased release of NO_x during chemical or electrical stimulation and the increased content of cyclic GMP in the stimulated tissue.[21,23] Histochemical study and the study by Bredt et al.[24] have demonstrated the presence of perivascular nerve fibers containing NADPH diaphorase or NO synthase immunoreactivity in cerebral arteries. Therefore, neurally induced relaxations in cerebral arteries from humans, monkeys, dogs, and cows are mediated by NO possibly released from vasodilator nerves (thus, called "nitroxidergic"[25]), which activates soluble guanylate cyclase and increases the production of cyclic GMP in smooth muscle. There is no distinct variation in the arterial response of mammals so far tested, except for the fact that bovine basilar arteries are insensitive to nicotine.

Conclusion

Mechanical responses to dopamine and histamine are quite different in human and Japanese monkey vs dog cerebral arteries. The difference is associated with the differences in the balance of vasoconstrictor and vasodilator responses mediated by α and DA_1 receptors, respectively, for dopamine and the H_1 subtype (smooth muscle), and H_1 (endothelium) and H_2 subtypes, respectively, for histamine. Norepinephrine-induced contractions are mediated by α_1-adrenoceptors in the human, monkey, and cow, and by α_2 subtypes in the dog arteries. Cerebral vasodilation mediated by

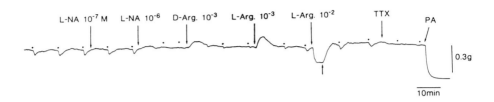

MONKEY MIDDLE CEREBRAL ARTERY — Transmural stimulation, 5Hz
L-nitro-arginine (L-NA)

Fig. 4. Relaxant responses to 5 Hz transmural electrical stimulation of a monkey middle cerebral artery strip before and after treatment with N^G-nitro-L-arginine (L-NA), D-arginine (D-Arg.), L-arginine (L-Arg.), and tetrodotoxin (TTX, $3 \times 10^{-7}M$). The strip was partially contracted with $PGF_{2\alpha}$. Dots above the tracing represent the application of electrical stimulation. The upward arrow means a supplemental dose of $PGF_{2\alpha}$ to raise the tone. PA = $10^{-4}M$ papaverine.

NO in these mammals in response to nerve stimulation is quite similar, suggesting that the vasodilator nerves play an important role in the regulation of cerebral vascular resistance and blood flow in a variety of mammals, including humans. Recent in vivo study supports this hypothesis.

References

1 Toda, N. (1983) *J. Pharmacol. Exp. Ther.* **226**, 861–868.
2 Hayashi, S., Park, M. K., and Kuehl, T. J. (1985) *J. Pharmacol. Exp. Ther.* **235**, 113–121.
3 Ayajiki, K. and Toda, N. (1990) *Eur. J. Pharmacol.* **191**, 417–425.
4 Medgett, I. C. and Langer, S. Z. (1983) *Naunyn-Schmiedeberg's Arch. Pharmacol.* **323**, 24–32.
5 Toda, N. (1983) *Am. J. Physiol.* **245**, H930–H936.
6 Toda, N. (1983) *Experientia* **39**, 1131–1132.
7 Toda, N. and Hatano, Y. (1979) *Eur. J. Pharmacol.* **57**, 231–238.
8 Iorio, L. C., Barnett, A., Leitz, F. H., Houser, V. P., and Korduba, C. A. (1983) *J. Pharmacol. Exp. Ther.* **226**, 462–468.
9 Toda, N. (1976) *Br. J. Pharmacol.* **58**, 121–126.
10 Toda, N. (1990) *Am. J. Physiol.* **258**, H311–H317.

[11] Moore, P. K., al-Swayeh, O. A., Chong, N. W. S., Evans, R. A., and Gibson, A. (1990) *Br. J. Pharmacol.* **99,** 408–412.

[12] Toda, N., Okamura, T., and Miyazaki, M. (1984) *Eur. J. Pharmacol.* **106,** 291–299.

[13] Toda, N. (1975) *J. Pharmacol. Exp. Ther.* **193,** 376–384.

[14] Lee, T. J. F., Su, C., and Bevan, J. A. (1975) *Experientia* **31,** 1424–1426.

[15] Duckles, S. P., Lee, T. J. F., and Bevan, J. A. (1977) *Neurogenic Control of Brain Circulation* (Owman, C. and Edvinsson, L., eds.), Pergamon, New York, pp. 133–141.

[16] Toda, N. (1982) *Am. J. Physiol.* **243,** H145–H153.

[17] Toda, N. and Ayajiki, K. (1990) *Am. J. Physiol.* **258,** H983–H986.

[18] Toda, N. (1981) *Br. J. Pharmacol.* **72,** 281–283.

[19] Toda, N. and Okamura, T. (1991) *J. Cardiovasc. Pharmacol.* **17(Suppl. 3),** S234–S237.

[20] Okamura, T., Inoue, S., and Toda, N. (1989) *Br. J. Pharmacol.* **97,** 1258–1264.

[21] Toda, N. and Okamura, T. (1990) *Biochem. Biophys. Res. Commun.* **170,** 308–313.

[22] Toda, N. and Okamura, T. (1990) *Am. J. Physiol.* **259,** H1511–H1517.

[23] Toda, N. and Okamura, T. (1991) *J. Pharmacol. Exp. Ther.* **258,** 1027–1032.

[24] Bredt, D., Hwang, P. M., and Snyder, S. H. (1990) *Nature (Lond.)* **347,** 768–770.

[25] Toda, N. and Okamura, T. (1992) *News Physiol. Sci.* **7,** 148–152.

Chapter 23

Regulation of the Circulation of the Brain

A Systemic Approach

Mauro Ursino

Introduction

The term cerebrovascular regulation is only apparently simple to define. It is employed in physiological literature to denote the strong capacity of the cerebrovascular bed to adequately adjust cerebral blood flow (CBF) to the most various and rapidly changing external perturbations. Among the physiological or pathological disturbances that the cerebrovascular bed must be able to face during human or animal life, mention can be made of alterations in arterial or intracranial pressure (ICP), body postural changes, variations in brain metabolism, and changes in blood gas content.

The problem of how the cerebrovascular bed can cope with all these perturbations is still far from being completely understood despite the great amount of experimental results that have been gathered in recent years. However, a major conclusion seems to emerge from the critical examination of recent physiological literature: A unique or predominant mechanism able to explain the greater part of cerebral autoregulation does not currently exist. There is no doubt that CBF and its regulation are the result of the equilibrium between many concomitant factors that affect cerebral hemodynamics simultaneously and superimpose themselves in

From *The Human Brain Circulation*, R. D. Bevan and J. A. Bevan, eds.
©1994 Humana Press

very complex ways. In recent studies,[1-5] the author proposed the concept that a systemic approach should be used by physiologists in analyzing the overall system that regulates brain hemodynamics. According to this point of view, we can follow three main steps to achieve a general model of intracranial hemodynamics:

1. Determination of the elementary subsystems involved in cerebrovascular control and their mutual interactions.
2. Mathematical description of each subsystem on the basis of anatomical, physical–chemical, and physiological considerations.
3. Analysis of the overall system's behavior in a closed-loop condition, i.e., in a condition in which all subsystems simultaneously interact and superimpose their respective influences.

In the following, in order to reach a systemic analysis of cerebrovascular hemodynamics, we shall start by examining the behavior of the controlled system, i.e., the cerebrovascular bed. Then, we shall describe the main feedback regulatory mechanisms that are believed to work on it to maintain adequate blood flow delivery to brain tissue and examine their reciprocal interactions. Finally, we shall move to a wider point of view, including also the relationships between intracranial pressure and cerebrovascular control mechanisms, and their clinical implications in pathological subjects.

The Cerebrovascular Bed

In applications of the automatic control theory, one usually starts the analysis by examining the properties of the controlled system, that is, the system in the absence of any feedback regulatory action. In brain hemodynamics, the controlled system is composed of the cerebrovascular bed extending from the intracranial arteries down to the dural sinuses. A detailed study of its properties is of crucial importance since, as we shall see later, the action of cerebrovascular feedback mechanisms cannot be properly understood without considering the main biophysical laws that govern the equilibrium of brain vessels.

A fundamental characteristic of the cerebrovascular bed consists of its segmental heterogeneity. This means that the behavior and the functional role of cerebral vessels significantly change in moving downstream along the cerebrovascular pathway. Let us focus attention on the very simplified electric analog of Fig. 1, composed of the series arrangement of six distinct segments. The hemodynamics of each segment is roughly schematized using the parameter hydraulic resistance, which represents pressure drop (hence energy dissipation) per unit of blood flow. Generally, an approximate expression for vascular resistance is computed using the Hagen-Poiseuille equation:

$$R = 8 \mu l / (\pi r^4) \tag{1}$$

where μ, r, and l are blood viscosity, inner vessel radius, and vessel length, respectively.

According to Eq. (1), resistance can be lowered either by decreasing blood viscosity or increasing vessel radius. Although the effect of hemodilution and blood hematocrit changes on CBF has been extensively studied in recent reports,[6] the fundamental way in which the cerebrovascular control system operates consists of modifying the inner radius, r, at specific locations along the cerebrovascular pathway.

The first portion of the cerebrovascular bed includes the basal arteries of the Circle of Willis. They have a significant role in redistributing the available blood flow toward ischemic brain areas, whereas their function in the active control of cerebrovascular resistance is still debated. The subsequent four segments describe the pressure drops occurring in large, medium, and small pial arteries, and in intracerebral arterioles, respectively. According to present knowledge, these segments are responsible for CBF control. Moreover, they exhibit significant differences in their active responses to physiological stimuli. In particular, there are two main differences that deserve particular attention: (1) the active response of proximal segments seems to be mainly elicited by pressure changes, whereas distal arterioles appear to be especially affected by local alterations in oxygen delivery to brain tissue; and (2) the maximum vasodilatory capacity is rather modest in large pial arteries (20–30% of the normal caliber), but significantly increases in moving downstream of the cerebrovascular bed (up to about 100% at the arteriole level).

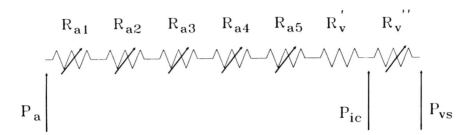

Fig. 1. Electric analog of the cerebrovascular bed used to study segmental heterogeneity in cerebrovascular control. R_{a1}–R_{a5}: resistances per tissue unit weight from basal and large pial arteries to small intracerebral arterioles. $R_v = R_v' + R_v''$: resistance per tissue unit weight of the capillary-venous cerebrovascular bed. R_v': venous resistance upstream of the collapsing section, R_v'': venous resistance of the collapsing lateral lakes and bridge veins. P_a, P_{vs}, and P_{ic}: arterial, venous-sinus, and intracranial pressures, respectively.

The first of these two aspects can be understood only by studying the fundamental nature of feedback mechanisms involved in CBF control. However, the second point can be clarified by simply looking at the mechanical properties of the blood vessel wall.

Vessel biomechanics are generally studied starting from the well-known Laplace law, which establishes the condition for the equilibrium of forces in radial direction. We have:

$$P_i r - P_o(r + h) = T = T_e + T_m \qquad (2)$$

where P_i and P_o are the intravascular and extravascular pressures, respectively, and h is wall thickness.

The left-hand member of Eq. (2) represents the force per unit length acting from inside to outside of the vessel. In steady-state conditions, this must be equilibrated to wall tension, T. The latter is the result of two main contributions: an elastic tension, T_e, which describes the mechanical properties of elastic and collagen fibers as well as of the relaxed smooth muscle, and an active tension, T_m, which represents the force per unit length exerted by smooth muscle active contraction.

Let us now look at what Eq. (2) means from the viewpoint of blood flow regulation. In particular, we want to show how, by modifying active smooth muscle tension, the control mechanisms may succeed in altering inner vessel radius and hence, hydraulic resistance and blood flow.

To this end, two examples of the elastic and active characteristics of brain vessels are shown in Fig. 2, with reference to a large pial artery and a small arteriole. These curves were obtained via mathematical simulation, starting from real experimental data.[7]

A remarkable aspect of vessel biomechanics is that intravascular pressure (hence the left-hand member of Eq.[2]) significantly decreases when moving from large arteries (where it is about 80–85 mmHg) down to arterioles (40–45 mmHg). This means that, as is evident in Fig. 2, proximal arteries in normal conditions are characterized by a working point associated with quite large values of wall strain and quite large stretching of collagen fibers. For this reason, large pial arteries in vivo exhibit only modest vasodilation even in response to complete smooth muscle relaxation. A different situation becomes evident if we move downstream in the cerebrovascular bed (Fig. 2, right panel). Small pial arteries and arterioles, in fact, because of their different normal working point, may exhibit strong vasodilation (more than 100% of their caliber), whereas their constrictory capacity is much more modest. However, it is worth noting that proximal segments contribute to about 30% of the overall cerebrovascular resistance under normal conditions.[8] As a consequence, even the modest vasodilatory capacity that these segments exhibit may be sufficient to account for a significant portion of CBF regulation during mild arterial hypotension.

The situation illustrated in Fig. 2, however, is not fixed, but may significantly vary if the initial working point of the cerebrovascular bed is altered owing to physiological or pathological stimuli. By way of example, Fig. 2 shows the case when, as a consequence of a vasodilatory stimulus (maybe functional hyperemia, hypoxia, or hypercapnia), cerebral vessels dilate when their working point shifts right in the radius-tension characteristic. In such conditions, the occurrence of further vasodilatory stimuli may produce only a lower increase in vessel caliber, i.e., the vascular bed behaves as if it has lost part of its regulatory capacity. As we shall see in a subsequent section, in a similar way, the existence of upper and

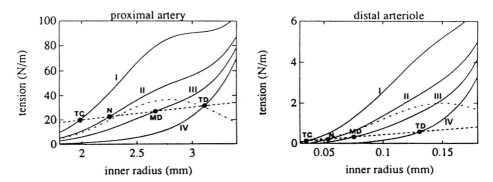

Fig. 2. Patterns of elastic (curve IV) active (-.) and total (curve II) wall tension for a proximal pial artery and a distal arteriole computed in normal conditions using original equations starting from real data (see ref. 7). In the same figure, the value of wall tension computed using Laplace law (Eq. [1]) is also shown (--). The intersection between this curve and total wall tension provides the normal equilibrium point (N). Moreover, in the same figure, the pattern of total wall tension is also presented for the case of moderate smooth muscle relaxation (curve III) and total smooth muscle constriction (curve I). The corresponding equilibrium points shift to MD (moderate dilation) and TC (total constriction), respectively. Finally, TD represents the equilibrium point when the smooth muscle is completely relaxed (total dilation). Note that proximal pial arteries exhibit a modest vasodilatory capacity (<30% of their normal caliber), whereas the maximum dilatatory capacity of small arterioles is as high as 125% of their normal caliber.

lower limits of autoregulation, and the shifting of these limits produced by external stimuli can be understood simply by looking at the tension-radius characteristics of consecutive cerebrovascular segments.

Let us now complete our analysis of the controlled system by examining the behavior of the last segment of Fig. 1, i.e., the venular-venous portion. According to recent results,[9] the active response of cerebral venules appears to be rather modest compared with that of the arterial and arteriolar segments. Hence, venous segments seem to be only minimally involved in CBF control. However, the role of the venous cerebrovascular bed changes as ICP rises, since, in this case, a portion of the cerebral veins tends to collapse with a

behavior similar to that of a Starling resistor. This may be characterized through the following main properties:

1. When intracranial pressure rises, the terminal portion of the venous
   cerebrovascular bed (bridge veins and lateral lakes) collapses or nar-
   rows at its entrance into the dural sinuses. Hence, venous resistance
   increases at its distal end.
2. As a consequence of the venous resistance increase, pressure in the
   large cerebral veins rises to a value a few mmHg higher than that of
   intracranial pressure. Hence, large veins remain open despite intracranial hypertension.
3. In the above conditions, CBF does not depend on the difference between
   systemic arterial pressure (SAP) and dural sinus pressure, but on the
   difference between SAP and ICP.

Looking at Fig. 1, we can subdivide cerebral venous resistance
into the series arrangement of two segments. The first, whose intravascular pressure is always higher than ICP, represents the open
cerebral veins. Its resistance is approximately constant over a broad
range of ICP values. The second represents the collapsing lateral
lakes and bridge veins, and its resistance progressively increases
with increasing ICP (*see* Ursino[10] for a more detailed mathematical
description).

Finally, from the electric analog of Fig. 1, we can write:

$$CBF = (SAP - ICP)/(R_{a1} + R_{a2} + R_{a3} + R_{a4} + R_{a5} + R_v') \tag{3}$$

where R_v' represents the hydraulic resistance of open veins
upstream of the collapsed section. CBF regulation mainly occurs
by modifying the arterial-arteriolar resistances $R_{a1} - R_{a5}$, in accordance with Eqs. (1) and (2).

The previous biophysical analysis synthetizes the main aspects
of cerebral circulation in a very simplified way that, however, is
sufficiently accurate for most physiological and clinical applications. The main limitation of this analysis is the assumption that, at
each level of intracranial pressure, the cerebrovascular bed reaches
a unique, stable, equilibrium condition, associated with a well-
defined degree of terminal venous collapse and a well-defined
degree of arterial-arteriolar dilation. The possible occurrence of
unstable phenomena, characterized by periodic vessel occlusions

and reopenings and by blood volume fluctuations, is also of importance, but its analysis requires the use of more complex mathematical approaches. At present, we are not aware of any detailed biophysical analysis of cerebral venous stability, whereas stability of the arterial-arteriolar vascular bed will be briefly studied in the last section of this chapter, in connection with the problem of ICP influences on regulatory mechanisms.

The Physiological Nature of Feedback Regulatory Mechanisms

As discussed above, the fundamental control of cerebral hemodynamics in response to external stimuli consists of modulating the degree of smooth muscle tension, especially at the arterial-arteriolar level. The present section will examine the possible physiological nature of the feedback mechanisms involved in this regulation and give the main elements necessary for their mathematical description. Finally, it will show how mechanisms can interact in complex ways in vivo, and what functional role each of them may play in the various manifestations of cerebrovascular control.

As a general rule, in order to reproduce the action of a feedback regulatory mechanism, one needs to collect several different pieces of information. These can be described as follows:

1. Knowledge of the stimulus able to trigger the mechanism action.
2. Knowledge of the effectors of the regulation, that is, those portions of the controlled system on which the mechanism exerts its influence.
3. The mechanism gain, i.e., the strength of its action.
4. The mechanism dynamics, which describe the time pattern of the regulatory response following a given perturbation. The simplest way to describe dynamics is by assigning the time constant. Recall that after a time-constant period, the mechanism has exerted about two-thirds of its complete action.

Traditionally, three main types of feedback regulatory mechanisms are considered in the physiological literature, i.e., the myogenic, the chemical-metabolic, and the neurogenic.

The Myogenic Mechanism

According to the myogenic hypothesis,[11] vascular smooth muscle would possess the intrinsic capacity to constrict in response to an increase in wall tension (i.e., in vivo, in response to a transmural pressure increase) and to relax in response to wall tension decrease. This mechanism might be involved in CBF control during arterial pressure and ICP changes.

In the past, the idea that the myogenic mechanism was the main one responsible for cerebral autoregulation was rather common among physiologists. Several recent studies, however, have cast serious doubts on this assumption:

1. Experiments performed by increasing venous pressure, at the same time maintaining ICP constant, show that CBF is well regulated despite the transmural pressure increase.[12] Only when metabolic influences are eliminated via oxygen superinfusion does arteriolar vasoconstriction become evident and CBF starts to decrease during venous hypertension.[13] These experiments indicate that the myogenic mechanism plays a secondary role in the control of cerebral hemodynamics with respect to other flow-dependent mechanisms, probably chemical–metabolic in nature.

2. In vitro experiments performed on cerebral arteries[14] and arterioles[15] subjected to transmural pressure alterations indicate that the strength of the myogenic reaction, at least in brain vessels, is rather modest. An example of myogenic response, measured by Osol and Halpern in a rat cerebral artery is shown in Fig. 3 together with the corresponding mathematical simulation. Note that the percentage decrease in vessel caliber per mmHg of transmural pressure increase observed in these experiments (–0.06%) can explain just a few percent of the overall CBF control during arterial pressure variations.

Probably, the main function of the myogenic mechanism is that of preventing large transmural pressure changes from causing excessive passive variations in vessel caliber, thus equalizing brain vessels to almost rigid tubes. The time pattern of this mechanism can be well reproduced using a time constant of 1–2 min (*see* Fig. 3). The possible involvement of a rate-dependent component of the myogenic response in brain vessels, similar to that observed in other vascular beds,[16] does not find, at present, any relevant experimental confirmation.

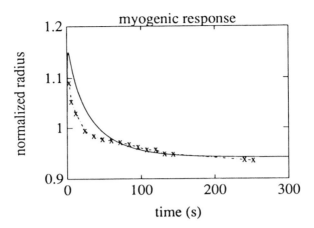

Fig. 3. Myogenic response of a basal cerebral artery measured in vitro by Osol and Halpern[14] in response to a 50-mmHg increase in transmural pressure (crosses). The continuous line represents the same response obtained via mathematical simulation.[3]

The Chemical Mechanism

In the chemical feedback mechanism, smooth muscle tension and, hence, vessel caliber and vascular resistance are affected by the concentration of vasoactive substances in the perivascular space. Many vasodilatory chemical agents involved in tissue metabolism might contribute to matching blood flow to the local tissue metabolic demand: among the others O_2, CO_2, H^+, adenosine, K^+, Ca^{2+} and osmolarity.

A few recent experimental results indicate that the main stimulus able to elicit chemical mechanism action is oxygen demand by brain tissue.[17] However, oxygen would not act on smooth muscle tension directly; rather, its action would be mediated by secondary metabolites produced in brain tissue during hypoxia.

A worthwhile characteristic of the chemical regulatory mechanism is its significant time heterogeneity. Several substances, in fact (mainly potassium[18] and adenosine[19]), are known to accumulate in brain tissue within a few seconds from the onset of ischemia, and so may participate in the very first temporal phase of CBF regulation. Other substances, however (mainly acidosis[18]), are characterized by much slower time dynamics (time constant no lower than 5–10 min). Their role in cerebrovascular regulation is probably that of constituting an extreme defense during prolonged tissue hypoxia, when the action of other more rapid mechanisms is exhausted or has revealed itself inadequate to maintain sufficient tissue perfusion. However, H^+ is believed to play a major role in brain vessel response to hypercapnia.[20] In this case, in fact, acidosis can very rapidly be produced in the tissue owing to the CO_2 hydration reaction.

The main effectors of chemical regulation are supposed to be small pial arteries and arterioles. In fact, these vessels directly face brain tissue, and so can be reached by vasoactive metabolites through diffusion processes.

There is wide agreement that the chemical mechanism may play a pivotal role in CBF control during functional hyperemia and changes in blood gas content. By contrast, its role during brain autoregulation to perfusion pressure changes is still questioned.

In the author's opinion, the chemical flow-dependent mechanism does not play a relevant role in the central autoregulation range (i.e., when SAP lies in the range 70–130 mmHg) provided alternative pressure-dependent mechanisms are active and maintain CBF constant despite the perfusion pressure variations. By contrast, if these mechanisms are weakened or impaired, or if the limits of autoregulation are approached, CBF starts to vary, and so, chemical feedback mechanisms are put into action. This problem will be examined in greater detail below, when the interaction among different feedback mechanisms will be simulated.

The Neurogenic Mechanism

Until a few years ago, most physiologists thought that neural fibers had a minimal role in the control of cerebral hemodynamics. This point of view, however, has been changing in recent years, thanks to two main new findings:

1. As demonstrated by Baumbach and Heistad,[21] the lack of evident steady-state CBF alterations following sympathetic stimulation is not a consequence of the minimal influence of neural fibers on brain vessels, but is rather imputable to the existence of antagonistic mecha-

nisms (probably chemical in nature), which mask the constrictory effect of sympathetic nerves through prompt dilation of distal arterioles. Accordingly, authors who measured CBF with dynamic means[22,23] observed that sympathetic (or parasympathetic) stimulation causes an initial 20–30% CBF decrease (or an initial CBF increase, respectively). However, within 1 min, an escape of blood flow from stimulation becomes evident, able to restore a fairly normal CBF level despite protracted stimulation.

2. In the past decade, vasodilatory parasympathetic fibers were shown to reach cerebral arteries especially through the VII cranial nerve and the greater superior petrosal nerve. Stimulation of these nerves was known to produce just modest CBF increments.[23] However, more recent results have shown that cholinergic fibers reach brain vessels also from the sphenopalatine ganglion and the otic and carotid ganglia.[24,25] Moreover, stimulation of the sphenopalatine ganglion was found to elicit a significant increase in cortical blood flow.[26]

The most rigorous way to study the neurogenic mechanism action consists of directly measuring the changes in brain vessel caliber following stimulation of neural fibers. There are, at present, various results showing that sympathetic stimulation causes a modest decrease in vessel caliber (about 10–12%) at the level of proximal cerebrovascular segments (large and medium pial arteries), whereas it has only minimal effects on more distal arterioles.[27,28] Sympathetic vasoconstriction occurs with a time constant of about 20 s (*see* Fig. 4), and is able to produce a 20–25% increase overall cerebrovascular resistance and a comparable decrease in CBF. Hence, maximum activation of sympathetic nerves might explain a significant portion of cerebral autoregulation during moderate arterial hypertension (i.e., when SAP lies in the range 100–130 mmHg).

At present we are not aware of any recent experimental result in which brain vessel dilation is measured after stimulation of vasodilatory fibers. However, the results of some experiments in which dilation of large and medium pial arteries is studied after topical application of acetylcholine or vasoactive intestinal peptide,[29] or during moderate arterial hypotension,[8] make it reasonable to formulate the hypothesis,[3] that vasodilatory fibers affect proximal cerebrovascular segments in a way similar to that of vasoconstrictory sympathetic fibers.

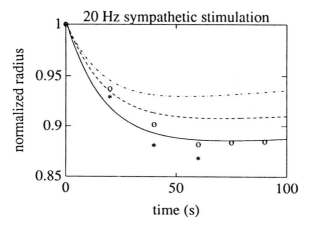

Fig. 4. Effect of 20 Hz sympathetic stimulation on the radius of medium (_.), large (--), and very large (continuous line) pial arteries obtained via mathematical simulation.[3] Open circles and asterisks denote the experimental points obtained by Kuschinsky and Wahl[27] on a large pial artery.

The stimulus able to trigger the action of the neurogenic mechanism is still not perfectly known. It is possible that neural fibers are activated by changes in transmural pressure at the level of the major brain arteries, through afferent information coming from local baroreceptor areas. As will be shown below, introduction of this hypothesis in our mathematical model allows the experimental dilation of proximal vessels, observed in the central autoregulation range, to be well explained *(see below)*.

Finally, the possible influence of additional less-explored neural factors on CBF (such as regulation by intrinsic nerves) will be briefly discussed in a subsequent subsection devoted to a brief review of possible new mechanisms.

The Interaction Among Physiological Mechanisms

The concepts described above lead us to formulate a simplified multifeedback mathematical model of cerebrovascular regulation, aimed at understanding the main interactions among mechanisms involved in CBF control and in assessing their reciprocal role. A block diagram describing the main aspects of this model is shown in Fig. 5.

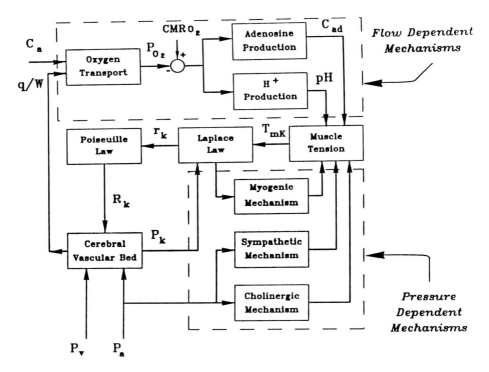

Fig. 5. Block diagram that describes the main relationships among the subsystems involved in cerebrovascular control. C_a: oxygen concentration in arterial blood; pH, C_{ad}: tissue acidosis and tissue adenosine concentration; P_{O2}, $CMRO_2$: oxygen tension in brain tissue and tissue oxygen consumption rate; q/W: cerebral blood flow per tissue unit weight; P_a, P_v: arterial and venous pressures; T_{mk}, r_k, R_k, P_k: smooth muscle tension, inner radius, hydraulic resistance per tissue unit weigth, and transmural pressure at the k-th segment of the arterial-arteriolar cerebrovascular bed.

According to our model, the main features of cerebrovascular regulation can be delineated as follows:

1. Pressure-dependent neural mechanisms affect the proximal segments of the cerebrovascular bed. They are especially influential in the central autoregulation range.
2. Chemical flow-dependent factors affect the distal (arteriolar) segments. They are significantly involved in functional hyperemia and hypoxia. Moreover, they participate in CBF autoregulation, especially in the lower pressure range.

3. The pressure-dependent myogenic mechanism has the main function of counteracting passive changes in vessel caliber. This is of great value in improving the mechanical properties of arterial-arteriolar segments.

The following will examine a few examples of the interaction among feedback regulatory mechanisms in vivo, through the use of computer mathematical simulation.

Normal Autoregulation

As a first example, let us consider the time pattern of inner radii in two different cerebrovascular segments, simulated in the steady-state conditions following different levels of arterial hypotension and hypertension. As is clear from Fig. 6, during moderate arterial pressure changes, the autoregulatory response is dominated by the active adjustments of proximal arterial segments, which are mainly neurogenic in nature. By contrast, during deep hypotension, the chemical flow-dependent dilation of distal arterioles becomes dominant. The simulation results of Fig. 6 are then compared with those obtained by Kontos et al. in the cat.[8] From this comparison, it can be noted that an evident limitation of this model is the insufficient dilation of small arteries and arterioles. At present, in fact, the author is not aware of any physiological mechanism able to explain the large and rapid arteriolar dilation occurring in the brain in vivo.

Finally, in Fig. 7, the pattern of tissue adenosine vs arterial pressure is shown. As is clear from this figure, adenosine content in the brain remains pretty constant until blood pressure is lowered to about 80 mmHg, when it significantly increases. This result is in accordance with experimental findings[30] and demonstrates that metabolic factors are especially involved in the low-pressure range of autoregulation.

Artificial Sympathetic Stimulation

In Fig. 8, the effect of stimulating sympathetic fibers on CBF is shown. An escape of blood flow from stimulation is evident in this figure, caused by the antagonistic effect of vasodilatory chemical factors, which accumulate in the arteriolar perivascular space as a consequence of the initial CBF decrease. However, the escape phenomenon simulated with this model is rather modest

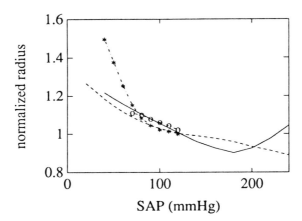

Fig. 6. Pattern of normalized inner radius vs systemic arterial pressure in a large (continuous line) and small (dotted line) pial artery, simulated with the model described in Ursino.[3] In the same figure, the experimental data obtained by Kontos et al.[8] in the cat are also shown (open circles: large pial artery; asterisks: small arteriole).

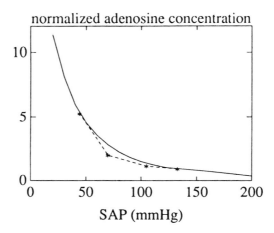

Fig. 7. Pattern of brain adenosine concentration vs systemic arterial pressure simulated via author's mathematical model[3] (continuous line), and experimentally measured by Winn et al.[30] in the rat (asterisks). All values are normalized with respect to the value at 123 mmHg.

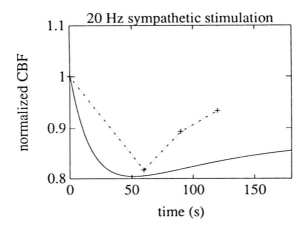

Fig. 8. Time pattern of normalized CBF simulated with the model described in Ursino[3] in response to a protracted 20 Hz stimulation of sympathetic fibers (continuous line). Crosses represent the experimental points obtained by Sercombe et al.[22] in analogous conditions.

compared with the real one. This result, too, indicates that the dilation of distal arterioles predicted by the simulation model is largely insufficient.

Effect of Vasodilatory Stimuli on the Autoregulation Plateau

Finally, Fig. 9 presents the pattern of CBF vs arterial pressure (autoregulation) obtained with the model first by assuming that the cerebrovascular bed is normally reactive, and then by assuming that the cerebrovascular bed is initially dilated owing to the previous application of a vasodilatory stimulus. As is clear from this figure, application of a vasodilatory stimulus on cerebral circulation increases the CBF level, but at the same time, reduces the width of the autoregulation plateau until, because of excessive vasodilation, autoregulation can be completely lost. This is the situation that can be experimentally and clinically encountered during hypoxia, hypercapnia, or after application of some pressure drugs (*see* ref. 31).

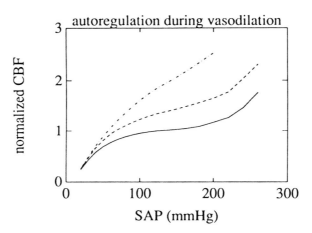

Fig. 9. Pattern of normalized CBF vs systemic arterial pressure (autoregulation) simulated with the model described in Ursino,[3] first assuming normal cerebrovascular reactivity (continuous line) and then assuming that the cerebrovascular bed is initially moderately (- -) or strongly (- .) dilated. Note the progressive disappearance of the autoregulation plateau.

The Need for New Mechanisms: Hypotheses for Future Studies

The results of previous simulation studies demonstrate that, although a unique predominant mechanism does not exist in cerebrovascular control, the interaction among various factors simultaneously operating on cerebral vessels may be able to explain a significant amount of CBF regulation in various physiopathological conditions. However, significant differences do still exist between these predictions and real experimental data. A critical analysis of these differences may help physiologists to understand where new mechanisms can be searched for and what their functional role may be.

The most evident difference between present theoretical knowledge and experimental data concerns the active response of small pial arteries and arterioles (both as to their strength and time constant), although even the response of more proximal cerebrovascular segments is in part underestimated. At present, we can only speculate about possible new mechanisms responsible for these differences:

1. The author included the action of only two vasodilatory factors, adenosine and H^+. It may be possible that some new metabolic factors, still to be discovered, contribute significantly to the strong arteriolar vasodilation experimentally observed in vivo. Otherwise, it can also be supposed that sufficient description of arteriolar vasodilation may be achieved by simply including the action of all vasoactive metabolites presently known (K^+, Ca^{2+}, osmolarity, direct O_2 and CO_2 effect, prostaglandins, and so forth) without supposing the existence of any new hypothetical substance. In the latter case, arteriolar vasodilation would be the result of the interaction among manifold minor factors, all to be considered together.

2. Some authors, in past decades, discussed the idea that the cerebral circulation is regulated by intrinsic nerve fibers, which might sense local alterations and rapidly regulate intraparenchymal vessel tone.[32] Although this is a very promising new concept, which might contribute to the understanding of many still unsolved aspects of cerebrovascular control, the author is not aware, at present, of sufficient experimental data able to support this hypothesis.

3. Blood flow might alter vessel tone and, hence, vascular resistance not only by modifying the concentration of vasodilatory factors in the perivascular space, but also by acting directly on the inner surface of the artery. Recent working hypotheses[33] assume that flow-induced shear stresses act either on the vascular endothelium or directly on smooth muscle cells through a cellular mechanism alternative to the myogenic one.

4. Many recent results demonstrate that the endothelium may contribute to cerebral vascular responses via the release of both relaxing and constrictory factors (*see* ref. 31). By way of example, the vasodilatory response to acetylcholine is known to be mediated by the production of an endothelium-derived relaxing factor. Moreover, recent data document the role of endothelium in mediating the response of cerebral vessels to transmural pressure changes[34] and, maybe, also to changes in blood flow.[35] It is, thus, possible that differences in the regulatory responses of brain vessels, and contradiction among experimental results, may be a consequence of a different status of the endothelium. To the author's knowledge, the endothelium does not contribute to a specific original feedback mechanism, but rather acts as an intermediate transducer able to mediate both pressure and flow autoregulatory responses.

Clinical Implications
of Cerebral Blood Flow Regulation in Humans

Most of the experimental data presented in this work were obtained through animal experimentation, because of evident ethical and practical reasons. Nevertheless, the existence of strong, rapid cerebrovascular regulation is well documented even in human subjects either by means of the noninvasive transcranial Doppler technique[36] or of positron emission tomography. In particular, transcranial Doppler monitoring of blood flow velocity in basal intracranial arteries indicates that, in healthy humans, the autoregulatory response to arterial pressure changes occurs with a time constant of a few seconds,[36] comparable to that observed by Kontos et al. in the cat.[8] It is worth noting that none of the traditional mechanisms examined until now seem able to explain such a rapid vessel response.

Autoregulation is known to be disturbed or impaired in many pathological conditions, such as brain tumor, space-occupying lesions, or head injury.[31] The exact reason for autoregulation loss in these patients is not known yet.

According to the systemic approach used throughout the present work, a loss of CBF regulatory capacity can be imputed either to damage of the controlled system (i.e., cerebral vessels) or of the feedback mechanisms involved in brain hemodynamic control.

The first situation is usually referred to as "vasoparalysis" in clinical literature. As is clear from examination of Fig. 2, vasoparalysis may occur when smooth muscle in arteries and arterioles is completely relaxed, and so cannot further respond to external vasoactive stimuli. Alternatively, damage of the smooth muscle contractile machinery (as occurs after an abrupt intravascular pressure increase) or disturbances in the endothelium may be of major significance in the loss of cerebrovascular response.

Alterations in the normal feedback mechanisms may include tissue acidosis, extracellular potassium increase (both affect the normal functioning of the chemical feedback mechanism and may be indicative of a dysfunction of brain tissue), or alterations in cerebrovascular neural pathways. Basically, if autoregulation is disturbed because of damage in a cerebrovascular segment, we may expect the active response in that segment to be lost whatever the external stimulus applied. By contrast, disturbance in a feedback regulatory mechanism may produce more contradictory results, depending on the role that the mechanism plays in response to the external perturbations. As an example of the latter behavior, we recall that, in some patients who exhibit diffuse loss of autoregulation, the cerebrovascular response to arterial CO_2 changes is still preserved,[37] i.e., autoregulation appears to be more vulnerable than other cerebrovascular controls. An explanation for this finding can be hypothesized by looking at the systemic model of Fig. 5. As discussed earlier, the neurogenic mechanism may be significantly involved in the autoregulation response, at least in the central pressure range, whereas it probably plays a minor role in functional hyperemia and in the response to O_2 and CO_2 arterial tension changes. If, in a patient with cerebral disease, the neural feedback mechanisms are damaged while other mechanisms (such as the chemical ones) are still functioning, we may have a disturbance in autoregulation with other regulatory responses working properly or being only moderately affected.

Another interesting clinical aspect of the cerebrovascular control is that the autoregulation plateau is not constant, but shifts toward higher pressures in hypertensive subjects.[31] Activation of sympathetic nerves is thought to play a major role in the acute phase of this phenomenon.[31] The sympathetic mechanism, in fact, is able to produce an increase in the vascular resistance of proximal cerebrovascular segments,[38] resulting in maintaining a normal CBF level even at higher pressure values. However, as shown in Fig. 10 by means of mathematical simulation, this effect is very modest if it is not accompanied by structural vascular changes, which increase the maximum smooth muscle active tension. These changes might include wall thickening and muscular hypertrophy.

Finally, it was considered of the greatest clinical value to examine the relationship between the action of cerebrovascular control mechanisms and ICP changes, because of the paramount importance that this relationship may have in the treatment of severely ill neurosurgical patients. As is well known, brain circula-

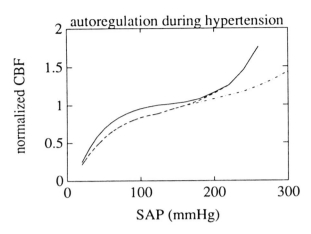

Fig. 10. Pattern of normalized CBF vs systemic arterial pressure (autoregulation) simulated with the model described in Ursino,[3] first assuming normal cerebrovascular reactivity (continuous line), then assuming that proximal segments are initially contracted owing to sympathetic activation (- -), and finally assuming that sympathetic activation occurs in a condition of chronic muscular hypertrophy (- .). The latter phenomenon was simulated by allowing smooth muscle to reach a maximum contractile tension higher than that reported for normal vessels. Note that only in the latter case, a normal CBF level may be warranted even in chronic hypertensive subjects.

tion occurs within a closed space, the overall volume of which must remain constant. This implies that any volume increase occurring within the cranial cavity (either resulting from vasodilation or injection of an external fluid) must be compensated by a decrease in all the remaining volumes. There are two fundamental ways by which the craniospinal system can cope with a volume load: The first, called volume storage, depends on the small elasticity of compressible structures present within the skull and may also reflect possible volume displacements along the spinal axis. According to this mechanism, an additional volume load is immediately stored within the cranio-spinal system via a compression and dislocation of other intracranial structures, and via an ICP increase.

The second mechanism, which can be called volume compensation, is based on the circulation of cerebrospinal fluid (CSF). During intracranial hypertension, the amount of CSF reabsorbed by dural sinuses increases in an effort to restore a more normal ICP level. In healthy humans, with preserved CSF outflow, volume compensation occurs with a time constant of 30 s or 1 min. However, this process may become incredibly slow in pathological conditions, characterized by impaired CSF outflow.

A fundamental point to be recognized is that ICP and the action of cerebrovascular control mechanisms are linked through a positive feedback loop. As discussed above, in fact, perfusion pressure in the brain is equal to the difference SAP-ICP. Moreover, transmural pressure of brain vessels also decreases when increasing the ICP level. As a consequence, all the regulatory feedback mechanisms (either elicited by transmural pressure changes or sensitive to the status of brain perfusion) may start to operate following an ICP rise, causing a significant vasodilation in all arterial-arteriolar segments. Cerebral vasodilation, in turn, occurs within a closed space and so causes a further delayed ICP increase.

In patients having preserved CSF outflow, the existence of a positive feedback loop may have only minor influence, since ICP changes are rapidly buffered by CSF dynamics. Interaction between ICP and cerebrovascular control, however, may have dramatic effects in patients with impaired CSF outflow, especially when the intracranial elasticity and storage capacity are also reduced.[39]

By way of example, let us examine the pattern of ICP measured in two severely head-injured patients (Fig. 11). Both curves describe the response to the so-called bolus injection test, as proposed originally by Marmarou and coworkers.[40] This consists of rapidly injecting a very small amount of fluid into the cranial cavity (up to 2 mL) and measuring the consequent ICP time pattern. The first of the two patients (Fig. 11, left panel) exhibits a monotonic ICP response, i.e., ICP first rises owing to fluid injection and then progressively returns toward baseline thanks to progressive CSF reabsorption. By contrast, the second patient exhibits an anomalous response, characterized by a secondary delayed ICP increase that develops well beyond the end of the injection period. Using an original mathematical model of intracranial dynamics,[39] we succeeded in explaining these contradictory ICP patterns. In particular, the first pattern (Fig. 11, left panel) can be explained assuming

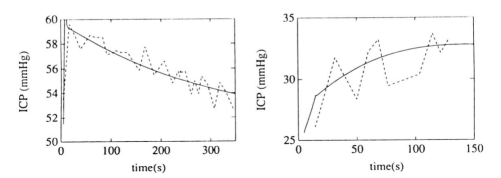

Fig. 11. Time pattern of intracranial pressure in two head-injured patients following the injection of 2 mL of fluid into the ventricular space. Dotted lines represent real clinical results. The continuous lines were obtained by means of computer simulation using the model described in Ursino and Di Giammarco.[39] The first ICP pattern is typical of patients having impaired autoregulation. The second can be imputed to the active blood volume changes induced by the action of CBF control mechanisms in patients with preserved autoregulation.

that, in this class of patients, autoregulation is impaired, so cerebral vessels behave passively during the ICP rise. By contrast, the parodoxical ICP increase evident in the second group of patients (Fig. 11, right panel) can be imputed to the active vasodilation of brain vessels in a condition of functioning autoregulation. This vasodilation is elicited by the intracranial hypertension, and the consequent reduction in both transmural and perfusion pressures. The previous example demonstrates that, by observing the ICP pattern, we can discriminate between head-injured patients who maintain preserved autoregulation and those whose autoregulation is impaired. This classification may be of the greatest value for the choice of the most correct treatment.

Finally, another striking consequence of the positive feedback loop existing between ICP and the action of cerebrovascular control mechanisms is that, in certain pathological conditions, intracranial dynamics may become instable.[39] Instability manifests itself with the development of self-sustained periodic fluctuations in ICP and in the other main cerebral hemodynamic quantities. A simu-

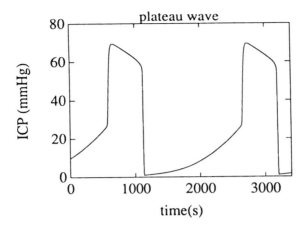

Fig. 12. Spontaneous self-sustained ICP oscillations (plateau waves) obtained with the model described in Ursino and Di Giammarco,[39] with reference to a patient having impaired CSF outflow and reduced craniospinal storage capacity.

lated example of such oscillations, obtained with the model described in Ursino and Di Giammarco,[39] is shown in Fig. 12, with reference to a patient with impaired CSF outflow and reduced intracranial elasticity. Note that the pattern of ICP shown in this figure closely resembles, both in frequency and shape as well as in amplitude, the so-called Lundberg plateau waves, frequently observed in neurosurgical patients in similar pathological conditions.[41] The model imputes these oscillations to active changes in cerebral blood volume, induced by autoregulatory mechanisms, when these changes occur within an intracranial space with reduced compensatory capacity (impaired CSF outflow and low craniospinal elasticity).

Final Remarks

The ambition of the present work was not to describe exactly how the complex system regulating cerebral blood flow actually works in animals or humans or to formulate definitive hypotheses on the role of the various mechanisms involved in this regulation.

The progress in physiological research is so rapid, and so many new data have been recently gathered that present knowledge probably will be outdated in the not too distant future.

The purpose of the systemic approach is another: i.e., to describe the way different factors can interact in vivo to constitute a complex, strongly controlled, multifeedback system. Knowledge of these interactions has a general validity, which goes well beyond the significance of any single particular hypotheses on which the model has been built.

In recent years, an enormous amount of experimental findings, collected on the most various aspects of cerebrovascular control, has remained uncorrelated, and only rare attempts have been performed to insert these data into a more comprehensive vision of overall cerebral hemodynamics. In other words, the enormous amount of analytical investigations is not accompanied, at present, by adequate synthetic studies.

The systemic point of view presented in this work, together with its necessary modeling aspects, offers the main advantage of providing a general framework in which manifold different experimental data can be synthetized and different knowledge unified. It is hoped that this approach may be stimulating to physiologists and clinicians, and contribute to broadening our understanding of the complexity with which overall hemodynamics operate both in physiological and pathological conditions.

Acknowledgment

This work was in part supported by the Italian National Council for Research (CNR).

References

[1] Ursino, M., Di Giammarco, P., and Belardinelli, E. (1989) *IEEE Trans. Biomed. Eng.* **36**, 183–191.

[2] Ursino, M., Di Giammarco, P., and Belardinelli, E. (1989) *IEEE Trans. Biomed. Eng.* **36**, 192–201.

[3] Ursino, M. (1991) *IEEE Trans. Biomed. Eng.* **38**, 795–807.

[4] Ursino, M. (1991) *CRC Crit. Rev. Biomed. Eng.* **18**, 255–288.

[5] Ursino, M. and Belardinelli, E. (1991) *Comments Theor. Biol.* **2**, 211–237.

[6] Hudak, M. L., Jones, M. D., Popel, A. S., Koehler, R. C., Traystman, R. J., and Zeger, S. L. (1989) *Am. J. Physiol.* **257,** H912–H917.

[7] Gore, R.W. and Davis, M. J. (1984) *Ann. Biomed. Eng.* **12,** 511–520.

[8] Kontos, H. A., Wei, E. P., Navari, R. M., Levasseur, J. E., Rosenblum, W. I., and Patterson, J. L. (1978) *Am. J. Physiol.* **234,** H371–H383.

[9] Auer, L. M. and Ishiyama, N. (1986) *Intracranial Pressure VI* (Miller, J. D., Teasdale, G. M., Rowan, J. O., Galbraith, S. L., and Mendelow, A. D., eds.), Springer-Verlag, Berlin, pp. 399–403.

[10] Ursino, M. (1988) *Ann. Biomed. Eng.* **16,** 379–401.

[11] Johnson, P. C. (1980) *Handbook of Physiology. The Cardiovascular System: Vascular Smooth Muscle* (Bohr, D. F., Somlyo, A. P., and Sparks, H. V., eds.), American Physiological Society, Bethesda, MD, pp. 409–442.

[12] Wagner, E. M. and Traystman, R. J. (1985) *Ann. Biomed. Eng.* **13,** 311–320.

[13] Wei, E. P. and Kontos, H. A. (1984) *Circ. Res.* **55,** 249–252.

[14] Osol, G. and Halpern, W. (1985) *Am. J. Physiol.* **249,** H914–H921.

[15] Dacey, R. G. and Duling, B. R. (1982) *Am. J. Physiol.* **243,** H598–H606.

[16] Grande, P. O., Lundvall, J., and Mellander, S. (1977) *Acta Physiol. Scand.* **99,** 432–447.

[17] Kontos, H. A., Wei, E. P., Raper, A. J., Rosenblum, W. I., Novari, R. M., and Patterson, J. L. (1978) *Am. J. Physiol.* **234,** H582–H591.

[18] Heuser, D. (1978) *Cerebral Vascular Smooth Muscle and its Control* (Purves, M. J., ed.), Elsevier, Amsterdam, pp. 339–348.

[19] Winn, H. R., Rubio, R., and Berne, R. M. (1979) *Circ. Res.* **45,** 486–492.

[20] Kontos, H. A., Raper, A. J., and Patterson, J. L. (1977) *Stroke* **8,** 358–360.

[21] Baumbach, G. L. and Heistad, D. D. (1983) *Circ. Res.* **52,** 527–533.

[22] Sercombe, R., Lacombe, P., Aubineau, P., Mamo, H., Pinard, E., Reynier-Rebuffel, A. M., and Seylaz, J. (1979) *Brain Res.* **164,** 81–102.

[23] Pinard, E., Purves, M. J., Seylaz, J., and Vasquez, J. V. (1979) *Pflug. Arch.* **379,** 165–172.

[24] Hara, H., Hamill, G. S., and Jacobowitz, D. M. (1985) *Brain Res. Bull.* **19,** 179–188.

[25] Suzuki, N., Hardebo, J. E., and Owman, C. (1990) *J. Cereb. Blood Flow Metab.* **9,** 204–211.

[26] Seylaz, J., Hara, H., Pinard, E., Mraovitch, S., MacKenzie, E. T., and Edvinsson, L. (1988) *J. Cereb. Blood Flow Metab.* **8,** 875–878.

[27] Kuschinsky, W. and Wahl, M. (1975) *Circ. Res.* **37,** 168–173.

[28] Auer, L. M. (1986) *Neural Regulation of Brain Circulation* (Owman, C. and Hardebo, J. E., eds.), Elsevier, Amsterdam, pp. 497–513.

[29] Hara, H., Jansen, I., Ekman, R., Hamel, E., MacKenzie, E. T., Uddman, R., and Edvinsson, L. (1989) *J. Cereb. Blood Flow Metab.* **9,** 204–211.

[30] Winn, H. R., Morii, S., and Berne, R. M. (1985) *Ann. Biomed. Eng.* **13,** 321–328.

[31] Paulson, O. B., Strandgaard, S., and Edvinsson, L. (1990) *Cerebrovasc. and Brain Metab. Rev.* **2**, 161–192.

[32] Nakai, M., Iadecola, C., Ruggiero, D., Tucker, L. W., and Reis, D. J. (1983) *Brain Res.* **260**, 35–49.

[33] Bevan, J. A. and Joyce, E. H. (1990) *Am. J. Physiol.* **258**, H663–H668.

[34] Harder, D. R. (1987) *Circ. Res.* **60**, 102–107.

[35] Rubanyi, G. M., Romero, J. C., and Vanhoutte, P. M. (1986) *Am. J. Physiol.* **250**, H1145–H1149.

[36] Aaslid, R., Lindegaard, K., Sorteberg, W., and Nornes, H. (1989) *Stroke* **20**, 45–52.

[37] Paulson, O. B., Olesen, J., and Christensen, M. S. (1972) *Neurology* **22**, 286–293.

[38] Baumbach, G. L., Mayhan, W. G., and Heistad, D. D. (1986) *Neural Regulation of Brain Circulation* (Owman, C. and Hardebo, J. E., eds.), Elsevier, Amsterdam, pp. 607–615.

[39] Ursino, M. and Di Giammarco, P. (1991) *Ann. Biomed. Eng.* **19**, 15–42.

[40] Marmarou, A., Schulman, K., and La Morgese, J. (1975) *J. Neurosurg.* **43**, 523–534.

[41] Lundberg N. (1960) *Acta Psychiat.* **36**, 1–193.

Chapter 24

Vascular Tissue Preservation Techniques

Else Müller-Schweinitzer

Introduction

Pharmacological studies on isolated blood vessels generally require freshly obtained tissues. These are usually taken from various animals, although results obtained from human tissue would be the most accurate and predictable for human pharmacology. Human tissue can be obtained from surgery and autopsy, but besides obtaining human material, the main problem is the diversity of tissue types available and the irregularity of supply. However, when available, often much more material is supplied than can be used within a few hours. Isolated tissues have a very short life-span, and experiments should commence as soon as possible, if not immediately, after removal from the body, but this is not always convenient. Hence, the advantages of a simple and reliable storage method for ensuring the supply of adequate vascular preparations for pharmacological studies are readily apparent.

Cold Storage of Vascular Tissue

Isolated vascular tissue can be stored for several days in physiologic salt solution at 2–8°C, and be used in pharmacological experiments. However, storage of blood vessels in the cold produces several species- and time-dependent progressive changes in their physiologic characteristics and their responses to drugs.

From *The Human Brain Circulation*, R. D. Bevan and J. A. Bevan, eds.
©1994 Humana Press

Cold Storage-Induced Changes

The most consistent changes observed in blood vessels after cold storage for 5–9 d is a degeneration of nerve endings as assessed by attenuated responses to transmural electric stimulation of coronary arteries from cattle[1] and guinea pig,[2] and/or by reduced norepinephrine (NE) content and ^{3}H-NE uptake in rabbit aorta[3,4] and portal veins.[5,6] Apparently controversial results on the contractile responsiveness to receptor-mediated agonists of various blood vessels reflect both species differences and time dependency of changes occurring during prolonged cold storage. Considerable species differences have been observed when the NE sensitivity of portal veins from rabbit, guinea pig, and rat was tested after 5–9 d of storage at 2–4°C.[5,6] Perfused branches of the femoral artery from dogs were sensitized to the stimulant activity of α-adrenoceptor agonists and 5-HT when stored for 24 h at 6°C,[7] whereas the sensitivity to these agonists appeared unchanged when the same vessels from dogs[8,9] or monkeys[10] had been stored for 3–7 d at 4°C. The same applies for cold-stored canine auricular arteries[11] and cattle coronary arteries,[1] which had been stored for 5–6 d at 4°C. Naturally, the phenomenon of cold storage-induced sensitization of vascular smooth muscle is transient in nature. Hence, rabbit aortae develop increased sensitivity to NE and epinephrine when stored for up to 7 d at 2–6°C,[3,12,13] but this phenomenon is reversed when the storage time is extended to 10–14 d.[4,12]

Contrary to that observed with receptor-mediated contractile responses, cold storage of skeletal muscle arteries from both dog[8,9] and monkey[10] and of rabbit aortae[4,12] leads consistently to significant suppression of the contractile responses to potassium chloride (KCl). Furthermore, it has been observed that cold-stored rabbit aortae, although supersensitive to NE, are subsensitive to calcium, i.e., they require a higher extracellular calcium concentration to develop the same tension as fresh aortae.[13] Several observations support the contention that cold storage of vascular smooth muscle induces depolarization of the cell membrane. Evidence for this comes from the finding that in cold-stored vascular smooth muscle, the tissue Na^+ and Ca^{2+} content is markedly increased, whereas the K^+ content is significantly decreased.[6,7,13] Even after 2 h of equilibration in normal Ringer solution at 37°C, when Na^+ content is normalized, the K^+ content is still significantly diminished.[13] Moreover, administration of external K^+ decreases the $^{45}Ca^{2+}$ influx into cold-stored portal veins, suggesting that cold storage alters the Na^+-K^+ balance by inhibiting the electrogenic Na^+ pump.[6] Recently, direct evidence for cold storage-induced depolarization of smooth muscle cells has been presented by the finding that in cold-stored guinea pig coronary arteries the resting membrane potential in the smooth muscle cells increases from –60 to –47 mV.[2]

In conclusion, cold storage is a simple method of storing isolated blood vessels for a short time period. However, both degeneration of nerve terminals and depolarization of the cell membrane will modify progressively their physiologic and functional characteristics.

Cryopreservation of Vascular Tissue

Mechanisms of Freezing Injury

Freezing of living mammalian cells without cryoprotective additives generally induces severe cell damage, and few if any cells survive.[14–18] During cooling to subzero temperatures, water tends to flow out of the cell and freeze externally. Microscopic observations have shown that cells do indeed shrink during freezing. If cooled too fast, cells are injured by the formation of intracellular ice crystals; if cooled too slowly, however, cells will be injured by the "solution effect," i.e., by changes in the composition of extra- and intracellular solutions, since the concentration of extracellular salts in the residual unfrozen medium increases as ice is formed.[15] As a consequence of changes in both temperature and concentration, cell membranes become leaky to cations and permeable to substances (e.g., to sucrose) that normally do not enter the cell.[16] In addition, evidence has been presented that the fraction of water that remains unfrozen is damaging, since it gives rise to crushing of the cells within the ice masses.[19]

Cryoprotective Additives

It is assumed that permeating cryoprotective agents such as dimethyl sulfoxide (DMSO) and glycerol, by entering the cell, replace some water, thereby protecting the cell from damage during freezing.[17] The cryoprotecting activities of various agents, such as DMSO, glycerol, N-methylacetamide, dimethylacetamide, N-methylformamide, dimethylformamide, and polyethylene glycol 400, have been tested in canine saphenous veins taking the maximal response to NE as a parameter for the postthaw recovery. The best postthaw recovery, about 60% of that produced by unfrozen veins, was obtained with venous segments that had been frozen slowly in fetal calf serum containing 1.8M DMSO.[20–22]

Nonpermeating cryoprotectants, such as sucrose and hydroxyethyl starch, function at the outer surface of the cell. They are suggested to stabilize the cell volume by retaining more liquid water at low temperatures, thereby reducing the external electrolyte concentration.[15] Both types of cryoprotecting agents act directly at the level of cell membrane, yet their protective action may be synergistic. Indeed, addition of 0.1M sucrose to a DMSO-containing cryomedium promotes the postthaw recovery of blood vessels, such as canine saphenous veins and porcine coronary arteries, although sucrose alone does not exhibit any noticeable cryoprotecting activity.[23]

Cryomedia

For many cell types, it is important to have serum or other high-molecular-weight polymers in the cryomedium. This has been demonstrated recently for endothelial cells in canine coronary arteries that had been frozen in Krebs-Henseleit solution (KH) containing 20% FCS and 1.8M DMSO. Omission of FCS from the cryomedium resulted in significant morphological changes and functional attenuation of the endothelial cells, although both the contractile and the endothelium-independent relaxant responses of the smooth muscle cells were unchanged.[24] However, considerable species differences appear to exist. Figure 1 shows concentration–response curves to substance P, the effect of which is strictly endothelium-dependent,[25] in pig circumflex coronary arteries that

Pig circumflex coronary artery

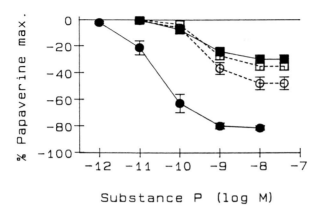

Fig. 1 Relaxant responses to substance P of rings from porcine circumflex coronary arteries stimulated with 3 μM PGF$_{2\alpha}$ without (●) and after cryopreservation at –196°C in fetal calf serum (FCS, ■), Krebs-Henseleit solution (KH, ○), and in KH with 50% FCS (□), containing 1.8M DMSO and 0.1M sucrose as cryoprotectants. The effects are expressed as percentages of the maximum response to papaverine, and the bars represent means ± SEM. For each point, n = 14. Method according to ref. 23.

had been frozen in various cryomedia, i.e., FCS, KH, and KH with 50% FCS, containing 1.8M DMSO and 0.1M sucrose. In these experiments, optimal postthaw recovery was obtained with pig coronary arteries that had been frozen in a medium without FCS. The same applies for smooth muscle contractile responses to PGF$_{2\alpha}$ and endothelium-independent relaxant responses to isoprenaline of pig circumflex coronary arteries that were better preserved in tissues that had been frozen in a medium without FCS (Fig. 2). However, here again considerable species differences exist. In contrast to that observed with pig coronary arteries, optimal postthaw recovery of both contractile responses to NE and relaxant responses to aminophylline of human pulmonary arteries were obtained with tissues that had been frozen in media containing at least 50% FCS (unpublished).

Pig circumflex coronary artery

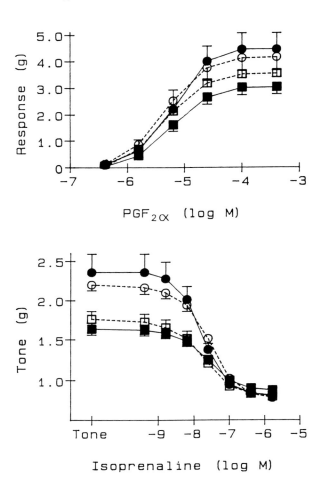

Fig. 2. Contractile responses to prostaglandin $F_{2\alpha}$ (PGF$_{2\alpha}$, top) and relaxant responses to isoprenaline during stimulation with 3 µM PGF$_{2\alpha}$ in the
presence of 10 nM ketanserin (bottom), of rings from porcine circumflex
coronary arteries without (●) and after cryopreservation at −196°C in fetal
calf serum (FCS, ■), Krebs-Henseleit solution (KH, ○), and in KH with 50%
FCS (□), containing 1.8M DMSO and 0.1M sucrose as cryoprotectants. The
effects are expressed in grams. Tone indicates the PGF$_{2\alpha}$-induced active tone
in addition to the existing passive preload. The bars represent means ± SEM.
For each point, $n = 8$–20. Method according to ref. 23.

Freezing Procedure

The optimal cooling rate not only depends on the type of cryoprotecting agent, but it also differs from cell to cell and is primarily dependent on (1) the water permeability of the cell membrane and (2) the surface-area-to-volume ratio of the cell. The presence of many different cell types within a tissue or organ implies, therefore, that no one freezing/thawing procedure can satisfy them all.[17] Moreover, in many peripheral arteries, cells are quite densely packed together, which may also reduce cell survival. Veins and pulmonary vessels are considerably less compact and often show better postthaw recovery than peripheral arteries. To minimize the effects of freezing damage, tissues are generally equilibrated with the cryoprotective medium before being slowly frozen. For most mammalian cells, the optimal cooling rate lies between 0.3 and 10°C/min. Once a sample is cooled to about −70°C, it can be transferred directly into liquid nitrogen (−196°C) and stored there indefinitely until use.

Thawing Procedure

In general, a rapid rate of warming that limits the growth of ice crystals in the frozen samples is desirable. As ice is converted into free water, cells are exposed to an extracellular hypotonic solution. Moreover, the dehydrated cells must now rehydrate in order to remain in osmotic equilibrium. Serum or other high-molecular-weight polymers in the medium may reduce the damaging effect of the dilution shock.[15] Before use, the frozen samples are thawed rapidly by placing the ampules for 2.5 min in a 37°C water bath. The vascular tissues are then rinsed in a dish containing Krebs-Henseleit solution to dilute the cryoprotective agent. With isolated mammalian cells, often a stepwise dilution protocol is used in order to avoid osmotic shock, which may kill cells when returned to isotonic solution. With isolated blood vessels, such as canine saphenous veins and rat portal veins, that had been frozen in fetal calf serum containing 1.8*M* DMSO, this procedure, did not improve the postthaw recovery (unpublished).

Hence, many factors during the freezing/thawing process, such as cryoprotective additives, cryomedium, temperature, and rate of addition and removal of the cryoprotectant(s), as well as the rate of cooling and rewarming, may modify the postthaw recovery of cryopreserved tissues. Optimal combination between cryoprotectants and cooling/thawing rates has to be derived largely by a process of trial and error for each tissue type.

Postthaw Recovery

Effects of Ion Transport

When frozen/thawed vessels are suspended in Krebs-Henseleit solution, in most instances, the initial preload is followed by a transient contraction before the smooth muscle relaxes, suggesting a transient depolarization. On the other hand, in frozen/thawed canine saphenous veins, contractile responses and $^{45}Ca^{2+}$ uptake during both depolarization or α_2-adrenoceptor stimulation are well preserved and similar to that observed with unfrozen veins. Moreover, a significant correlation between $^{45}Ca^{2+}$ uptake and contractile responses during stimulation by KCl or guanfacine in the absence and presence of various calcium channel blockers suggests that cryopreservation of smooth muscle cells from dog saphenous veins does not alter the Ca^{2+} transport.[26] By contrast, in frozen/thawed human pulmonary arteries, a potassium channel opener, such as cromakalim, SDZ PCO400, or RP 49356, proved to be significantly less potent than in unfrozen vessels,[27] suggesting that in certain vascular tissues, the freezing/thawing process may induce some depolarization of the smooth muscle cell membranes.

Enzyme Activity and Biomechanical Properties

After cryopreservation of human and canine veins, both the monoamine oxidase activity[28,29] and the endogenous prostaglandin synthesis[28,30–32] are well preserved. However, despite unchanged collagen synthesis and elastic properties of venous tissue,[33,34] the evidence suggests that under arterial hemodynamic conditions, the compliance of cryopreserved canine veins is significantly reduced.[30]

Adrenergic Nerve Endings

Adrenergic nerve endings appear to be well preserved after cryopreservation. Evidence for this comes from experiments with rabbit ear arteries that had been immersed in newborn calf serum containing 1.8*M* DMSO and stored at –70°C. After thawing, the contractile responses to electric field stimulation of these arteries are similar to those elicited in unfrozen tissues.[35] In addition, determination of basal and stimulation-induced tritium overflow after preincubation with ³H-NE of canine saphenous vein strips has shown that cryopreservation does not alter the absolute tritium overflow during sustained electrical stimulation, yet the basal outflow from frozen/thawed vein strips is slightly higher than that observed with strips from fresh veins.[22]

Endothelial Cell Function

Relaxant responses to various hormones and neurotransmitters are known to be mediated by the release of endothelium-derived relaxing factor(s) (EDRF)[36] and represent a useful tool to assess the viability of vascular endothelial cells after cryopreservation. Using this method, it has been demonstrated that endothelium-mediated relaxant responses to acetylcholine of a rabbit central ear artery and its main side branch are well preserved after storage for several days at –70°C while suspended in newborn calf serum containing 1.8*M* DMSO.[35] The same applies for the endothelium-dependent relaxant responses of both human[37] and porcine[23,38] coronary arteries following cryostorage at –75 and –196°C. For some arteries, such as canine circumflex coronary, it appears to be important to have serum in the cryomedium, to provide protection for the endothelial cells.[24] However, as shown in Fig. 1, with pig circumflex coronary arteries, optimal postthaw endothelial cell function can be obtained when the arteries are frozen in KH containing 1.8*M* DMSO and 0.1*M* sucrose without FCS. Yet the substance P-induced endothelium-dependent relaxation[25] was considerably weaker in the frozen/thawed arteries as compared to unfrozen tissues. Canine veins may release both endothelium-derived relaxing and contracting factors,[39] and it has been shown that even in autogenous venous grafts, the endothelium of cryopreserved veins can release both relaxing and contracting factors.[40]

Smooth Muscle Cell Function

Functional changes of smooth muscle cells following cryopreservation have been estimated by measuring responses to numerous contracting agonists and/or endothelium-independent vasodilators in isolated blood vessels from various species such as dogs,[21,23,24,26,28,40–42] pigs,[23,38] rabbits,[35] and humans.[21,27,29,37] Generally, a good functional postthaw recovery was obtained with vessels that had been immersed in media containing 1.8–2.1M DMSO, slowly frozen to −70°C, and stored at −70 to −196°C. After thawing, in most of these blood vessels, the maximum contractile force was found to be diminished when compared to that produced by unfrozen tissues. However, there was always a very good correlation when the affinities for different agonists on frozen/thawed and unfrozen vessels were compared. Thus, highly significant correlations of pD_2 values for various agonists on fresh and frozen/thawed canine basilar arteries,[28] pig circumflex coronary arteries,[38] human pulmonary vessels,[27] and human saphenous veins[29] have been demonstrated (Fig. 3). Furthermore, the affinity parameters (pA_2 and pD'_2 values) for all receptor antagonists investigated up to now proved to be unchanged after cryopreservation. The same is true for calcium channel blockers tested against KCl and guanfacine in canine saphenous veins.[26]

Summary

Despite the relevance of human isolated tissue to human pharmacology, its use is still very much the exception rather than the rule. The major reason for this is that the supply of fresh human material is both irregular and unpredictable, and once removed from the patient, it has a very short life-span.

Storage of isolated blood vessels in physiologic salt solution at 4°C induces rapid and progressive changes of physiologic and functional properties within a few days. Cryopreservation and storage at −196°C of isolated blood vessels offers the prospect of

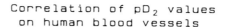

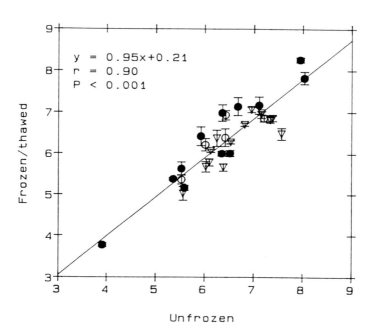

Fig. 3. Correlation between drug potencies as assessed by the pD_2 values, for various agonists determined on unfrozen (abscissa scale) and frozen/thawed (ordinate scale) human saphenous veins (∇), human basilar arteries ($\bigcirc$), and human pulmonary arteries ($\blacksquare$). Data were compared by linear regression analysis. The correlation coefficient and regression for the correlation are indicated.

indefinite storage of the material with only damage associated with the freezing and thawing process. Despite certain problems, such as maintenance of the endothelial function and some reduction in contractile force, the main biochemical properties, uptake mechanisms, and affinities of most agonists and antagonists have been shown to be well preserved after cryopreservation. Hence, this technique offers clear potential for ensuring the supply of vascular material for pharmacological studies.

References

1 Kalsner, S. and Quillan, M. (1989) *J. Pharmacol. Exp. Ther.* **249**, 785–789.

2 Keef, K. D. and Kreulen, D. (1988) *Circ. Res.* **62**, 585–595.

3 Shibata, S., Hattori, K., Sakurai, I., Mori, J., and Fujiwara, M. (1971) *J. Pharmacol. Exp. Ther.* **177**, 621–632.

4 Varma, D. R. and McCullough, H. N. (1969) *J. Pharmacol. Exp. Ther.* **166**, 26–34.

5 Hughes, J. and Vane, J. R. (1970) *Br. J. Pharmacol.* **39**, 476–489.

6 Kaiman, M. and Shibata, S. (1987) *Blood Vessels* **15**, 217–230.

7 Murphy, J. C., Carrier, O., and Shadi, J. (1973) *Am. J. Physiol.* **225**, 1187–1191.

8 Sinanovic, O. and Chiba, S. (1987) *Arch. Int. Pharmacodyn. Ther.* **287**, 146–157.

9 Sinanovic, O. and Chiba, S. (1987) *Eur. J. Pharmacol.* **143**, 353–360.

10 Sinanovic, O. and Chiba, S. (1988) *Jpn. J. Pharmacol.* **46**, 237–246.

11 Ito, T. and Chiba, S. (1985) *Arch. Int. Pharmacodyn. Ther.* **275**, 13–21.

12 Shibata, S. (1969) *Circ. Res.* **14**, 179–187.

13 Carrier, O., Jr., Murphy, J. C., and Tenner, T. E. (1973) *Eur. J. Pharmacol.* **24**, 225–233.

14 Litvan, G. G. (1972) *Cryobiology* **9**, 182–189.

15 Mazur, P. (1977) *The Freezing of Mammalian Embryos* (Elliott, K. and Whelan, J., eds.), Elsevier, Amsterdam, pp. 19–42.

16 Pegg, D. E. (1976) *J. Clin. Path.* **29**, 271–285.

17 Pegg, D. E. (1985) *Progress in Transplantation* (Morris, P. J. and Tilney, N. L., eds.), Churchill Livingstone, Edinburgh, pp. 69–105.

18 Pegg, D. E. (1987) *The Biophysics of Organ Cryopreservation* (Pegg, D. E., and Karow, A. M., Jr., eds.), Plenum, New York, pp. 117–140.

19 Schneider, U. and Mazur, P. (1987) *Cryobiology* **24**, 17–17.

20 Müller-Schweinitzer, E. (1988) *Folia Haematol, Leipzig* **115**, 405–410.

21 Müller-Schweinitzer, E. (1988) *TIPS* **9**, 221–223.

22 Müller-Schweinitzer, E. and Tapparelli, C. (1987) *Neuronal Messengers in Vascular Function* (Nobin, A., Owman, C., and Arneklo-Nobin, B., eds.), Elsevier (Biomedical Division), Amsterdam, pp. 105–110.

23 Müller-Schweinitzer, E. and Ellis, P. (1992) *Naunyn-Schmiedeberg's Arch. Pharmacol.* **345**, 594–597.

24 Ku, D. D., Willis, W. L., and Caulfield, J. B. (1990) *Cryobiology* **27**, 511–520.

25 Gulati, N., Mathison, R., Huggel, H., Regoli, D., and Beny, J. L. (1987) *Eur. J. Pharmacol.* **137**, 149–154.

26 Ebeigbe, A. B., Müller-Schweinitzer, E., and Vogel, A. (1988) *Brit. J. Pharmacol.* **94**, 381–388.

27 Ellis, P. and Müller-Schweinitzer, E. (1991) *Br. J. Pharmacol.* **103**, 1377–1380.

28 Müller-Schweinitzer, E. and Tapparelli, C. (1986) *Naunyn Schmiedeberg's Arch. Pharmacol.* **332,** 74–78.

29 Müller-Schweinitzer, E., Tapparelli, C., and Victorzon, M. (1986) *Brit. J. Pharmacol.* **88,** 685–687.

30 Showalter, D., Durham, S., Sheppeck, R., Berceli, S., Greisler, H., Brockman, K., Makaroun, M., Webster, M., Steed, D., Siewers, R., and Borovetz, H. (1989) *Surgery (St. Louis)* **106,** 652–659.

31 Louagie, Y. A., Legrand-Monsieur, A., Lavenne-Pardonge, E., Remacle, C., Delvaux, P., Maldague, P., Buche, M., Ponlot, R., and Schoevaerdts, J.-C. (1990) *J. Cardiovasc. Surg.* **31,** 92–100.

32 Passani, S. L., Angelini, G. D., Breckenridge, I. M., and Newby, A. C. (1988) *Eur. J. Cardiothorac. Surg.* **2,** 233–236.

33 Brockbank, K. G. M., Donovan, T. J., Ruby, S. T., Carpenter, J. F., Hagen, P.-O., and Woodley, M. A. (1990) *J. Vasc. Surg.* **11,** 94–102.

34 L'Italien, G. J., Maloney, R. D., and Abbott, W. M. (1979) *J. Surg. Res.* **27,** 239–243.

35 Thompson, L., Duckworth, J., and Bevan, J. (1989) *Blood Vessels* **26,** 157–164.

36 Furchgott, R. F. and Zawadzki, J. V. (1989) *Nature* **288,** 373–376.

37 Ku, D. D., Winn, M. J., Grigsby, T., and Caulfield, J. B. (1992) *Cryobiology* **29,** 199–209.

38 Schoeffter, P. and Müller-Schweinitzer, E. (1990) *J. Pharm. Pharmacol.* **42,** 646–651.

39 Furchgott, R. F. and Vanhoutte, P. M. (1989) *FASEB J.* **3,** 2007–2018.

40 Elmore, J. R., Gloviczki, P., Brockbank, K. G. M., and Miller, V. M. (1991) *J. Vasc. Surg.* **13,** 584–592.

41 Weber, T. R., Dent, D. L., Lindenauer, S. M., Allen, E., Weatherbee, L., Spencer, H. H., and Gleich, P. (1975) *J. Surg. Res.* **18,** 247–255.

42 Dent, T. L., Weber, T. R., Lindenauer, S. M., Ascher, N., Weatherbee, L., Allen, E., and Spencer, H. H. (1974) *Surg. Forum (Philadelphia)* **25,** 241–243.

Chapter 25

In Vitro Small Artery Methodology

Joseph E. Brayden

Introduction

In the past 10 years, techniques for the study of small blood vessels in vitro have been applied by numerous investigators. As a result, a substantial library of information about resistance artery function has been developed.[1] Data are now available regarding the anatomical, pharmacological, physiological, biochemical, and pathophysiological properties of resistance arteries isolated from many different vascular beds and from numerous species, including humans. The rationale underlying these studies has been the recognition that the determinants and regulators of peripheral vascular resistance can be understood only by direct study of very small blood vessels. This chapter will describe some of the techniques available for the study of such vessels in vitro and will describe current applications of these techniques in studies designed to identify basic mechanisms of vascular control.

In Vitro Techniques
for Study of Resistance Artery Function
Myograph Techniques
Isometric Force Measurements

The contributions of many investigators have led to the development of the currently available techniques for the study of resistance artery function. Bevan and Osher[2] were among the first

From *The Human Brain Circulation*, R. D. Bevan and J. A. Bevan, eds.
©1994 Humana Press

to explore the possibility of extending existing techniques for the study of isometric force development in large arteries to a level appropriate for the examination of the resistance vasculature. These techniques were further refined by Mulvany and Halpern[3] in 1976 and have been described in detail.[4] In this method, short segments of artery are attached to a force transducer and to a displacement device via small diameter wires threaded through the vascular lumen. Resting tension can be adjusted by separating the two wires, and isometric force development in response to agonists or other interventions, such as shear stress or wall distension, can be monitored (*see* Fig. 1). Using this approach, one can study arteries with resting diameters as small as 60–80 µm.[5]

Isolated Pressurized Arteries

A second major technical advance in the effort to obtain information about the function of small blood vessels was the development of techniques for the study of isolated, pressurized arteries. This may be a more physiologically relevant configuration in comparison to the wire-mount system mentioned above, because vessels can be exposed to physiological transmural pressures and assume a shape more like that experienced in vivo. Using these techniques, the effects of pressure changes as well as the effects of fluid flow through the lumen of the blood vessel can be assessed. Duling and colleagues[6] made a significant contribution in development of this technique, and this approach has since been modified and refined by others.[7] In this approach, arteries are isolated and cannulated at one end with a micropipet (*see* Fig. 2). This pipet is connected to a pressurization reservoir, and blood in the lumen can be removed by elevating pressure slightly to initiate flow through the vessel. The distal end of preparation is then cannulated with a second pipet that can be sealed or left open depending on the nature of the study. Transmural pressure can then be adjusted to any chosen level, and arterial diameter can be monitored using a video dimension analyzer. Using this methodology, analysis of arteries as small as 30–40 µm in lumen diameter has been reported.[6]

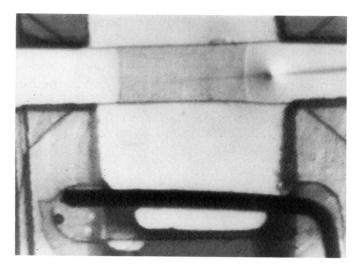

Fig. 1. A rabbit cerebral artery mounted in a myograph for recording of isometric force and membrane potential. The artery is supported by two fine tungsten wires (20 μm in diameter) attached to lucite blocks. An "L-shaped" platinum wire for electrical stimulation of perivascular nerves can be seen at the bottom of the photograph. A glass microelectrode for intracellular recording of membrane potential is shown entering the bath from the right and contacting the artery near the center of the segment. Arterial segment length is 1.3 mm.

Other Techniques

Numerous other techniques have been successfully applied to the study of small blood vessels, in some instances forming a valuable adjunct to the in vitro techniques described above. Microvessels have been studied for many years using light and electron microscopy techniques adapted for analysis of very small samples.[8] Techniques for the biochemical analysis of small vascular segments are also available, and have included study of contractile and connective tissue proteins[9] and of regulatory mechanisms in membrane fractions isolated from resistance arteries.[10] In addition, techniques for studying ion flux by isotope methodologies can now be applied successfully to small blood vessels mounted in the myograph systems described above.[11]

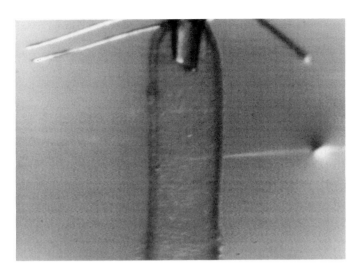

Fig. 2. Photograph of a pressurized middle cerebral artery isolated from a rabbit. The artery is tied to a glass micropipet (pipet and nylon sutures can be seen at top of photo) that is connected to a pressurization reservoir. Microelectrode for membrane potential recordings enters the bathing solution from the right. Arterial lumen diameter is 125 μm.

Whereas studies of isolated, intact arteries have provided much useful mechanistic information about arterial function, such information often can be supplemented and greatly expanded by focusing on the behavior of individual cells (i.e., endothelial, smooth muscle) that reside within the vascular wall. Techniques for isolation of endothelial and vascular smooth muscle cells involving enzymatic digestion of the blood vessel wall have been applied to large arteries for a number of years, and recently, this approach has been extended to include the resistance vasculature.[12] A variation on this theme has been the simultaneous measurement of ion-channel activity and calcium influx in isolated cells.[13]

Specific Applications
of Small Artery In Vitro Techniques

Specific applications of the techniques described above have provided valuable information about the mechanisms of control of tone in the resistance vasculature and will now be briefly discussed.

Hypertension and the Resistance Vasculature

Use of the Mulvany/Halpern myograph has provided extensive information about the physiology and biophysics of force generation in resistance arteries, and has allowed detailed analysis of the vascular changes associated with the development and maintenance of hypertension. Numerous abnormalities of vascular function in small arteries from hypertensive animals and humans have been identified using this technique. Fundamental alterations in vascular structure,[8,14] neuronal activity,[14,15] contractility,[9,14] excitation-contraction coupling,[14] and endothelial cell function (*see below*), to note just a few observations, have been identified in resistance arteries isolated from hypertensives. Experiments of this type have provided a comprehensive picture of the vascular changes that occur in association with hypertension as well as the efficacy of antihypertensive agents to reverse some of the detrimental effects of elevated blood pressure.

Membrane Potential and Vascular Regulation

The important role of membrane potential as a mechanism of vasoconstriction and vasodilation in small blood vessels has been clearly demonstrated using a variety of in vitro techniques. For instance, membrane depolarization has been shown to be an important mechanism of myogenic tone in resistance arteries, and alterations of membrane potential induce significant changes in the degree of tone.[16–18] Tone in small arteries is very sensitive to removal of extracellular calcium[19] and is reduced or abolished by calcium-entry blockers,[18,20] indicating the central importance of voltage-dependent calcium channels in this response.[12] More recently, integrative studies involving measurements of membrane potential, diameter, and single-ion channel activity by patch-clamp analysis have demonstrated a key role for large-conductance calcium-activated potassium channels in regulation of myogenic tone in small cerebral and coronary arteries.[18] These potassium channels act in a negative feedback pathway to balance the strong depolarizing response to increases in transmural pressure in these arteries.

Endothelial Function in Resistance Arteries

Endothelial function in small blood vessels, both under normal conditions and in samples taken from animals with various cardiovascular diseases, has been examined. For instance, Tesfamariam and Halpern[21] noted that endothelium-dependent vasodilation was reduced in pressurized mesenteric resistance arteries isolated from hypertensive animals as compared to controls. Similar observations were reported for resistance arteries isolated from hypertensive animals and mounted in the Halpern/Mulvany myograph.[22,23] Hyperpolarization of vascular smooth muscle in response to endothelium-dependent vasodilators has been observed in small arteries, and is equivalent to or greater than that seen in large arteries.[24,25] Several unique features of the responses in small arteries have been noted and include a more sustained hyperpolarization in some arteries,[24,25] but a distinct absence of responsiveness to EDHF or pharmacological hyperpolarizing vasodilators in certain regions of the microcirculation of the brain.[24,26] Endothelium-dependent hyperpolarizing responses are reduced in resistance arteries isolated from hypertensive rats compared to normotensives.[27]

Neural Regulation of Resistance Arteries

Another area where the approaches outlined above have been successfully applied relates to the mechanisms of neurally mediated changes in vascular tone in small blood vessels.[28] Analysis of the effects of adrenoceptor antagonists on neurally evoked electrical and mechanical responses of resistance arteries has demonstrated the potential role for a nonclassical adrenoceptor in these tissues.[5,29] In addition, a role for nonclassical neurotransmitter substances, such as neuropeptide Y and ATP, as regulators of resistance arterial tone has been suggested by studies employing the resistance artery myograph techniques outlined above.[28,30] Mechanisms of neurogenic vasodilation also have been elucidated using these techniques. For example, Brayden and Bevan[31] demonstrated the possible role for VIP as a mediator of neurogenic vasodilation of cerebral arteries. Neild and colleagues[32] have shown a neurogenic cholinergic vasodilator system in mesenteric arterioles using a video dimension analyzer system of their own design.

Combined Force/Diameter and Fluorometric Techniques

Various imaging techniques, which until very recent years have been applied primarily to cultured or freshly isolated single vascular smooth muscle cells, have been adapted to the study of isolated, intact resistance arteries. For instance, using a fluorescent label (BCECF) that is sensitive to changes in pH, Aalkjaer and Mulvany[33] have shown clearly that intracellular pH is altered during contraction or relaxation of resistance arteries. Fluorescent calcium indicators have been employed both in isometrically configured arteries and pressurized resistance arteries to provide fundamental information about the changes in intracellular calcium that occur in small blood vessels during various forms of stimulation.[34-36]

Ion Channels

Results of the studies described above have been supported and expanded on using techniques for analysis of ionic currents and single-channel activity in cells isolated from small arteries. For instance, Hirst and colleagues have measured calcium currents in voltage-clamped segments of cerebral arterioles.[37] Quayle et al.[12] have described the properties of single calcium channels in smooth muscle cells isolated from resistance-sized cerebral arteries of the rat. These studies indicate the feasibility of studying ion channels in cells isolated from small arteries.

Studies of Human Cerebral Arteries

Arteries isolated from the human cerebral circulation demonstrate some of the same properties that have been observed in arteries from laboratory animals. For instance, pressurized human middle cerebral arteries taken at autopsy had resting membrane potentials at low pressure (5 mmHg) of about –60 mV. When pressurized, such arteries depolarized and developed myogenic tone. At high pressure (120 mmHg), the arteries were highly depolarized, and there was evidence of rhythmic electrical activity (Fig. 3).

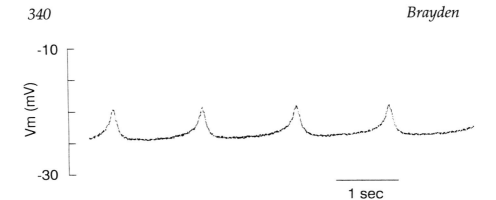

Fig. 3. Membrane depolarization and spiking activity in a branch of human middle cerebral artery. The artery was pressurized to 120 mmHg. Myogenic tone was present at this pressure. The changes in membrane potential were associated with small oscillations in diameter.

In another series of experiments, human arteries were mounted for recording membrane potential and isotonic force development, and responses to electrical field stimulation were studied in some of the arteries. As can be seen in Fig. 4, electrical stimulation induced a large depolarization that was associated with a transient contraction. Both the electrical and the mechanical responses were abolished by tetrodotoxin, but neither guanethidine nor benextrimine had significant effects on these responses. These limited data would suggest that human cerebral arteries express some of the same physiological activity as has commonly been observed in cerebral arteries isolated from laboratory animals.

Conclusions

In vitro techniques are currently available for the study of arteries as small as 30–40 μm in diameter. With the range of methods available, an integrated approach to the study of resistance artery function, from single-channel to intact tissue, is possible, and as a result, many of the unique features of the resistance vasculature are presently emerging. Over the next few years, this should

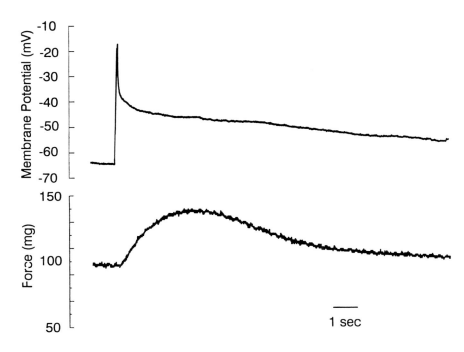

Fig. 4. Excitatory junction potential and contraction of wire-mounted human middle cerebral artery. Electrical stimulation was applied via platinum wires placed on either side of the arterial segment. A single electrical pulse (0.3-ms duration, 80 V) induced a large, transient depolarization followed by a secondary depolarization that was sustained for more than 10 s.

result in rapid progress toward a comprehensive understanding of the peripheral vasculature in health and disease.

References

[1] Mulvany, M. J. and Aalkjaer, C. (1990) *Physiol. Rev.* **70,** 921–961.
[2] Bevan, J. A. and Osher, J. V. (1972) *Agents Actions* **2,** 257–260.
[3] Mulvany, M. J. and Halpern, W. (1976) *Nature* **260,** 617–618.
[4] Mulvany, M. J. and Halpern, W. (1977) *Circ. Res.* **41,** 19–26.
[5] Owen, M. P., Quinn, C., and Bevan, J. A. (1985) *Am. J. Physiol.* **249,** H404–H414.
[6] Duling, B. R., Gore, R. W., Dacey, R. G., and Damon, D. N. (1981) *Am. J. Physiol.* **241,** H108–H116.
[7] Halpern, W., Mongeon, S. A., and Root, D. T. (1984) *Smooth Muscle Contraction* (Stephens, N. L., ed.), Dekker, New York, pp. 427–456.

8 Lee, R. M. K. W., Forrest, J. B., Garfield, R. E., and Daniel, E. E. (1983) *Blood Vessels* **20**, 72–91.

9 Brayden, J. E., Halpern, W., and Brann, L. R. (1983) *Hypertension* **5**, 17–25.

10 Kwan, C.-Y. (1991) *The Resistance Vasculature* (Bevan, J. A., Halpern, W., and Mulvany, M. J., eds.), Humana, Totowa, NJ, pp. 281–304.

11 Aalkjaer, C. and Mulvany, M. J. (1985) *J. Physiol. Lond.* **362**, 215–231.

12 Quayle, J. M., McCarron, J. G., Asbury, J. R., and Nelson, M. T. (1993) *Am. J. Physiol.* **264**, H470–H478.

13 Benham, C. D. (1989) *J. Physiol. Lond.* **419**, 689–701.

14 Aalkjaer, C., Heagerty, A. M., Petersen, K. K., Swales, J. D., and Mulvany, M. J. (1987) *Circ. Res.* **61**, 181–186.

15 Whall, C. W., Meyers, M. M., and Halpern, W. (1980) *Blood Vessels* **17**, 1–15.

16 Harder, D. R. (1984) *Circ. Res.* **55**, 197–202.

17 Brayden, J. E. and Wellman, G. C. (1989) *J. Cereb. Blood Flow Metab.* **9**, 256–263.

18 Brayden, J. E. and Nelson, M. T. (1992) *Science* **256**, 532–535.

19 Cauvin, C., Saida, K., and Vanbreemen, C. (1984) *Blood Vessels* **21**, 23–31.

20 Quayle, J., McCarron, J. G., Halpern, W., and Nelson, M. T. (1990) *Biophys. J.* **57**, 301a (abstract).

21 Tesfamariam, B. and Halpern, W. (1988) *Hypertension* **11**, 440–444.

22 Demey, J. G. and Gray, S. D. (1985) *Prog. Appl. Microcirc.* **8**, 181–187.

23 Diederich, D., Yang, Z., Buhler, F. R., and Luscher, T. F. (1990) *Am. J. Physiol.* **258**, H445–H451.

24 Brayden, J. E. (1991) *Circ. Res.* **69**, 1415–1420.

25 Garland, C. J. and McPherson, G. L. (1992) *Br. J. Pharmacol.* **105**, 429–435.

26 McCarron, J. G., Quayle, J. M., Halpern, W., and Nelson, M. T. (1991) *Am. J. Physiol.* **261**, H287–H291.

27 Brayden, J. E. (1991) *Circulation* **84(Suppl. III)**, S25 (abstract).

28 Neild, T. O. and Brayden, J. E. (1991) *The Resistance Vasculature* (Bevan, J. A., Halpern, W., and Mulvany, M. J., eds.), Humana, Totowa, NJ, pp. 217–240.

29 Hirst, G. D. S. and Neild, T. O. (1981) *J. Physiol. Lond.* **313**, 343–350.

30 Morris, J. L. and Murphy, R. (1988) *J. Auton. Nerv. Syst.* **24**, 241–249.

31 Brayden, J. E. and Bevan, J. A. (1986) *Stroke* **17**, 1189–1192.

32 Neild, T. O., Shen, K. Z., and Surprenant, A. (1990) *J. Physiol. Lond.* **420**, 247–265.

33 Aalkjaer, C. and Mulvany, M. J. (1988) *Prog. Biochem. Pharmacol.* **25**, 150–158.

34 Bukoski, R. (1990) *J. Hypertension* **8**, 37–43.

35 Jensen, P. E., Mulvany, M. J., and Aalkjaer, C. (1992) *Pfluegers Arch. Physiol.* **420**, 536–543.

36 Meininger, G. M., Zawieja, D. C., Falcone, J. C., Hill, M. A., and Davey, J. P. (1991) *Am. J. Physiol.* **261**, H950–H959.

37 Hirst, G. D. S., Silverberg, G. D., van Helden, D. F. (1986) *J. Physiol. Lond.* **371**, 289–304.

Chapter 26

Molecular Aspects of Endothelial Function in Hemostasis, Inflammation, and Thrombosis

Kenneth K. Wu

Introduction

The vascular endothelium is composed of a monolayer of endothelial cells lining the entire vasculature. Although the role that these cells play in maintaining blood fluidity was recognized in the mid-19th century,[1] mechanisms by which they maintain blood fluidity remained elusive for the next 100 years until the early 1970s, when endothelial cells were successfully maintained in culture[2,3] and a number of important molecules were isolated and characterized. Some of these molecules play a major role in maintaining blood fluidity and the patency of blood vessels. During the past decade, we have witnessed an explosion of new information concerning endothelial function. Our concepts on the endothelium have been converted from what was perceived to be a biochemically inert cell into the current view that it is a multifunctional tissue capable of generating a myriad of biologically active and physiologically important compounds involving a wide variety of physiological functions, including maintaining patent cerebral blood vessels.

The molecules described below are based on work performed on cultured cells prepared from different sources of blood vessels and different animal species. Despite the diversity of vascular

From *The Human Brain Circulation*, R. D. Bevan and J. A. Bevan, eds.
©1994 Humana Press

sources and animal species, the biochemical characteristics and functions of molecules produced by these endothelial cells are strikingly similar. It is reasonable to assume that cerebral vascular endothelium may possess similar molecular characteristics as endothelial cells from other sources. However, further studies are needed to determine whether cerebral microvascular endothelium may possess unique functional and biochemical characteristics.

Endothelial cells synthesize a myriad of molecules that may be transported to the cell surface, secreted into the extracellular milieu, or stored in intracellular granules and secreted on stimulation. Some molecules are constitutively expressed, whereas others are induced by exogenous stimuli. This chapter will focus on two types of molecules: (1) constitutively expressed molecules involved in maintaining blood fluidity and hemostasis, and (2) inducible molecules participating in inflammatory reactions.

Endothelial Cells and Patency of Blood Vessels

Key Protective Molecules

The vascular endothelial cell possesses several important antithrombotic properties that are considered to be responsible for maintaining blood fluidity and preventing thrombus formation on the vascular wall. These antithrombotic properties are ascribed to specific molecules that are synthesized by vascular endothelial cells. These molecules include:

1. Prostacyclin.
2. Plasminogen activators.
3. Thrombomodulin.
4. Heparin-like molecules.
5. Surface ecto-enzymes.
6. Endothelium-dependent relaxing factor (EDRP).

The molecular characteristics are given below, and their physiological roles are summarized in Table 1.

Prostacyclin

Prostacyclin (PGI_2) is a metabolite of arachidonic acid with potent biological activities.[4] It inhibits platelet activation, secretion, and aggregation, and maintains vascular relaxation. Its anti-

Table 1

A Brief Summary of Key Protective Molecules Produced by Endothelial Cells

Molecules	Biochemical action	Function
Surface-bound		
Thrombomodulin (TM)	Thrombin binding	TM bound thrombin cleaves protein C to generate activated protein C, which with protein S as its cofactor inactivates coagulation factors Va and VIIIa
Heparin-like molecules	Cofactor for antithrombin III	Facilitates antithrombin binding to and neutralizes the activity of thrombin and other activated coagulation factors
Ecto-ADPase	Degrades ADP	ADP is a major mediator of platelet activation and aggregation, ecto ADPase inactivates ADP, thereby reducing platelet aggregation potential
Secreted		
Prostacyclin	Stimulates platelet and smooth muscle cell adenylate cyclase with cAMP accumulation	Inhibits platelet activation and relaxes vascular smooth muscle cells
Endothelium-dependent relaxing factors (EDRF, nitric oxide)	Stimulates vascular smooth muscle cell, platelet guanylate cyclase, and cGMP accumulation	Relaxes vascular smooth muscle cells and acts synergistically with prostacyclin to inhibit platelet activation
Tissue plasminogen activator (tPA)	Catalyzes the conversion of plasminogen to plasmin, which digests fibrin	Lysis of fibrin clots

thrombotic and vasodilating activities are potentiated by endothelium-dependent relaxing factor (EDRF, nitric oxide). The endothelial cell is the major source of PGI_2 biosynthesis.[5] Its synthesis is stimulated by shear stress, physiological agonists, and pathologic insults. The synthesized PGI_2 is released extracellularly, and acts in a paracrine manner on platelets and smooth muscle cells. The mechanism of PGI_2 action is receptor-mediated stimulation of intracellular cyclic AMP.[4]

PGI$_2$ is not stored in the cell. It is synthesized and released when cells are under physiological or pathologic stimulation.[5-7] Cell stimulation leads to an increase in the intracellular calcium level, which activates phospholipase A_2. Phospholipase A_2 catalyzes the deacylation of arachidonic acid (AA) from the second (sn-2) position of membrane phospholipids, notably phosphatidylcholine (PC). Arachidonic acid may be liberated from phospholipids by an alternate pathway where phospholipase C catalyzes the conversion of phosphatidylinositol (PI) to diacylglycerol and inositol trisphosphate, and diacylglycerol lipase catalyzes the release of arachidonic acid from diacyglycerol. The released arachidonic acid is converted into prostaglandin G_2 (PGG_2) and then PGH_2 by a bifunctional enzyme, PGH synthase (also called cyclooxygenase). PGH_2 is a common precursor for formation of PGI_2, PGE_2, $PGF_{2\alpha}$, and PGD_2. The pathway for converting AA into PGI_2 and prostaglandins is termed the cyclooxygenase pathway. The released AA is also converted to 15-hydroxyeicosatetraenoic acid (15-HETE) in the endothelial cell via the lipoxygenase pathway. In vitro experiments in cultured endothelial cells show that PGI_2 is the predominant form of eicosanoids generated during endothelial cell activation.

PGI$_2$ synthesis is tightly regulated at each of the three enzymatic steps.[8,9] Phospholipase A_2 governs the initial rate of synthesis, whereas PGH synthase determines the capacity for PGI_2 production. PGH synthase turns over rapidly. Moreover, it undergoes "suicidal" autoinactivation during catalysis. The capacity for PGI_2 synthesis is, hence, dependent on the steady-state level of PGH synthase.[10] Inflammatory cytokines, such as IL-1, are capable of inducing *de novo* synthesis of PGH synthase, thereby causing a sustained production of PGI_2 for several hours.[10] By contrast, agonists, such as thrombin, histamine, and ionophore A23187, which do not induce *de novo* synthesis of PGH synthase and hence cannot maintain the cellular PGH synthase levels during catalysis, stimulate PGI_2 production only for a short time reaching a plateau in 30 min.[11] Prostacyclin (PGI) synthase also undergoes autoinactivation during catalysis and probably plays an important part in regulating PGI_2 synthesis.[12]

PGI_2 is also produced by a transcellular metabolic pathway through which PGH_2 produced by one cell (platelets) is converted into PGI_2 by another cell (endothelial cells and lymphocytes).[13,14] It has been shown that interaction of platelets with the damaged vessel wall leads to PGI_2 formation by this mechanism.[15] Multiple mechanisms of PGI_2 synthesis have important implications in thrombosis, atherosclerosis, and inflammation.

PGI_2 is unstable. Its half-life is estimated to be 3–4 min in aqueous solution, but is prolonged by plasma proteins, primarily albumins.[16,17] It is hydrolyzed to the chemically stable and biologically inactive metabolite, 6-keto-$PGF_{1\alpha}$ ($6KPGF_{1\alpha}$). $6KPGF_{1\alpha}$ is further metabolized to 2,3 donor $6KPGF_{1\alpha}$, which is considered valuable for estimating in vivo PGI_2 synthesis.[18]

Thrombomodulin

Thrombomodulin (TM) is a glycoprotein constitutively expressed on the luminal surface of endothelium.[19] Thrombin generated on the vessel wall binds TM, and the bound thrombin cleaves a peptide from protein C and converts it into an enzymatically active protein C (aPC).[20] Activated protein C is a potent anticoagulant. With protein S as a cofactor, aPC degrades coagulation factors V_a, and VIII_a, thereby limiting coagulation activity.

Heparin-Like Molecules

Thrombin occupies a central position in coagulation and hemostasis. It is a potent proteolytic enzyme responsible for converting fibrinogen to fibrin, activating factor VII, and also activating a number of other procoagulant factors. Moreover, through its binding to a specific receptor on platelets, it activates platelets and induces platelet secretion and aggregation. Thrombin activity is neutralized by at least two mechanisms: (1) neutralization by plasma antithrombins and (2) inactivation by binding to thrombomodulin. Two plasma antithrombin proteins have been clearly defined: (1) antithrombin III (AT-III) and (2) heparin cofactor II. The neutralizing properties of both molecules require heparin or its analogs as a cofactor.[21] Heparin enhances the binding affinity of AT-III for thrombin. The endothelial cell is capable of synthesizing and expressing biologically active heparin-like molecules on its luminal surface.[22] These membrane-associated heparin molecules appear to have a major physiological function in maintaining blood fluidity.

Plasminogen Activators

Plasminogen activators are enzymes that catalyze the conversion of plasminogen to plasmin. Plasmin is a potent proteolytic enzyme that lyses fibrin clot. Plasminogen activators are, hence, crucial for fibrinolysis. At least two types of plasminogen activators—tissue type (tPA) and urokinase (uPA)—have been characterized. Physiologically, tPA plays a critical role in plasmin generation at the site of fibrin formation and consequently in the lysis of thrombi. Normal endothelial cells produce and release tPA continuously to maintain a steady-state blood level of tPA. In the absence of fibrin formation, tPA has only a weak activity on plasma plasminogen, and only negligible plasmin is generated. Moreover, tPA activity is checked by a specific inhibitor, i.e., plasminogen activator inhibitor-1 (PAI-1), which binds tPA and neutralizes its activity.[23] PAI-1 is also synthesized in endothelial cells.[24] Balance between tPA and PAI-1 production and release appears to be critical for maintaining a normal fibrinolytic potential.

Surface Ecto-Enzymes: ADPase

The endothelial cell surface possesses a number of enzymes, notably ADPase, ATPase, and angiotensin-converting enzyme. ADPase is considered to be of physiological importance because of its ability to degrade ADP. ADP is stored in the dense granules of platelets and is released on platelet activation. It is a major mediator of platelet aggregation and a contributor to vasoconstriction.[25]

Endothelium-Derived Relaxing Factor (EDRF)

Nitric oxide (NO) is a major, if not the only EDRF. Its synthesis is catalyzed by nitric oxide synthase (NOS). At least two types of NO synthase have been cloned from bovine and human endothelial cells.[26,27] NO synthase catalyzes the conversion of L-arginine into citrulline and NO. NO produced by endothelial cells diffuses into the smooth muscle cells lying underneath the endothelial cells. Its smooth muscle relaxing action is mediated by increasing cyclic GMP formation in the cell. NO acts synergistically with PGI_2 in inhibiting platelet activation and smooth muscle cell relaxation. Recent studies indicate that NO is produced by other cells, including neurons and macrophages, and has diverse biological activities and physiological functions.[28]

Maintenance of Blood Fluidity

Circulating blood contains a myriad of cells, proteins, and other biologically active molecules. Blood cells, such as platelets and granulocytes, are prone to aggregation and adhesion. Plasma proteins, particularly the coagulation factors, have the propensity for forming blood clots.[29–31] The circulating blood, however, stays fluid even when the blood vessel is severely damaged. In fact, blood fluidity is a prerequisite for survival. What maintains blood fluidity? This was considered to be a fundamental question that received much attention and debate in the 19th century. Ingenious experiments at that time pointed out the importance of the endothelial lining in maintaining blood fluidity.[1] Advances in the past decade have provided solid evidence to support these earlier observations. Moreover, advances at the molecular level have begun to shed light on its biochemical mechanisms. At quiescent states or under minor insults, blood fluidity is maintained by steady blood flow, and negative cell-surface charges fortified by potent inhibitory molecules expressed by the endothelium. Since the coagulation system and platelet activation are interdependent and mutually amplifying, once platelets and coagulation are activated, the reaction is increasingly magnified and becomes perpetual unless they are controlled by inhibitory molecules. Recent studies using sensitive immunoassays for coagulation peptides provide convincing evidence for a low-grade coagulation activation in healthy human subjects.[31] These findings imply that the defense molecules are in constant operation to keep coagulation and platelet activation in check. As described above, a majority of the inhibitory molecules are derived from the vascular endothelium. Their key actions are listed in Table 1. These molecules are constitutively expressed either on the luminal surface of the endothelium or released into the adjacent site. Of particular interest is thrombomodulin, which is not an active inhibitory molecule *per se*, but by binding to thrombin, it enables thrombin to cleave protein C and generate activated protein C (aPC). aPC and its cofactor protein S inactivate factor Va and VIIIa, thereby decelerating the reaction rate of coagulation.[20] Once thrombin is bound to TM, it is eventually degraded. TM, therefore, serves as a surface molecule not only for thrombin-induced aPC formation, but also for neutralizing one of the most potent and important mediators of fibrin formation and platelet aggregation. Thrombin appears to occupy a central position in coagulation and platelet activation. It catalyzes the final stage of fibrin formation, and is an extremely potent agonist for platelet activation and aggregation. In the presence of heparin-like molecules, it is bound to antithrombin-III, and the complex is cleared. It is also neutralized by heparin cofactor II. Hence, there exist at least three types of molecules that neutralize this powerful mediator of coagulation and platelet aggregation. Through its binding to thrombomodulin, it downregulates its own production.

Prostacyclin and nitric oxide are produced in minute quantities normally, and because of the extremely short half-life of these molecules in circulation, they act in a paracrine fashion. They act synergistically on platelets, reducing platelet adhesion to damaged vascular wall and inhibiting platelet activation and aggregation. NO also acts synergistically with PGI_2, in relaxing vascular smooth muscle. These two molecules are critical for preventing platelets from interacting with the vascular endothelium and for maintaining a normal vascular tone.

Endothelial Cells and Hemostasis

Normal Hemostasis

These defense molecules also play a critical role in rendering blood fluid even in the presence of blood vessel severance. When a blood vessel is severed, hemostatic plugs are formed by complex cell–cell, protein–protein, and protein–cell interactions and reactions. The initiating event is triggered by the exposure of subendothelial tissues following the depletion of the endothelial lining. The subendothelial materials, notably collagen, activate platelets and serve as an anchor tissue for platelet adhesion. Platelet adhesion is critical for the subsequent platelet aggregation. Platelet adhesion is mediated by von Willebrand factor (VWF), a multimeric molecule synthesized by vascular endothelial cells and mega-karyocytes.[32] It is synthesized as a prepro-VWF monomer that undergoes several steps of posttranslational modification and multimerization to form the active mature multimer of about 20 million mol wt.[33] In endothelial cells, it is constitutively synthesized, stored in Weibel-Palade bodies, and released into the plasma to maintain a stable plasma level adequate for hemostasis. In plasma, the multimeric vWF undergoes degradation to yield a spectrum of lower-molecular-weight multimers that are eventually cleared. Demultimerization is thought to be the result of the action of pro-teases, but the identity of these proteases remains unknown. The high-molecular-weight VWF multimers are thought to be the active component.

VWF is a putative platelet adhesive molecule. The exact mechanism by which it mediates platelet adhesion to damaged vascular wall has not been entirely elucidated. It is certain, however, that platelet adhesion requires its binding to platelet membrane glycoprotein Ib-IX complex.[34] It has been suggested that the VWF multimer serves as a bridge molecule between platelets and subendothelial matrix by binding to its platelet GPIb-IX receptor on one end and to the matrix receptor on the other.[35] Recent studies indicate that under shear stress, VWF is the primary ligand for platelet aggregation.[36] The important role that VWF plays in platelet adhesion and aggregation in vivo is supported by increased bleeding tendency when VWF is reduced.

Subendothelial matrix contains substances that activate coagulation and platelets. Tissue factor in the matrix serves as a cofactor for factor VII/VIIa-dependent coagulation activation.[37] Collagen and probably other yet unidentified substances in the subendothelial matrix convert platelets from metabolically quiescent to active cells. The activated platelets undergo rapid membrane, cytoskeletal, and metabolic changes. As a result of cell membrane phospholipid rearrangements, the outer membrane becomes a binding site for factor Va and factor VIIIa whereby coagulation reaction is accelerated and generation of thrombin is enhanced.[29,30] Membrane glycoprotein IIb-IIIa complex undergoes conformational changes and, consequently, becomes an effective receptor for fibrinogen binding, which leads to platelet aggregation.[38] Activation of cytoskeletal proteins in platelets results in centralization and secretion of dense granules and α granules. Adenosine diphosphate (ADP) and serotonin from the dense granules, in turn, activate adjacent platelets and induce platelet aggregation. Collagen, thrombin, and several other agonists are capable of activating platelet phospholipase A_2, which catalyzes the liberation of arachidonic acid (AA), and the liberated AA is converted into thomboxane A_2 (TXA_2).[39] TXA_2 causes further platelet activation and secretion. Hence, the initial activation by collagen is followed by amplification of platelet activation and recruitment of new platelets into formation of an increasingly large mass. Activation of platelets fortifies thrombin generation and fibrin formation, and thrombin, in turn, causes platelet activation and aggregation. The interdependent and mutually enhancing relationship between platelets and coagulation leads to the formation of a growing mass of platelets enmeshed in fibrin. These explosive and perpetual reactions must be kept in check. Otherwise, the platelet-fibrin clot would propagate and eventually occlude the entire blood vessel. Multiple mechanisms participate in controlling the propagation of clots, and these mechanisms are not entirely known. However, the molecules discussed earlier play major roles in controlling the growth of the hemostatic plug and thrombus. These molecules probably work concurrently and synergistically to reduce platelet activation, aggregation, and recruitment, and to suppress coagulation reaction. PGI_2 and NO act in concert to inhibit platelet secretion and aggregation, and to prevent vasospasm, whereas ecto-ADPase on the endothelial surface degrades ADP, thereby reducing further platelet aggregate formation. Thrombomodulin-bound thrombin activates protein C, and the activated protein C digests factor Va and VIIIa, whereas heparin-like molecules on the endothelial surface serve as the cofactor for antithrombin-mediated inactivation of thrombin, factor Xa, factor IXa, and factor XIa. Recent studies indicate that endothelial cells produce tissue-factor pathway inhibitor (TFPI), which inactivates factor VIIa-TF.[40] These inhibitory molecules act at different sites of the coagulation cascade to ensure that thrombin generation, as well as the level of activated coagulation factors, is under tight control and fibrin formation is checked.

Thrombosis

Loss of these defense molecules owing to extensive vascular damage, such as atherosclerosis, results in the development of massive mural thrombus, causing obstruction of arteries leading to catastrophic tissue ischemia and infarction. Emboli may arise from carotid arteries, and cause intracerebral arterial occlusion and thrombotic stroke.

Perturbation of endothelium by endotoxins (lipopolysaccharide, LPS), cytokines, and possibly other types of insults may lead to drastic functional changes without overt morphological evidence of endothelial damage. These insults may suppress the expression of defense molecules and induce the expression of procoagulant molecules, converting the endothelium from an "antithrombotic" tissue to a "pro-thrombotic" tissue. Since loss of the defense molecules may contribute significantly to development of vascular diseases, a new therapeutic strategy to restore and/or enhance the endothelial cell antithrombotic properties by gene transfer is being developed.[41-44] Retroviral and adenoviral vectors have been used to transfer and strongly express the desired genes into vascular endothelial or smooth muscle cells. For example, to enhance tPA production, tPA gene has been inserted into a retroviral or adenoviral vector wherein the viral genome responsible for viral replication and capsid formation is removed. In their places, reporter genes such as β-galactosidase (β-gal), and neomycin-resistant genes are inserted. Replication-defective viral particles are generated by incubating the viral vectors with a packaging cell line wherein the viral genome has been inserted into the chromosomes of the cultured cell line. The packaging cell line is incapable of producing viral particles because it lacks the DNA signal for assembling the viral capsids. When the packaging cell line is transfected with the viral vector carrying the desired gene to be transferred, replication-defective viral particles are produced. The viral particles that possess intact capsid proteins are amphotropic, and can effectively infect vascular endothelial or smooth muscle cells. The desired gene along with powerful retroviral promoter (long terminal repeat, LTR) and neomycin-resistant gene are incorporated onto the host cell chromosome and become a transcription unit. In vitro cultured cell experiments and the implantation of autologous endothelial cells on stents in in vivo experiments confirmed the validity of increasing tPA production by this approach. The protective action and antithrombotic efficacy of this approach remain to be established. We have recently inserted PGHS-1 gene into a retroviral vector BAG[45] and generated replication-defective viral particles carrying this gene in a ψCRIP packaging cell line.[46] We then infected a cultured endothelial cell line, EA.hy926, with this vector and showed that by increasing PGHS enzyme expression, there was a marked increase in PGI_2 synthesis.[47] Work is now in progress to evaluate the effects of overexpressing the PGHS gene, and consequently enhanced PGI_2 synthesis on carotid intimal hyperplasia and thrombosis.

Endothelial Cells and Inflammation

Acute inflammation is characterized by infiltration of neutrophils, monocytes-macrophages, and lymphocytes. Release from these activated leukocytes of proteases, cytokines, and lipid mediators is responsible for most of the inflammatory reactions. A critical step in inflammation is the migration of these leukocytes from intravascular to extravascular space. Quiescent endothelium confines the leukocytes within the lumen of blood vessels. During inflammation, receptors for leukocyte adhesive molecules (integrins) are rapidly expressed on the endothelial cell surface.[48] Expression of endothelial cell adhesive molecules (CAMS) permits the binding of leukocyte integrins and adhesion of leukocytes to the endothelial cell surface. Leukocyte-endothelial cell adhesion is followed by migration and/or transgression of these cells into the extracellular space.

A number of endothelial cell adhesive molecules have been identified and characterized.[48] Based on their similarity to known molecules, they are categorized into two major groups: (1) immunoglobulin (Ig) gene superfamily and (2) selectin family. Belonging to group 1 are ICAM-1, ICAM-2, and VCAM-1, and to group 2 are P-selectin (GMP140 or PADGM), E-selectin (ELAM-1), and L-selectin. All the molecules except ICAM-2 are not expressed constitutively on the endothelial cell surface. On stimulation by inflammatory mediators, they are expressed either by *de novo* protein synthesis or through translocation from stored granules. P-selectins are stored in the Weibel-Palade bodies of endothelial cells, which are translocated to the plasma membrane, after which P-selectins are secreted following stimulation by thrombin and inflammatory mediators. E-selectin, ICAM-1, and VCAM-1 are not presynthesized and stored, but are synthesized on stimulation.

These newly expressed receptors recognize specific ligands on leukocyte membranes. Several ligands have been purified and characterized. The specificity and selectivity of ligand–receptor interactions in inflammation are not entirely clear. Recent studies indicate that neutrophil adhesion is mediated at least in part by binding of neutrophil membrane integrins CD11/CD18, notably LFA-1 (CD11A/CD18) to endothelial cell surface ICAM-1. The adhesion process is likely to be more complicated and may involve multiple ligand–receptor interactions.

Release of P-selectin adhesive molecules to the endothelial cell surface is considered to be responsible for the rapid transgression of neutrophils. The ligand for P-selectin is not clearly defined, but several molecules have been identified and are being characterized.[49]

IL-1 stimulates endothelial cells to produce inflammatory mediators, such as PGE_2, PGI_2, and platelet activating factor (PAF). Microvascular endothelial cells may differ from arterial and venous endothelial cells in their capacity for generating eicosanoids. PGE_2 appears to be the predominant product of some microvascular endothelial cells, such as those from the foreskin, whereas PGI_2 is the major product of larger vessels. The brain microvascular endothelial cells generate a substantial quantity of PGI_2. The mechanism by which IL-1 stimulates PGE_2 and PGI_2 formation in cultured endothelial cells has been elucidated. IL-1 not only activates phospholipase A_2 and releases arachidonic acid, but also induces *de novo* synthesis of PGH synthase. Since PGH synthase undergoes autoinactivation during catalysis, the capacity for PGE_2/PGI_2 synthesis is governed by the steady-state level of this enzyme. By inducing synthesis of this enzyme, IL-1 induces a prolonged stimulation and a higher capacity for the synthesis of these inflammatory eicosanoids than other agonists. Both PGE_2 and PGI_2 contribute to inflammatory responses, and may contribute to vascular hyperplasia and early atherosclerosis since these pathological lesions exhibit features similar to classic acute inflammation.

Inflammatory cytokines produced by activated monocytes–macrophages and lymphocytes exert profound effects on endothelial cell functions.[50] Several of the endothelial cell functions induced by cytokines have direct relevance to inflammation. Expression of adhesive molecules on cell surfaces has been described above. Neutrophils, monocytes, and lymphocytes are attracted to the endothelium. Adhesive molecules on leukocyte surfaces, notably LFA-1 and Mac-1, bind to endothelial cell-surface adhesive molecules, i.e., ICAM-1, which triggers further cellular changes eventually leading to migration of leukocytes through the endothelial layer. The transgressed macrophages and lymphocytes and the endothelial cells are stimulated to synthesize cytokines, which in turn induce the production and release of inflammatory mediators from endothelial cells, fibroblasts, and macrophages. This positive regulatory loop is considered to be the key mechanism for chronic inflammation and probably also for intimal fibromuscular hyperplasia.

Summary

Endothelial cells are biochemically active, capable of expressing an array of biologically active and physiologically important molecules. A major role of these molecules is to maintain patency of blood vessels and blood fluidity. Insults to the endothelium may lead to derangement in the expression of these defense molecules and expression of new molecules that promote blood cell adhesion and vasospasm. The brain comprises mostly microvascular endothelium. Although a wealth of knowledge has been accumulated over the past decade with respect to endothelial cell function and has been valuable for understanding brain physiology and biochemistry, it remains to be determined whether brain microvascular endothelium has unique characteristics and whether it contributes to region-specific function of brain. Work in this area has been hampered by difficulty in obtaining homogenous cultured cells from cerebral microvasculature and particularly cells from different regions of the brain. It is hoped that there will soon be technical breakthroughs leading to the successful culture of cerebral microvascular endothelial cells to allow better characterization of their specific functions.

Acknowledgments

The author wishes to thank Teri Trevino for secretarial assistance. The work is supported by grants from the National Institutes of Health (NS-23327 and HL-18584).

References

[1] Cirillo, V. T. (1983) *J. Med. Soc. NJ* **80,** 535–539.

[2] Jaffe, E. A., Nachman, N. L., Becker, C. G., and Minick, G. R. (1973) *J. Clin. Invest.* **52,** 2745–2756.

[3] Gimbrone, M. A., Jr., Cotran, R. S., and Folkman, J. (1973) *J. Cell Biol.* **60,** 674–683.

[4] Moncada, S. and Vane, J. R. (1979) *Pharmacol. Rev.* **30,** 293–331.

[5] Weksler, B. B., Ley, C. W., and Jaffe, E. A. (1978) *J. Clin. Invest.* **62,** 923–930.

[6] Baenziger, N. L., Force, L. E., and Becherer, P. R. (1980) *Biochem. Biophys. Res. Comm.* **92,** 1435–1440.

7   Rossi, V., Breviario, F., Ghezzi, P., Dejana, E., and Mantovani, A. (1985) *Science* **229**, 171–176.

8   Needleman, P., Turk, J., Jakshik, B. A., Morrison, A. R., and Leftowith, J. B. (1986) *Ann. Rev. Biochem.* **55**, 69–102.

9   Smith, W. L., Marnett, L. J., and DeWitt, D. L. (1991) *Pharmacol. Ther.* **49**, 157–179.

10 Maier, J. A. M., Hla, J., and Maciag, T. (1990) *J. Biol. Chem.* **265**, 10,805–10,808.

11 McIntire, T. M., Zimmerman, G. A., Satoh, K., and Prescott, S. M. (1985) *J. Clin. Invest.* **76**, 271–280.

12 DeWitt, D. L. and Smith, W. L. (1983) *J. Biol. Chem.* **258**, 3285–3293.

13 Marcus, A. J. (1990) *Meth. Enzymol.* **187**, 585–598.

14 Wu, K. K. and Papp, A. C. (1990) *Meth. Enzymol.* **187**, 578–584.

15 FitzGerald, G. A., Smith, B., Pederson, R. M., and Brash, A. R. (1984) *N. Engl. J. Med.* **310**, 1065–1068.

16 Tsai, A.-L., Hsu, M.-J., Patsch, W., and Wu, K. K. (1991) *Biochim. Biophys. Acta* **1115**, 131–140.

17 Lucas, F. U., Skrinska, V. A., Chisolm, G. M., and Hesse, B. L. (1986) *Thromb. Res.* **43**, 379–387.

18 FitzGerald, G. A., Pedersen, A. K., and Patrono, C. (1983) *Circulation* **67**, 1174–1177.

19 Dittman, W. A. and Majerus, P. W. (1990) *Blood* **75**, 329–336.

20 Esmon, C. T. (1987) *Science* **235**, 1348–1352.

21 Marcum, J. A. and Rosenberg, R. D. (1985) *Biochem. Biophys. Res. Comm.* **126**, 365–372.

22 Stone, A. L. Beeler, D., Oosta, G., and Rosenberg, R. D. (1982) *Proc. Natl. Acad. Sci. USA* **79**, 7190–7194

23 Loskutoff, D. J. and Edgington, T. S. (1977) *Proc. Natl. Acad. Sci. USA* **74**, 3903–3907.

24 Schleef, R. R., Bevilacqua, M. P., Swadey, M., Gimbrone, M. A., Jr., and Loskutoff, D. *J. Biol. Chem.* **26**, 5797–5803.

25 Marcus, A. J., Safieu, L. B., Hajjak, A., Ulman, H. L., Islam, N., Boekman, M. J., and Eirra, A. M. (1991) *J. Clin. Invest.* **88**, 1690–1696.

26 Sessa, W. C., Harrison, J. K., Barber, C. M., Zeng, D., Durieux, M. E., D'Angelo, D. D., Lynch, K. R., and Peach, M. J. (1992) *J. Biol. Chem.* **267**, 15,274–15,276.

27 Janssens, S. P., Shimouchi, A., Quertermous, T., Bloch, D. B., and Bloch, K. D. (1992) *J. Biol. Chem.* **267**, 14,519–14,522.

28 Bredt, D. S., Hwang, P. M., and Snyder, S. H. (1990) *Nature* **347**, 768–770.

29 Roberts, H. R. and Lozier, J. N. (1992) *Hosp. Pract.* **27(1)**, 97–116.

30 Furie, B. and Furie, B. C. (1988) *Cell* **53**, 505–518.

31 Rosenberg, R. D. (1987) *The Molecular Basis of Blood Diseases* (Stamatoyanopoulos, G., ed.), W. B. Saunders, Philadelphia, PA, pp. 534–574.

32 Ruggeri, Z. M. and Zimmerman, T. S. (1987) *Blood* **70**, 895–904.

[33] Handin, R. I. and Wagner, D. D. (1989) *Prog. Hemost. Thromb.* **9,** 233–259.

[34] Fox, J. E. B., Aggerveck, L. P., and Berndt, M. C. (1988) *J. Biol. Chem.* **263,** 4882–4890.

[35] Fauvel, F., Grant, M. E., Legrand, Y. J., Souchon, H., Tobelem, G., Jackson, D. S., and Caen, J. P. (1983) *Proc. Natl. Acad. Sci. USA* **80,** 551–554.

[36] Houdijk, W. M. P., Sakasiassen, K. S., Nievelstein, P. F. E. M., and Sixma, J. J. (1985) *J. Clin. Invest.* **75,** 531–540.

[37] Edgington, T. S., Mackman, N., Brand, K., and Ruf, W. (1991) *Thromb. Haemost.* **66,** 67–79.

[38] Bennet, J. S., Shattil, S. J., Power, J. W., and Gartner, T. K. (1988) *J. Biol. Chem.* **263,** 12,948–12,953.

[39] Samuelsson, B., Goldyne, M., Granstrom, E., Hamberg, M., Hammarstrom, S., and Malmsten, C. (1987) *Ann. Rev. Biochem.* **47,** 997–1029.

[40] Broze, G. J., Jr. (1992) *Hosp. Pract.* **27(3),** 71–104.

[41] Nabel, E. G., Plautz, G., and Nabel, G. J. (1991) *JACC* **17,** 189B–194B.

[42] Wilson, J. M., Birinyi, L. K., Salomon, R. N., Libby, P., Callow, A. D., and Mulligan, R. C. (1989) *Science* **244,** 1344–1346.

[43] Dichek, D. A., Neville, R. F., Zwiebel, J. A., Freeman, S. M., Leon, M. B., and Anderson, F. (1989) *Circulation* **80,** 1347–1353.

[44] Lim, C. S., Chapman, G. D., Gammon, R. S., Muhlstein, J. B., Bauman, R. P., Stack, R. S., and Swain, J. L. (1991) *Circulation* **83,** 2007–2011.

[45] Price, J., Turner, D., and Cepko, C. (1987) *Proc. Natl. Acad. Sci. USA* **84,** 156–160.

[46] Mann, R., Mulligan, R. C., and Baltimore, D. (1983) *Cell* **33,** 153–159.

[47] Xu, X.-M., Sanduja, S. K., Ohashi, K., Wang, L.-H., and Wu, K. K. *J. Clin. Invest.* **91,** 1843–1849.

[48] Osborn, L. (1990) *Cell* **62,** 3–6.

[49] Moore, K. L., Stults, N. L., Diaz, S., Smith, D. F., Cummings, R. D., Varki, A., and McEver, R. P. (1992) *J. Cell. Biol.* **118,** 445–456.

[50] Pober, J. S. and Cotran, R. S. (1990) *Physiol. Rev.* **70,** 427–451.

Chapter 27

The Role of 21-Aminosteroids in Cerebral Ischemia and Reperfusion

Mark A. Helfaer, Jeffrey R. Kirsch, and Richard J. Traystman

Introduction

Damage associated with cerebral ischemia occurs during the ischemic event as well as after the commencement of reperfusion. Reperfusion injury may be caused by a compromise in perfusion owing to diminished blood pressure as occurs, for example, with heart failure, or an elevation of intracranial pressure, as in cerebral edema. In the cascade of deleterious events following ischemia and reperfusion, a final pathway of lipid peroxidation may be entered. This pathway, if interrupted, could potentially halt subsequent injury. The 21-aminosteroids are agents that demonstrate the ability to inhibit lipid peroxidation.

Pathophysiology Leading to Lipid Peroxidation in Brain Following Ischemia and Reperfusion

Oxygen radicals are believed to be important initiators of lipid peroxidation associated with ischemia and reperfusion.[1,2] In brief, oxygen radical production may result from an overreduced electron-transport chain during ischemia.[3] During ischemia, there is calcium influx into cells, which presumably sets the stage for production of oxygen radicals during reperfusion. During reperfusion,

From *The Human Brain Circulation*, R. D. Bevan and J. A. Bevan, eds.
©1994 Humana Press

breakdown products of arachidonic acid,[4] adenosine,[5] or a mechanism involving leukocytes[6,7] have been elucidated as mediators of oxygen radical production. Superoxide is one oxygen radical that, although not as reactive as other radical species, can be produced by these processes and either results in direct injury[8,9] or can react with other species to produce more injury. In the presence of a metal catalyst (e.g., ferrous ion, but not ferric ion), superoxide can be converted to the more reactive hydroxyl radical by Fenton chemistry. Hydroxyl radicals react with almost every type of molecule found in living cells.[10]

Recently, a nitric oxide mechanism has been proposed to explain the sequence of events leading to radical mediated brain injury. Nitric oxide is produced during conversion of arginine to citrulline by nitric oxide synthase in endothelium, astrocytes, and neurons.[11] Increased nitric oxide production presumably occurs during ischemia via a mechanism that involves release of excitatory amino acids and stimulation of excitatory amino acid receptors.[12] Although nitric oxide itself does not appear to be toxic to the brain, reaction with superoxide produced during ischemia and reperfusion may result in formation of peroxynitrites,[13] which have a reactivity similar to hydroxyl radicals.

Regardless of the source, these radical species may provoke iron-dependent lipid peroxidation where the unpaired electron of a radical attacks unsaturated fatty acids within the cell membrane.[10] In short, a hydroxyl-like radical is able to remove hydrogen from polyunsaturated fatty acids, creating a carbon centered radical that quickly reacts with oxygen to give a peroxy radical.[14] Peroxy radical can perpetuate the chain and convert itself into a lipid hydroperoxide. Lipid hydroperoxides can produce alkoxy and peroxy radicals in the presence of transition metal ions (e.g., iron) to yield carbonyl products. These radicals are highly reactive and may rapidly induce formation of conjugated dienes.[15,16] Lipid peroxidation is enhanced in in vitro systems by lactic acidosis;[17] however, that has not been substantiated in in vivo systems.[18] Evidence for lipid peroxidation can be obtained by measuring tissue levels of conjugated dienes or malonaldehyde.[19,20] More indirect evidence for lipid peroxidation in the brain following ischemia and reperfusion comes from detecting a change in endogenous levels of naturally occurring antioxidants.[21,22]

In the brain, lipid peroxidation has been demonstrated in in vitro preparations of anoxia and reoxygenation,[23,24] and in some[25-27] in vivo models of ischemia and reperfusion. There is a correlation of increased lipid peroxidation in regions with increased vulnerability to ischemia and reperfusion.[27] Thus, secondary injury can be ongoing long after the primary insult has been completed and explains the sometimes delayed deterioration that can occur following the insult. The importance of lipid peroxidation in the pathophysiology of brain injury from ischemia and reperfusion remains controversial. Information available to delineate the potential importance of lipid peroxidation comes from studies that have administered inhibitors of oxygen radical pathways, or specifically of lipid peroxidation, and determined if these agents prevent neurologic injury following transient cerebral ischemia.

Inhibitors of oxygen radicals have limited success as therapeutic agents. For example, exogenously administered superoxide dismutase alone does not diminish the hyperemia[28] or delayed hypoperfusion,[19] or improve neurologic outcome[30] following global ischemia and reperfusion. In the setting of focal cerebral ischemia, however, administration of superoxide dismutase has been associated with improved neurologic outcome.[8,9,31] Likewise, superoxide dismutase decreases the amount of delayed development of vasogenic brain edema following brain injury.[32] Some of the limitation of the therapeutic efficacy of superoxide dismutase may be the result of its poor ability to penetrate the blood–brain barrier.[33,34]

Several antioxidants have also been tested for therapeutic efficacy in the setting of ischemia and reperfusion. α-Tocopherol is a nonenzymatic inhibitor of oxygen toxicity,[35] which has been demonstrated to inhibit lipid peroxidation in brain tissue taken from animals exposed to ischemia and reperfusion.[36] Likewise, α-tocopherol administration is associated with decreased lipid peroxidation in vivo, improved recovery of electrical function, decreased brain edema, and improved neurologic outcome.[37-40]

Corticosteroids have been used in a variety of clinical situations, including cases of neurologic injury. Promising anecdotal evidence prompted many physicians to investigate the efficacy of steroids in cases of neurologic injury, including stroke, and traumatic brain and spinal cord injury. In some models of cerebral ischemia, steroids have been demonstrated to decrease the flux of ions and fluid that leads to cerebral edema.[41] However, in other models, steroids do not improve edema caused by ischemia.[42-44] Steroids are also not effective in decreasing brain injury from focal[45] or global[46] ischemia in patients.

Steroid therapy is associated with problematic side effects, such as hyperglycemia, catabolic states, and increased incidence of serious infections.[47-49] These confounding metabolic effects of the glucocorticoids need to be removed to unmask the salutary effects of the drugs.[50] Bolstered by the modest successes of high-dose methylprednisolone studies,[51] development of related drugs continued with this latter focus in mind. This modest efficacy of steroid therapy in neurologic injury was demonstrated at doses that were far in excess of those used clinically, which led to the speculation that the mechanism of action was one different from the antiinflammatory actions attributed to steroids. The drugs that have shown the most promise are those with the steroid moiety backbone, but substituted in the 21 position.

Characteristics of 21-Aminosteroids

The best-studied 21-aminosteroid is tirilazad mesylate (U74006F;21-[-4-2(2,6-di-1-pyrrolidinyl-4-pyrimidinyl)-1-piperazinyl]-16α-pregna-1,4,9(11)-triene-3,20-dione, monomethane sulfonate). In in vitro systems, tirilazad mesylate inhibits ACTH secretion in cultured pituitary cells.[52] In in vivo systems, tirilazad mesylate stimulates release of ACTH in adrenalectomized rats;[52] however, it has no effect on the pituitary-adrenal axis in normal rats. Chronic tirilazad mesylate administration is also not associated with hyperglycemia, alteration in electrolytes, or loss of body weight because of hormonally mediated myopathic effects.[53,54] Tirilazad mesylate administration has no effect on thymus weight and no reduction in phytohemagglutinin-stimulated T-cell proliferation, which has been interpreted to indicate that the drug does not cause significant immunosuppression.[53] Although 21-amino-steroids are not potent oxygen radical scavengers, one 21-aminosteroid, U74500A, decreases oxygen radical production by monocytes in normal patients and patients with multiple sclerosis,[55] as well as from polymorphonuclear leukocytes in normal patients.[56] Whereas decreased oxygen radical production by leukocytes may be beneficial for several pathologic states caused by excessive leukocyte activity, it may have deleterious immunological effects. The effects of tirilazad mesylate on oxygen radical production have not been investigated.

21-Aminosteroids and Neurologic Ischemia

The 21-aminosteroids tirilazad mesylate[57] and U78517F[58] have been shown to reverse the tendency toward intracellular accumulation of calcium following cerebral ischemia. By the above synthesis, the last common pathway of neurologic injury regardless of the initiating event is by lipid peroxidation. Therefore, inhibition of lipid peroxidation should be an efficacious way to ameliorate the damage in neurologic injury. Tirilazad mesylate inhibits lipid peroxidation in vitro by a mechanism independent of iron in much the same way as α-tocopherol inhibits lipid peroxidation. In contrast, U74500A also acts as an iron chelator. Endogenous substances within the brain that prevent lipid peroxidation, such as α-tocopherol, are consumed in the face of ischemia, but when treated with 21-aminosteroids, α-tocopherol levels are preserved.[59] With an in vitro analog to ischemia (i.e., combined oxygen-glucose deprivation), U74500A affords protection against cell death. This effect was less than the effect of NMDA antagonists, but was additive with the latter, suggesting that the mechanism afforded by 21-aminosteroids is not related to the NMDA receptor.[60]

Results of studies evaluating the therapeutic efficacy of tirilazad mesylate are consistent with what would be expected from its actions to prevent significant lipid peroxidation through some mechanism involving membrane function. For example, it may be expected that the salutary effects of tirilazad mesylate may be greater in paradigms with accentuated lipid peroxidation and in models that allow sufficient time during reperfusion for lipid peroxidation to occur.

When tirilazad mesylate is administered after 12.5 min of cardiac arrest,[61] there is no effect on delayed hypoperfusion or return of $CMRO_2$ 4 h following the insult. However, the investigators indicate that the cardiac resuscitation efforts in the drug-treated animals were conducted with greater ease. In spite of demonstrating no immediate short-term therapeutic efficacy of tirilazad mesylate in terms of blood flow and metabolism, other investigators have demonstrated improved neurological outcome following transient global ischemia. Following 10 min of normothermic ventricular fibrillation, dogs treated during resuscitation with tirilazad mesylate demonstrated an improved neurologic status and decreased mortality 24 h after ischemia. However, this improvement could not be demonstrated until 10 h after the insult.[54] It is not clear that diminished mortality in tirilazad-mesylate-treated animals (83 vs 33%) may be partially attributed to a neuroprotective effect of the drug rather than a nonneurological effect on the cardiovascular or the renal systems.[62] Pretreatment prior to reperfusion with tirilazad mesylate also improved neurologic outcome following 12 min of complete cerebral ischemia produced by elevation of intracranial pressure.[59] Forty-eight hours following this injury, all tirilazad-mesylate-treated animals had a normal neurologic outcome, in contrast to the placebo-treated animals, which had significant neurologic impairments. In a similar experimental paradigm, tirilazad failed to effect the pattern of postischemic cerebral blood flow and the return of high-energy phosphates and somatosensory-evoked potentials.[63]

The neuroprotective effects of the 21-aminosteroids are somewhat different in the setting of incomplete ischemia. For example, early reports[64] demonstrated attenuation of hypoperfusion 3 h after 5 min of near complete cerebral ischemia induced by neck tourniquet inflation in cats. However, arterial blood pressure and CBF were better maintained in drug-treated animals. Associated with this improved maintenance of CBF was an improved recovery of somatosensory-evoked potential amplitude in drug-treated animals. Pretreatment with tirilazad mesylate 30 min prior to 10 min of bilateral carotid occlusion with hemorrhagic hypotension

(50 mmHg) in rats afforded benefits at 24 and 72 h. The parameters demonstrating an improvement were magnetic resonance imaging in neocortex (but not hippocampus) on each day after the insult, which correlated with histopathologic findings on day 3.[65] These findings might be in part because tirilazad mesylate attenuates the cardiovascular deterioration, which follows 2 h of hemorrhagic hypotension.[66]

In rats, however, treatment with tirilazad mesylate prior to and following transient forebrain ischemia did not result in improved histopathologic outcome.[67] Following transient incomplete forebrain ischemia, tirilazad-treated animals demonstrated an improved rate of recovery of high-energy phosphates with no effect of drug treatment on ultimate metabolic, blood flow, or electrical recovery.[68,69] On the contrary, in the setting of hyperglycemia, when accentuated lipid peroxidation would be anticipated, treatment with tirilazad mesylate improves both the rate and the ultimate metabolic recovery of dogs subjected to incomplete global cerebral ischemia.[68]

Testing of 21-aminosteroids in the setting of focal cerebral ischemia has produced mixed results. Following 3 h of unilateral carotid artery occlusion, gerbils have improved survival 24 and 48 h after ischemia when treated with 10 mg/kg of tirilazad mesylate. Other animals that survived this insult had histologic evidence of protection with drug administration[70] after 24 h. Hall and Travis have demonstrated that tirilazad mesylate inhibits brain edema.[71] However, Young et al.[72] found that tirilazad mesylate could inhibit postischemic edema formation only if collateral flow was present. Utilizing a middle cerebral artery occlusion model in rats, treatment after the occlusion resulted in less ionic flux and edema formation 24 h after the occlusion.[72] On the contrary, Hoffman and colleagues reported no improvement in neurologic outcome score or histopathology for 3 d following unilateral carotid occlusion with hemorrhagic hypotension (30 mmHg) for 30 min[73] in rats. The lack of delivery of the drug during ischemia would explain the negative results of Hoffman et al.,[73] in which the ischemic insult (30 min of unilateral carotid occlusion coupled with hypotension to 35 mmHg) could prevent sufficient quantities of drug in the tissue during ischemia.

Some encouraging results examining the effects on spinal cord ischemia have been reported using a model of 25 min of infrarenal aortic clamping in rabbits. Pretreatment with 10 mg/kg of tirilazad mesylate 10 min prior to ischemia and 0.75 mg/kg every hour for 6 h following release of the crossclamp conferred significant neurologic protection. Specifically, five out of nine tirilazad-mesylate treated animals were neurologically normal whereas only one out of 10 of the vehicle-treated animals was normal.[7] The results of these studies evaluating the efficacy of 21-aminosteroids in models of ischemic nervous tissue are enticing, yet conflicting.

Conclusions

The protective effect of the 21-aminosteroids in cerebral ischemia may be based on the antiinflammatory properties or ability to inhibit lipid peroxidation. The antiinflammatory properties are similar to those of the glucocorticoid steroids, but without the hyperglycemic and catabolic effects. The antiinflammatory effects may be most clear in cases in which the drug inhibits edema formation and deleterious ion fluxes. The mechanism by which swelling and edema formation are inhibited may be the result of the ability of the drug to inhibit lipid peroxidation. Regardless of the mechanism, given the data of the agents investigated, 21-aminosteroid administration does not ameliorate all injury from ischemia. The aminosteriods are likely to play an important role in a multimodality approach[75] in the care of patients suffering from cerebral ischemia. These agents will be utilized in concert with other manipulations to preserve cardiovascular function as well as preventing the cascade of deleterious events that follow such injuries.

References

[1] Traystman, R. J., Kirsch, J. R., and Koehler, R. C. (1991) *J. Appl. Physiol.* **71,** 1185–1195.
[2] Kontos, H. A. and Wei, E. P. (1986) *J. Neurosurg.* **64,** 803–807.
[3] Cino, M. and Del Maestro, R. F. (1989) *Arch. Biochem. Biophys.* **269,** 623–638.
[4] Armstead, W. M., Mirro, R., Busija, D. W., and Leffler, C. W. (1988) *Am. J. Physiol.* **255,** H401–H403.

5   Patt, A., Harken, A. H., Burton, L. K., Rodell, T. C., Piermattei, D., Schorr, W. J., Parker, N. B., Berger, E. M., Horesh, I. R., and Terada, L. S. (1988) *J. Clin. Invest.* **81,** 1556–1562.

6   Kochanek, P. M., Dutka, A. J., and Hallenbeck, J. M. (1987) *Stroke* **18,** 634–637.

7   Hallenbeck, J. M., Dutka, A. J., Tanishima, T., Kochanek, P. M., Kumaroo, K. K., Thompson, C. B., Obrenovitch, T. P., and Contreras, T. J. (1986) *Stroke* **17,** 246–253.

8   Imaizumi, S., Woolworth, V., Fishman, R. A., and Chan, P. H. (1990) *Stroke* **21,** 1312–1317.

9   Matsumiya, N., Koehler, R. C., Kirsch, J. R., and Traystman, R. J. (1991) *Stroke* **22,** 1193–1200.

10 Halliwell, B. and Gutteridge, J. M. (1984) *Biochem. J.* **219,** 1–14.

11 Palmer, R. M. and Moncada, S. (1989) *Biochem. Biophys. Res. Commun.* **158,** 348–352.

12 Garthwaite, J., Garthwaite, G., Palmer, R. M., and Moncada, S. (1989) *Eur. J. Pharmacol.* **172,** 413–416.

13 Beckman, J. S., Beckman, T. W., Chen, J., Marshall, P. A., and Freeman, B. A. (1990) *Proc. Natl. Acad. Sci. USA* **87,** 1620–1624.

14 Bielski, B. H., Arudi, R. L., and Sutherland, M. W. (1983) *J. Biol. Chem.* **258,** 4759–4761.

15 Hasegawa, K. and Patterson, L. K. (1978) *Photochem. Photobiol.* **28,** 817–823.

16 Small, R. D., Scaiano, J. C., and Patterson, L. K. (1979) *Photochem. Photobiol.* **29,** 49–51.

17 Rehncrona, S., Hauge, H. N., and Siesjo, B. K. (1989) *J. Cereb. Blood Flow Metab.* **9,** 65–70.

18 Lundgren, J., Zhang, H., Agardh, C.-D., Smith, M.-L., Evans, P. J., Halliwell, B., and Siesjo, B. K. (1991) *J. Cereb. Blood Flow Metab.* **11,** 587–596.

19 Pryor, W. A., Stanley, J. P., and Blair, E. (1976) *Lipids* **11,** 370–379.

20 Dahle, L. K., Hill, E. G., and Holman, R. T. (1962) *Arch. Biochem. Biophys.* **98,** 253–261.

21 Rehncrona, S., Smith, D. S., Akesson, B., Westerberg, E., and Siesjo, B. K. (1980) *J. Neurochem.* **34,** 1630–1638.

22 Siesjo, B. K., Bendek, G., Koide, T., Westerberg, E., and Wieloch, T. (1985) *J. Cereb. Blood Flow Metab.* **5,** 253–258.

23 Kogure, K., Watson, B. D., Busto, R., and Abe, K. (1982) *Neurochem. Res.* **7,** 437–454.

24 Yoshida, S., Abe, K., Busto, R., Watson, B. D., Kogure, K., and Ginsberg, M. D. (1982) *Brain Res.* **245,** 307–316.

25 Watson, B. D., Busto, R., Goldberg, W. J., Santiso, M., Yoshida, S., and Ginsberg, M. D. (1984) *J. Neurochem.* **42,** 268–274.

26 Yoshida, S., Abe, K., Busto, R., Watson, B. D., Kogure, K., and Ginsberg, M. D. (1982) *Brain Res* **245**, 307–316.

27 Bromont, C., Marie, C., and Bralet, J. (1989) *Stroke* **20**, 918–924.

28 Helfaer, M. A., Kirsch, J. R., Haun, S. E., Moore, L. E., and Traystman, R. J. (1991) *Am. J. Physiol.* **261**, H548–H553.

29 Schurer, L., Grogaard, B., Gerdin, B., and Arfors, K. E. (1990) *Acta Neurochir.* **103**, 163–170.

30 Forsman, M., Fleischer, J. E., Milde, J. H., Steen, P. A., and Michenfelder, J. D. (1988) *Acta Anaesthesiol. Scand.* **32**, 152–155.

31 Liu, T. H., Beckman, J. S., Freeman, B. A., Hogan, E. L., and Hsu, C. Y. (1989) *Am. J. Physiol.* **256**, H589–H593.

32 Chan, P. H., Longar, S., and Fishman, R. A. (1987) *Ann. Neurol.* **21**, 540–547.

33 Petkau, A., Chelack, W. S., Kelly, K., Barefoot, C., and Monasterski, L. (1976) *Res. Commun. Chem. Pathol. Pharmacol.* **15**, 641–654.

34 Haun, S. E., Kirsch, J. R., Helfaer, M. A., Kubos, K. L., and Traystman, R. J. (1991) *Stroke* **22**, 655–659.

35 Tappel, A. L. (1972) *Ann. NY Acad. Sci.* **203**, 12–28.

36 Yoshida, S., Busto, R., Santiso, M., and Ginsberg, M. D. (1984) *J. Cereb. Blood Flow Metab.* **4**, 466–469.

37 Yamamoto, M., Shima, T., Uozumi, T., Sogabe, T., Yamada, K., and Kawasaki, T. (1983) *Stroke* **14**, 977–982.

38 Suzuki, J., Abiko, H., Mizoi, K., Oba, M., and Yoshimoto, T. (1987) *Acta Neurochir. (Wien.)* **88**, 56–64.

39 Yoshida, S., Busto, R., Santiso, M., and Ginsberg, M. D. (1984) *J. Cereb. Blood Flow Metab.* **4**, 466–469.

40 Fleischer, J. E., Lanier, W. L., Milde, J. H., and Michenfelder, J. D. (1987) *Stroke* **18**, 124–127.

41 Betz, A. L., and Coester, H. C. (1990) *Stroke* **21**, 1199–1204.

42 Plum, F. (1963) *Arch. Neurol.* **9**, 571–573.

43 Ito, U., Ohno, K., Suganuma, Y., Suzuki, K., and Inaba, Y. (1980) *Stroke* **11**, 166–172.

44 Siegel, B. A., Studer, R. K., and Potchen, E. J. (1972) *Arch. Neurol.* **27**, 209–212.

45 Patten, B. M., Mendell, J., Bruun, B., Curtin, W., and Carter, S. (1972) *Neurology (Minneapolis)* **22**, 377–383.

46 Jastremski, M., Sutton Tyrrell, K., Vaagenes, P., Abramson, N., Heiselman, D., and Safar, P. (1989) *JAMA* **262**, 3427–3430.

47 DeMaria, E. J., Reichman, W., Kenney, P. R., Armitage, J. M., and Gann, D. S. (1985) *Ann. Surg.* **202**, 248–252.

48 Deutschman, C. S., Konstantinides, F. N., Raup, S., and Cerra, F. B. (1987) *J. Neurosurg.* **66**, 388–395.

49 Robertson, C. S., Clifton, G. L., and Goodman, J. C. (1985) *J. Neurosurg.* **63**, 714–718.

50 Sapolsky, R. M. and Pulsinelli, W. A. (1985) *Science* **229**, 1397–1400.
51 Bracken M. B., Shepard, M. J., Collins, W. F., Holford, T. R., Young, W., Baskin, D. S., Eisenberg, H. M., Flamm, E., Leo-Summers, L., Maroon, J., Marshall, L. F., Perot, P. L., Piepmeier, J., Sonntag, V. K. H., Wagner, F. C., Wilberger, J. E., and Winn, H. R. (1990) *N. Engl. J. Med.* **322**, 1405–1411.
52 Burrin, J. M. and Hart, G. R. (1990) *J. Endocrinol.* **126**, 203–209.
53 Braughler, J. M., Chase, R. L., Neff, G. L., Yonkers, P. A., Day, J. S., Hall, E. D., Sethy, V. H., and Lahti, R. A. (1988) *J. Pharmacol. Exp. Ther.* **244**, 423–427.
54 Natale, J. E., Schott, R. J., Hall, E. D., Braughler, J. M., and D'Alecy, L. G. (1988) *Stroke* **19**, 1371–1378.
55 Fisher, M., Levine, P. H., Doyle, E. M., Arpano, M. M., Bergeron, D. A., Cohen, R. A., and Hoogasian, J. J. (1991) *Neurology* **41**, 297–299.
56 Fisher, M., Levine, P. H., and Cohen, R. A. (1990) *Stroke* **21**, 1435–1438.
57 Hall, E. D., Pazara, K. E., and Braughler, J. M. (1991) *Stroke* **22**, 361–366.
58 Hall, E. D., Pazara, K. E., Braughler, J. M., Linseman, K. L., and Jacobsen, E. J. (1990) *Stroke* **21(11 Suppl.)**, III83–III87.
59 Perkins, W. J., Milde, L. N., Milde, J. H., and Michenfelder, J. D. (1991) *Stroke* **22**, 902–909.
60 Monyer, H., Hartley, D. M., and Choi, D. W. (1990) *Neuron* **5**, 121–126.
61 Sterz, F., Safar, P., Johnson, D. W., Oku, K.-I. and Tisherman, S. A. (1991) *Stroke* **22**, 889–895.
62 Podrazik, R. M., Obedian, R. S., Remick, D. G., Zelenock, G. B., and D'Alecy, L. G. (1989) *Curr. Surg.* **46**, 287–292.
63 Helfaer, M. A., Kirsch, J. R., Hurn, P. D., Blizzard, K. K., Koehler, R. C., and Traystman, R. J. (1992) *Stroke* **23**, 1479–1486.
64 Hall, E. D. and Yonkers, P. A. (1988) *Stroke* **19**, 340–344.
65 Lesiuk, H., Sutherland, G., Peeling, J., Butler, K., and Saunders, J. (1991) *Stroke* **22**, 896–901.
66 Hall, E. D., Yonkers, P. A., and McCall, J. M. (1988) *Eur. J. Pharmacol.* **147**, 299–303.
67 Beck, T. and Bielenberg, G. W. (1990) *Brain Res.* **532**, 336–338.
68 Maruki, Y., Koehler, R. C., Kirsch, J. R., and Traystman, R. J. (1991) *J. Cereb. Blood Flow Metab.* **11**, S141.
69 Haraldseth, O., Gronas, T., and Unsgard, G. (1991) *Stroke* **122**, 1188–1192.
70 Linberg, J. V. (1987) *Adv. Ophthalmic. Plast. Reconstr. Surg.* **6**, 51–62.
71 Hall, E. D. and Travis M. A. (1988) *Brain Res.* **451**, 350–352.
72 Young, W., Wojak, J. C., and DeCrescito, V. (1988) *Stroke* **19**, 1013–1019.
73 Hoffman, W. E., Baughman, V. L., Polek, W., and Thomas, C. (1991) *J. Neurosurg. Anesthesiol.* **3**, 96–102.
74 Fowl, R. J., Patterson, R. B., Gewirtz, R. J., and Anderson, D. K. (1990) *J. Surg. Res.* **48**, 597–600.
75 Gisvold, S. E., Safar, P., Rao, G., Moossy, J., Kelsey, S., and Alexander, H. (1984) *Stroke* **15**, 803–812.

Chapter 28

Therapeutic Potential of L-Arginine, a Precursor of Nitric Oxide, in Focal Cerebral Ischemia

Eiharu Morikawa, Zhihong Huang, Sami Rosenblatt, Tazuka Yoshida, and Michael A. Moskowitz

Introduction

Nitric oxide (NO) is synthesized from the amino acid L-arginine by NO synthase, an enzyme present in cerebrovascular endothelium[1] and perivascular nerve fibers.[2] The synthesis of NO is calcium-dependent and requires NADPH. NO or a related thiol has been proposed as a mediator of endothelium-dependent relaxation.[3] NO may also be neurotoxic and may be a mediator of cytotoxic effects of glutamate both in vitro[4] and in vivo (*see* ref. 5 for a review). Both glutamate neurotoxicity and dilatation of blood vessels are important to the pathophysiology of focal cerebral ischemia, as is the NO-induced inhibition of platelet aggregation and adhesion.[6,7] Current studies were undertaken to compare the effects of inhibiting NO synthase with the effects of providing substrate for NO synthesis, L-arginine, during the first 24 h after focal brain ischemia.

From *The Human Brain Circulation*, R. D. Bevan and J. A. Bevan, eds.
©1994 Humana Press

Materials and Methods

Middle Cerebral Artery Occlusion

Models

The following three models of focal cerebral ischemia were used: model 1, proximal middle cerebral artery (MCA) occlusion as described by Tamura et al.[8] in Sprague Dawley (SD) or spontaneously hypertensive rats (SHR); model 2, distal MCA occlusion plus ipsilateral common carotid artery (CCA) occlusion (tandem CCA/MCA occlusion) in SHR described by Brint et al.,[9] model 3, distal MCA occlusion plus transient bilateral CCA occlusion in Long Evans (LE) rats as described by Chen et al.[10]

Brain surface landmarks for proximal and distal MCA occlusion were the medial edge of the lateral olfactory tract and the rhinal fissure, respectively. Thus, proximal occlusion interrupted flow proximal to the origin of the lateral lenticulostriate arteries yielding infarction in the striatum and cortex. Distal MCA occlusion, on the other hand, resulted in infarction within the neocortex. In all three models, the right MCA was occluded.

Anesthesia was induced and maintained by halothane, 3 and 1%, respectively, plus 70% nitrous oxide/balance oxygen. Rats were intubated (PE-240 polyethylene tubing) and mechanically ventilated. The right femoral artery was cannulated for continuous arterial blood pressure monitoring. Arterial blood was sampled intermittently for pH, Pa_{CO_2}, Pa_{O_2}, hematocrit, and plasma glucose. Respiratory parameters were adjusted as needed to maintain normal arterial blood gases. Rectal temperature was maintained normothermic by a Homeothermic Blanket Control Unit (Harvard Apparatus, Edenbridge, Kent, UK) preset to 37°C.

The distal or proximal segment of MCA was exposed as described previously[8,9] with minor modifications. Briefly, a 1-cm skin incision was placed approximately midway between the right outer canthus and anterior pinna. Temporalis muscle was incised and retracted to expose the squamous bone (distal) or the infratemporal fossa (proximal). A craniotomy (3 mm diameter) was created at the juncture of the zygoma and squamous bone (distal), or just anterior to the foramen ovale (proximal). The dura mater was opened with a fine curved needle.

In model 1, proximal MCA occlusion was completed either by double ligation (10-0 monofilament) and transection, or by electrocauterization after single ligation between the medial edge of lateral olfactory tract and the rhinal fissure. The latter method of occlusion yielded consistently larger infarcts as previously described.[11] In model 2, the right CCA was ligated (4-0 silk) first, followed by electrocauterization of the adjacent 2-mm vessel segment. The coagulated segment was then transected. In model 3, distal MCA occlusion was performed by double ligation (10-0 monofilament) and transection, combined with temporary (45 min) bilateral CCA occlusion with metallic clips.

After surgery, the rats were returned to their cages, allowed free access to food and water, and given a single injection of cefazolin, 50 mg, im.

Measurement of Infarct Volume

Unless otherwise mentioned, rats were killed by decapitation 24 h after vascular occlusion. To measure infarct volume, brains were removed and placed in ice-cold saline for 10 min and sectioned coronally into seven 2-mm slices in a rodent brain matrix. Slices were placed in 2% TTC (2,3,5-triphenyltetrazolium chloride monohydrate) (Sigma, St. Louis, MO) at room temperature for 30 min followed by 10% formalin overnight.[12] The area of infarction, outlined in white, was measured on the posterior surface of each section (Bioquant IV image analysis system, R and M Biometrics, Inc., Nashville, TN), and the infarct volume was calculated by numeric integration of the sequential areas.

Experimental Protocols

1. NO synthase inhibitors: Two treatment protocols using NO synthase inhibitors, N^G-nitro-L-arginine (L-NA) and N^G-nitro-L-arginine methyl ester (L-NAME) were used.
   a. L-NA, 1 mg/kg, was injected ip at 5 min, 3 and 6 h after MCA occlusion.
   b. L-NAME, 3 mg/kg, was injected ip at 5 min, 3, 6, 24, and 36 h after MCA occlusion and rats were sacrificed after 48 h of survival in this study. L-NA and L-NAME were obtained from Sigma

and were dissolved in saline at a concentration of 1.5 mg/mL. An equivalent volume of saline was used as control.
2. L-Arginine: Pretreatment and early posttreatment protocols were used.

In protocol 1, rats received L- or D-arginine, 300 mg/kg ip, at 16 and 3 h before and 5 and 120 min after MCA occlusion. In protocol 2, rats received 300 mg/kg of L-arginine by iv infusion over 10 min beginning 5 min after MCA occlusion and again ip 1 h after MCA occlusion.

L- and D-Arginine hydrochloride were obtained from Sigma. Three hundred milligrams of L- or D-arginine were dissolved in 1 mL of distilled water. Both solutions were adjusted to pH 7.0 with sodium hydroxide. An equivalent volume of saline was used for control animals.

Nitric Oxide Synthase Assay

To evaluate NO synthesis in the brain after treatment with L-arginine analogs, NO synthase activity was measured in the cerebellum by the conversion of [^{3}H]arginine to [^{3}H]citrulline as described by Bredt and Snyder.[13] On sacrifice, the cerebellum was removed, weighed, and homogenized in 2 mL of buffer (50 mM HEPES, 1 mM EDTA, pH 7.4). The sample was centrifuged at 3500 rpm (PR-2, International Equipment Co., Boston, MA) for 5 min, and the pellet discarded. The reaction mixture consisted of 100 μL of 50 mM HEPES, 1 mM EDTA, 1 mM NADPH, and 1 mM Ca^{2+} at pH 7.4; 25 μL of 100 nM [^{3}H]arginine (1 mCi/mL); and 25/50 μL of the supernatant. After incubation for 10 min at room temperature, the reaction was stopped by adding 2 mL of 20 mM HEPES and 2 mM EDTA at pH 5.5. The samples were placed over 1-mL columns of Dowex AG50WX-8 (Na$^+$ form) and eluted with 2 mL distilled water. Radioactivity was determined by liquid scintillation counting. NO synthase activity in the normal rat cerebellum was assayed in each experiment, and data were expressed as a percentage of normal activity in the cerebellum.

[^{3}H]Arginine (58.4 Ci/mmol) was obtained from New England Nuclear/DuPont (Boston, MA). Columns and AG50WX-8 (H$^+$ form) were obtained from Bio-Rad Laboratories (Richmond, CA), and the latter was converted to the Na$^+$ form by stirring with 1M sodium hydroxide. Buffer ingredients were obtained from Sigma.

Laser-Doppler Flowmetry

Preparation

Rats were placed in a stereotaxic frame, and the MCA occluded by a metallic clip (Zen clip, Ohwa Tsusho). A second craniotomy was made 4–6 mm lateral and –2 to 1 mm rostral to bregma, a region that corresponds to the transition between severely ischemic and mildly ischemic zones in this model.[14] A paper-thin layer of the skull was left intact, thus enabling the tip of the recording probe to remain dry throughout the measurement and avoiding epidural bleeding. The recording probe (0.8 mm diameter, P-433) attached to a laser-Doppler flowmeter (BPM 403A, Vasomedics, Inc., St. Paul, MN) was steadily advanced under stereotaxic control perpendicular to the cortical surface and away from large blood vessels until it touched the surface without indenting. Steady-state baseline measurements were obtained before CCA/MCA occlusion. rCBF after occlusion was expressed as a percentage of this baseline.[15] Preinfusion rCBF was recorded 2 and 5 min after MCA occlusion, and postinfusion rCBF was determined at 15-min intervals beginning 15 min after occlusion.

Experimental Protocol

Male SHRs were subjected to tandem CCA/MCA occlusion (as in model 2 above) and 5 min later, L-arginine (3, 30, 300 mg/kg), D-arginine (300 mg/kg), or an equivalent volume of saline was infused over 10 min at a rate of 0.1 mL/kg/min. To examine the effects of anesthesia on the L-arginine response, pentobarbital (65 mg kg^{-1} ip) was administered to four rats ventilated mechanically with room air instead of halothane/N$_2$O.

Closed Cranial Window

Twenty male Sprague-Dawley rats and four SHRs were anesthetized with sodium pentobarbital (50 mg/kg ip supplemented by 10 mg/kg ip every hour). The rats were paralyzed (pancuronium bromide 0.5–1.0 mg iv) and mechanically ventilated with O$_2$-supplemented room air; end-tidal Pa$_{CO2}$ was continuously monitored (Novametrix Medical Systems, Wallingford, CT) and maintained.

The skull was exposed through a linear midline incision from the occiput to the forehead. A left parietal craniotomy about 7×5 mm was made by a drill. The dura was incised and reflected. A metallic window equipped with three ports was placed over the exposed brain surface. The space under the window was filled with mock CSF (Na 156.5, K 2.95, Ca 2.5, Mg 1.33, Cl 138.7, HCO_3 24.6 [all in mEq/L], dextrose 66.5 mg/dL and urea 40.2 mg/dL; equilibrated with gas containing 10% oxygen, 5% CO_2, and the balance nitrogen; pH 7.33–7.38). The ICP was maintained constant by adjusting the height of the outflow tube to approx 6 cm H_2O.

The pial vessels were visualized using an intravital microscope (200× magnification; Leitz, Bensheim, Germany). A TV camera (Dage MTI Inc., CCD-72 series, Michigan City, IN) that was attached to the microscope transposed the picture onto a video monitor (Dage MTI Inc.) where the diameters of vessels were measured using a video measurement system (VIA-100, Boeckler Instruments, USA, Tuscon, AZ).

Baseline diameters were measured after allowing equilibration for 30 min. In 13 animals, measurements were made following L-arginine infusion (3, 30, and 300 mg/kg) over 10 min. In seven animals, L-NAME (1 μM) was superfused 20 min prior to L-arginine infusion. Data are expressed as a percentage of baseline diameter.

Statistical Analysis

Results are presented as means ± SEM. Paired or unpaired Student's *t*-test, as appropriate, was used to determine the statistical significance unless otherwise noted. $P < 0.05$ was taken as statistically significant.

Results

Physiologic Variables

There were no significant between-group differences in the monitored physiologic variables at the time of MCA occlusion or when blood flow or pial vessel diameter was measured (data not shown). A single injection of 3 mg/kg L-NAME ip raised MAP approx 10 mmHg (Fig. 1). However, there were no physiological

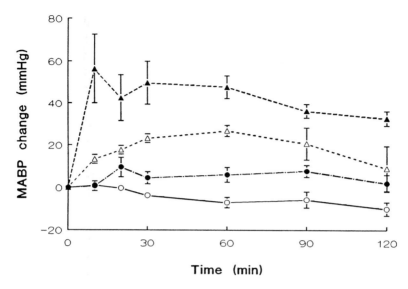

Fig. 1. Mean arterial blood pressure (MABP) after injecting either 100 mg/kg (filled triangle), 10 or 30 mg/kg (open triangle), 1 or 3 mg/kg (filled circle) of L-NAME or saline (open circle) ip. Error bars denote SEM. n = 3–6/group.

changes observed after 1 μM superfusion under the cranial window. Body temperature 2 h after MCA occlusion was not different between L- and D-arginine-treated animals (36.7 ± 0.2 and 36.9 ± 0.2°C, respectively).

Infarct Volumes

NO Synthase Inhibitors (Table 1)

Treatment with L-NA (1 mg/kg given 5 min, 3 and 6 h after occlusion) increased infarct volume by 67 and 68% in the Tamura and Chen model, respectively, as compared to saline-treated controls. Because of the large variance and small animal numbers, these differences did not reach statistical significance. However, statistical significance was reached after combining the cortical infarct data from the two studies (111 ± 14 [n = 17] vs 62 ± 17 mm³ [n = 16], p < 0.05).

Table 1
Cerebral Infarct Volume and Cerebellar NOS Activity
After L-NAME or L-NA Treatment in Models of Focal Ischemia

Model/strain	Group	Inf. vol., n		% NOS, n		
Tamura/SD	Saline	85 ± 37	(7)	95 ± 9	(5)	
	L-NA	142 ± 30	(8)	46 ± 11	(6)*	
Chen/LE	Saline	66 ± 13	(9)	98 ± 9	(8)	
	L-NA	111 ± 21	(9)	73 ± 16	(6)	
Tamura/SD	Saline	156 ± 27	(11)	97 ± 7	(10)	
	L-NAME	188 ± 19	(12)	42 ± 5	(11)*	
Chen/LE	Saline	109 ± 19	(6)	90 ± 4	(6)	
	L-NAME	109 ± 22	(7)	45 ± 8	(7)*	

Values are means ± SEM. *$p < 0.01$.
See text for dose and schedule of L-NA and L-NAME administration.

Treatment with 3 mg/kg L-NAME given 5 min, 3, 6, 24, and 36 h after occlusion enlarged the infarct volume by 21% in the Tamura model, but did not change the results in the Chen model. This increase, however, did not reach statistical significance even after experiments were combined.

Treatment with both L-arginine analogs significantly decreased cerebellar NO synthase activity at the time of sacrifice. However, there was no correlation between the reduction in activity and volume of cerebral infarction in any of the studies (data not shown).

L-Arginine (Table 2)

Pretreatment with L-arginine (300 mg/kg) reduced infarct volume by 15 and 31% in the Tamura and Brint models, respectively ($p < 0.05$). Furthermore, treatment initiated 5 min after occlusion decreased infarct volume by 28% ($p < 0.05$). By contrast, D-arginine (300 mg/kg) was without effect.

L-Arginine (300 mg/kg) reduced infarct volume by 35% in normotensive Sprague-Dawley rats when given 5 min after MCA occlusion ($p < 0.05$).

Laser-Doppler Flowmetry

Consistent with published observations,[14] rCBF decreased to approx 20% of baseline in dorsolateral cortex after CCA/MCA occlusion. This level was sustained throughout the 2-h recording

Table 2
Cerebral Infarct Volume in Models of Focal Ischemia
After L-Arginine Treatment

Model/strain	Protocol	Group	Inf. vol., n
Tamura/SHR	1	Saline	240 ± 7 (10)
		L-Arg	205 ± 7 (10)*
Brint/SHR	1	Saline	147 ± 12 (10)
		L-Arg	101 ± 9 (19)*
		D-Arg	167 ± 14 (10)
Brint/SHR	2	Saline	154 ± 9 (12)
		L-Arg	111 ± 12 (10)*
Tamura/SD	2	Saline	231 ± 13 (17)
		L-Arg	150 ± 12 (14)**

Values are means ± SEM. *$p < 0.05$, **$p < 0.01$.
See text for detail of protocols 1 and 2.

period. L-Arginine (300 mg/kg, iv infusion), but not an equivalent dose of D-arginine, significantly increased rCBF during this period ($p < 0.01$ by repeated-measures ANOVA followed by Fisher's least significant difference test) (Fig. 2). When mean rCBF values were compared before and after L-arginine infusion, 30 and 300 mg/kg increased rCBF from 17 ± 5 to 31 ± 8% ($n = 4$, $p < 0.05$) and from 22 ± 3 to 33 ± 4% ($n = 12$, $p < 0.01$), respectively. Pre- and posttreatment rCBF did not differ after saline (20 ± 5.3 to 18 ± 5.2%, $n = 6$), L-arginine, 3 mg/kg (18 ± 2.9 to 21 ± 3.5%, $n = 4$), or D-arginine, 300 mg/kg (21 ± 4.9 to 25 ± 4.9%, $n = 6$) (Fig. 3). Significant increases in response to L-arginine (300 mg/kg) were observed in pentobarbital-anesthetized rats (29 ± 6 to 44 ± 8%, $n = 4$, $p < 0.05$), thus excluding the possibility of an effect mediated by a specific anesthetic agent.

Pial Vessel Diameter

L-Arginine, 30 and 300, but not 3 mg/kg, increased pial vessel diameter following iv infusion (115 ± 3.2% [$n = 5$], 115 ± 2.2% [$n = 5$], and 101 ± 0.8% [$n = 3$], respectively, after 30 min) (Fig. 4). Pretreatment with L-NAME (1 µM) significantly attenuated the response to 30 and 300 mg/kg (104 ± 0.5% [$n = 3$] and 106 ± 0.9% [$n = 4$], $p < 0.05$ and 0.01, respectively) (Fig. 5).

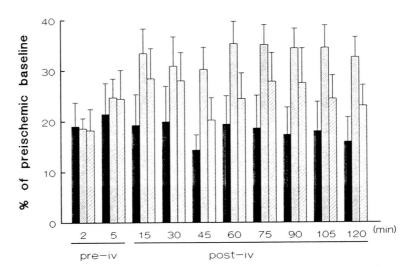

Fig. 2. rCBF as measured by laser-Doppler flowmetry in dorsolateral cortex after CCA/MCA occlusion. Saline (filled columns, $n = 6$), 300 mg/kg of L-arginine (fine-hatched column, $n = 12$), and D-arginine (coarse-hatched column, $n = 6$) were infused iv over 10 min beginning 5 min after MCA occlusion. Error bars denote SEM.

Discussion

Our studies demonstrate that parenteral administration of L-arginine, even if given after MCA occlusion, reduces focal infarct size in both normotensive and hypertensive animals. The mechanism probably relates to nitric oxide synthesis, resultant vasodilation, and increases in brain blood flow. Following MCA occlusion, L-arginine increased rCBF from below the ischemic threshold, that is, from about 20% of baseline, to more than 30%, which is approximately the threshold for infarction.[16] The increases in flow, observed within dorsolateral cortex, were sustained for at least 2 h (Fig. 2).

The response to L-arginine was not confined to the ischemic brain. L-Arginine infusion and superfusion (data not shown) increased pial vessel diameter in normal animals (Fig. 4). In this instance, vasodilation probably depended on NO synthase activity and NO synthesis, since L-NAME (1 μm) significantly reduced

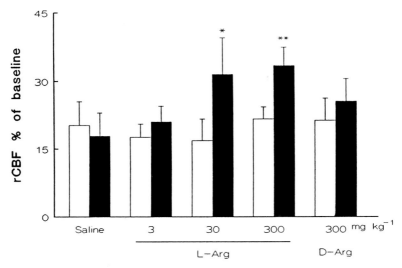

Fig. 3. Average rCBF in dorsolateral cortex before (open column) and after (filled column) iv infusion of L- or D-arginine or saline during CCA/MCA occlusion. *See text* for protocol. Error bars denote SEM. *$p < 0.05$, **$p < 0.01$ by paired Student's *t*-test.

the vasodilator response to L-arginine (Fig. 5). Decreased vasodilation may account for the enlarged infarcts after NOS inhibition and distal MCA occlusion,[17] and for the findings reported herein (Table 1).

At least three reports have described the beneficial effects of NO synthase inhibition on stroke outcome in rodents, however. In one study, protective effects were demonstrated using L-NA in a mouse MCA occlusion model.[18] In another, L-NA reduced the magnitude of brain injury in a hypoxic–ischemic neonatal rat model.[19] A third study in adult rats reported smaller infarcts with L-NAME after proximal MCA occlusion.[20] The apparent discrepancies may relate to differences in methodology. In all three studies, ventilation was spontaneous, $PaCO_2$ values (unreported) were almost certainly high, and baseline blood flows may have become correspondingly high. Although NO synthase inhibition reportedly blocks the blood flow response to elevated $PaCO_2$, it is not clear that the levels of inhibition achieved were sufficient to block

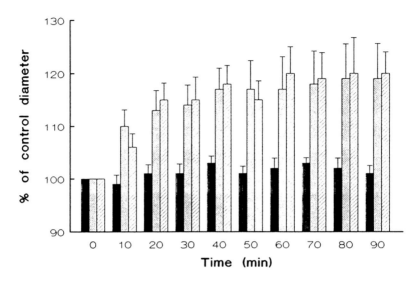

Fig. 4. Changes in pial vessel diameter (closed cranial window) with time in Sprague-Dawley rats after 3 (filled column), 30 (fine-hatched column), or 300 mg/kg (coarse-hatched column) of L-arginine iv infusion. Error bars denote SEM. $n = 3–5$/group.

the $PaCO_2$ response. We postulate that raised $PaCO_2$ masks the consequences of inhibiting NO synthesis within the cerebrovasculature and unmasks parenchymal effects of NO synthase inhibitors on NO neurotoxicity as suggested by Dawson and Snyder. The discrepant results may also reflect possible differences in the degree of NO synthase inhibition at the vessel wall vs brain parenchyma inasmuch as endothelial and brain NO synthase represent different NO synthase isoforms.[21] In this regard, it would be of interest to test and compare the effects of NO synthase inhibitors that do not cross the blood–brain barrier.

Under normal steady-state conditions, NO synthase may well be saturated with substrate.[22,23] However, when L-arginine becomes depleted or is in greater demand, or when the endothelium is damaged,[24–27] the reaction may become substrate-limited. Hence, in cholesterol-fed, but not normal rabbits, L-arginine infusion augmented endothelium-dependent vasodilation of hind limb vessels.[28] L-Arginine may stimulate NO synthesis when delivered to cerebral

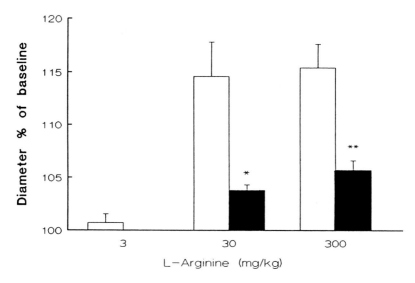

Fig. 5. Changes in pial vessel diameter (closed cranial window) 30 min after L-arginine iv infusion with (filled column) and without (open column) 1 μM L-NAME superfused 20 min before the amino acid. Baseline vessel diameters were 42 ± 4.2, 49 ± 3.7, and 40 ± 4.1 μm, respectively, for 3, 30, and 300 mg/kg of L-arginine; 34 ± 7 and 40 ± 9.9 μm, respectively, for 30 and 300 mg/kg of L-arginine with L-NAME pretreatment. L-NAME (1 μM) did not affect vessel diameter by itself. Error bars denote SEM. $*p < 0.05$, $**p < 0.01$ compared with L-arginine alone by unpaired Student's *t*-test.

vessels distal to an occlusion wherein blood flow and substrate delivery are low and demand for NO synthesis may be high. Responses in normal pial vessels, however, suggest that the enzyme may not be saturated with substrate. We wonder whether the lack of L-arginine-induced hemodynamic changes (e.g., changes in blood pressure) suggests some unique properties of NO synthase within rat cerebral vessels not shared by systemic vessels. Hence, the use of L-arginine as a cerebrovasodilator in humans merits further study.

Acknowledgments

We thank Ken Maynard for measuring NO synthase activity and Naoki Koketsu for the data from the Chen model. These studies were supported by Interdepartmental Stroke Program Project Grant NS 10828.

References

[1] Palmer, R. M. J., Ashton, D. S., and Moncada, S. (1988) *Nature* **333,** 664–666.

[2] Nozaki, K., Moskowitz, M. A., Maynard, K. I., and Koketsu, N. (1992) *Stroke* **23,** 76.

[3] Moncada, S., Palmer, R. M. J., and Higgs, E. A. (1991) *Pharmacol. Rev.* **43,** 109–142.

[4] Dawson, V. L., Dawson, T. M., London, E. D., Bredt, D. S., and Snyder, S. H. (1991) *Proc. Natl. Acad. Sci. USA* **88,** 6368–6371.

[5] Dawson, T. M., Dawson, V. L., and Snyder, S. H. (1992) *Ann. Neurol.* **32,** 297–311.

[6] Radomski, M. W., Palmer, R. M. J., and Moncada, S. (1987) *Biochem. Biophys. Res. Commun.* **148,** 1482–1489.

[7] Radomski, M. W., Palmer, R. M. J., and Moncada, S. (1987) *Br. J. Pharmacol.* **92,** 181–187.

[8] Tamura, A., Graham, D. I., McCulloch, J., and Teasdale, G. M. (1981) *J. Cereb. Blood Flow Metab.* **1,** 53–60.

[9] Brint, S., Jacewicz, M., Kiessling, M., Tanabe, J., and Pulsinelli, W. (1988) *J. Cereb. Blood Flow Metab.* **8,** 474–485.

[10] Chen, S. T., Hsu, C. Y., Hogan, E. L., Maricq, H., and Balentine, J. D. (1986) *Stroke* **17,** 738–743.

[11] Bederson, J. B., Pitts, L. H., Tsuji, M., Nishimura, M. C., Davis, R. L., and Bartkowski, H. (1986) *Stroke* **17,** 472–476.

[12] Kano, M., Moskowitz, M. A., and Yokota, M. (1991) *J. Cereb. Blood Flow Metab.* **11,** 628–637.

[13] Bredt, D. S. and Snyder, S. H. (1990) *Proc. Natl. Acad. Sci. USA* **87,** 682–685.

[14] Jacewicz, M., Brint, S., Tanabe, J., Wang, X., and Pulsinelli, W. (1990) *J. Cereb. Blood Flow Metab.* **10,** 903–913.

[15] Dirnagl, U., Kaplan, B., Jacewicz, M., and Pulsinelli, W. (1989) *J. Cereb. Blood Flow Metab.* **9,** 589–596.

[16] Jacewicz, M., Tanabe, J., and Pulsinelli, W. A. (1992) *J. Cereb. Blood Flow Metab.* **12,** 359–370.

[17] Yamamoto, S., Golanov, E. V., Berger, S. B., and Reis, D. J. (1992) *J. Cereb. Blood Flow Metab.* **12,** 717–726.

[18] Nowicki, J. P., Duval, D., Poignet, H., and Scatton, B. (1991) *Eur. J. Pharmacol.* **204,** 339–340.

[19] Trifiletti, R. R. (1992) *Eur. J. Pharmacol.* **218,** 197–198.

[20] Buisson, A., Plotkine, M., and Boulu, R. G. (1992) *Br. J. Pharmacol.* **106,** 766–767.

21 Lamas, S., Marsden, P. A., Li, G. K., Tempst, P., and Michel, T. (1992) *Proc. Natl. Acad. Sci. USA* **89,** 6348–6352.
22 Baydoun, A. R., Emery, P. W., Pearson, J. D., and Mann, G. E. (1990) *Biochem. Biophys. Res. Commun.* **173,** 940–948.
23 Bredt, D. S. and Snyder, S. H. (1990) *Proc. Natl. Acad. Sci. USA* **87,** 682–685.
24 Aisaka, K., Gross, S. S., Griffith, O. W., and Levi, R. (1989) *Biochem. Biophys. Res. Commun.* **163,** 710–717.
25 Gold, M. E., Bush, P. A., and Ignarro, L. J. (1989) *Biochem. Biophys. Res. Commun.* **164,** 714–721.
26 Rosenblum, W. I., Nelson, G. H., and Shimizu, T. (1992) *Am. J. Physiol.* **262,** H961–H964.
27 Schini, V. B. and Vanhoutte, P. M. (1991) *J. Cardiovasc. Pharmacol.* **17,** S10–S14.
28 Girerd, X. J., Hirsch, A. T., Cooke, J. P., Dzau, V. J., and Creager, M. A. (1990) *Circ. Res.* **67,** 1301–1308.

Chapter 29

Acute Vasospasm and Subarachnoid Hemorrhage

Role of Protein Kinase C

Ismail Laher and John A. Bevan

Introduction

The pathogenesis of cerebral vasospasm that occurs following the leakage of blood into the subarachnoid space is associated, at least in the early phase, with increased vascular sensitivity to a number of vasoconstrictors. A variety of agents present in red blood cells and platelets are proposed to initiate the nonspecific, increased vascular sensitivity that manifests as acute vasospasm. We propose that mediators that are released in concentrations subthreshold for vasoconstriction increase the intracellular sensitivity of events involved in Ca^{2+}-dependent excitation-contraction coupling. Consistent with this is the observation that the weak constrictor response to thrombin in rabbit cerebral arteries is greatly increased by the presence of activated platelets. Pretreatment of arteries with a relatively selective inhibitor of protein kinase C abolished the amplification caused by activated platelets. Additional evidence for an important role for protein kinase C is provided by direct measurements, indicating that the extent of vasospasm is correlated with the formation of diacylglycerol, the endogenous activator of protein kinase C, and that the level of membrane-bound, active protein kinase C is also increased in vasospasm. The partici-

From *The Human Brain Circulation*, R. D. Bevan and J. A. Bevan, eds.
©1994 Humana Press

pation of protein kinase C in the early phase of vasospasm thus represents a novel target for therapy in subarachnoid hemorrhage.

It has been reported that between 50 and 75% of subarachnoid hemorrhage (SAH) are caused by ruptured aneurysms.[1] Primary SAH owing to blood leaking into the subarachnoid space often leads to prolonged vasospasm of cerebral arteries located near the aneurysm.[2] It is this vasospasm that is considered to be a leading cause of death and disability in SAH patients. Based on evidence from animal models of SAH and supported by clinical findings, the pathogenesis of cerebral vasospasm associated with SAH can be divided into two stages, representing acute and chronic changes in vascular functioning and structure.[3,4] The vasospasm that occurs shortly after an aneurysm ruptures is transient in nature and reversed by commonly used vasodilators; this phase of vasospasm is not readily observed under clinical conditions and is largely a phenomenon studied in animal models of SAH.[5] Of greater concern is the vasospasm that develops several days after the hemorrhage and that lasts considerably longer; this phase of vasospasm is not readily treated with vasodilators and presents with significant clinical manifestations.[3,4] This chronic phase of vasospasm is associated with structural alterations in vascular morphology, including fibrosis, smooth muscle proliferation, and necrosis (*see* Chapter 30).[3,6] Alterations in vascular pharmacology have been most widely studied in the early, reversible phase of SAH and are the subject of this chapter.

Early Changes in Vascular Function

The frequency and severity of cerebral vasospasm are related to the presence of blood in the subarachnoid space.[7] Following intracranial bleeding, red blood cells and platelets accumulate in large numbers at the site of the aneurysm. A number of potent spasmogens are liberated from red blood cells and platelets, but efforts to assign a causative role to specific mediators in the pathogenesis of cerebral vasospasm have not been successful.[3–5] The pharmacological properties of some of the vasoactive agents found in red blood cells and platelets are briefly discussed below.

Hemolysis of Red Blood Cells

Following a ruptured aneurysm, red blood cells in the sub-arachnoid space undergo breakdown or hemolysis, thereby releasing their contents. The most potent spasmogen among these is oxyhemoglobin, a peptide consistently found to occur in high concentrations during SAH.[8] The rate of formation of oxyhemoglobin from lysed erythrocytes in the subarachnoid space closely parallels the development of vasospasm. Application of red blood cells or hemoglobin containing cytoplasm increased the vessel wall thickness of middle cerebral arteries; on the other hand, application of a platelet-rich fraction of white blood cells did not produce arterial thickening.[9] By studying the morphology of arteries following interaction with various components of red blood cells, Macdonald et al.[10] concluded that oxyhemoglobin is the agent most likely to be responsible for vasospasm following SAH with some contribution from bilirubin, the metabolite of hemoglobin. Oxyhemoglobin may be released in amounts sufficient to cause maximal contraction of cerebral arteries. Its breakdown product (methemoglobin) is converted to bilirubin in vivo and constricts cerebral arteries from a number of species, but causes only minor changes in luminal diameter of cerebral arteries in a primate model of SAH.[10] However, increases in levels of bilirubin are not always associated with cerebrovascular changes.[4]

During the spontaneous oxidation of oxyhemoglobin to methemoglobin, superoxide free radicals are also released. Oxyhemoglobin and lipid peroxides both cause vasoconstriction and structural damage in cerebral arteries,[10] such as necrosis of vascular smooth muscle cells, damage to nerve endings, and disruption of endothelial cell integrity.[3] Endothelium-dependent relaxation is impaired in vasospastic cerebral arteries during SAH.[11] By virtue of its ability to inhibit the effects of spontaneously released endothelial-derived relaxing factors, hemoglobin simultaneously augments the vasoconstrictor potency of other agents. Hemoglobin also inhibits response to calcium entry blockers in cerebral arteries, thereby decreasing the effectiveness of vasodilator mechanisms in SAH.[12]

Platelet Aggregation

Endothelial damage in cerebral arteries close to a ruptured aneurysm exposes the arterial lining to circulating platelets, ultimately leading to activation and aggregation of platelets within minutes or hours after SAH, and causing localized vasoconstriction. Platelets store vasoactive compounds, which they release by exocytosis following excitation-secretion coupling. This secretion forms a positive feedback system that potentiates the aggregation caused by the primary stimulus. Human platelets are a rich source of thromboxane A_2 and serotonin (5-HT), and also release other vasoactive agents, such as platelet-derived growth factors (PDGF), adenosine diphosphate, adenosine triphosphate, norepinephrine, epinephrine, dopamine, and small amounts of histamine. The main role of platelets is likely to be in the initiation of the early phase of vasospasm, since thromboxane A_2, 5-HT, and PDGF are compounds with limited bioavailability.[13] PDGF released by aggregating platelets promotes the migration and subsequent proliferation of smooth muscle cells to the medial layer of arteries, thus causing a reduced lumen diameter.[14]

Thromboxane A_2 has a half-life of less than a minute at body temperature and is hydrolyzed to its inactive metabolites, thromboxane B_2 and 6-keto prostaglandin $F_{1\alpha}$. During the first 3 d of a hemorrhage, platelet-rich plasma from patients with SAH have a reduced aggregability and thromboxane B_2 release compared to platelets from plasma of healthy individuals; with progressive deterioration, both platelet aggregability and thromboxane B_2 release increase markedly.[13] Platelet-derived thromboxane A_2 constricts cerebral arteries, and is twice as potent as serotonin in bovine and human cerebral arteries.[15] It is unlikely that polymorphonuclear leukocytes, lymphocytes, or the arterial wall produce significant amounts of thromboxanes, although a nonplatelet source, possibly neuronal, cannot be excluded in studies of the basilar artery of dogs.[16] It is possible that other eicosanoids with long-acting vasoconstrictor effects are also released from platelets, since levels of prostaglandin $F_{2\alpha}$, a potent and chemically stable constrictor that is actively transported from the cerebrospinal fluid, correlate with the development and severity of vasospasm in patients.[17]

Following the short-lasting release of thromboxane A$_2$, activated platelets then release serotonin whose vasoconstrictor activity is longer lasting. Serotonin exerts pronounced vasoconstrictor effects in cerebral arteries with little evidence of desensitization. Cerebral arteries of most species, including humans, are more sensitive to serotonin than are peripheral arteries. Serotonin has been proposed as a putative neurotransmitter in the cerebral circulation of rabbits, where it is likely to be taken up by adrenergic nerves after its release from platelets.[18]

Contractile Responses to Thrombin

Thrombin not only causes platelet aggregation, but also stimulates the formation of a fibrin clot during coagulation by activating the proteolytic cleavage of fibrinogen. Both thrombin and fibrinogen constrict cerebral arteries. Thrombin-induced contractions of cerebral arteries are characterized by a delayed onset and are generally of a sustained nature compared to tone owing to other vasoconstrictors, and are not readily reversed by most pharmacological receptor antagonists.[19] Whereas thrombin causes vasoconstriction in cerebral arteries from rabbits,[20] the predominant response in human cerebral arteries is an endothelial-dependent dilation.[19]

Receptor Synergism

The initial phase of vasospasm following SAH is unlikely to be caused by the action of one vasoconstrictor; the consensus is that acute vasospasm is the result of the interaction of various substances released by hemolyzing red blood cells, aggregating platelets, and factors associated with the coagulation cascade.[3–5] It is clear that a variety of mediators are continuously released during SAH at concentrations that are subthreshold for vasoconstriction. Thus, the extent of contraction in response to platelet-derived substances is greater than would be expected from the measured amounts of endogenously released substances, thereby suggesting mutual amplification. The ability of cerebrospinal fluid to amplify constrictor responses in human basilar artery segments is greatly enhanced when taken from patients with SAH.[21] In addition, when human platelets are activated with thrombin, contraction of the canine basilar artery results from the mutual amplification of the individual effects of the various agonists released by platelets, since supramaximal concentrations of serotonin or thromboxane A$_2$ antagonists are only partially effective.[22]

Acute increases in vascular sensitivity to a number of vasoconstrictors occur in cerebral arteries from animals with SAH. Arteries from animals with SAH are more sensitive to norepinephrine, serotonin, depolarization-induced contractions to K$^+$ and Ca^{2+}, prostaglandins, and superoxide free radicals.[3-5,23] Experiments in a rabbit model of SAH indicate that nonspecific increases in vascular sensitivity occur within 10 min of initiation of a hemorrhage in the absence of alterations in endothelium-dependent relaxations.[24] Injection of blood into the cisterna magna causes large increases in the levels of neuropeptide Y in the cerebrospinal fluid (CSF) of rabbits. Both neuropeptide Y and CSF from animals with SAH potentiate cerebral artery constriction to norepinephrine.[25]

Role of Protein Kinase C

It remains difficult to implicate a single spasmogen in the etiology of acute vasospasm.[3-5] Recordings of the sensitivity of cerebral blood vessels support the concept that exaggerated responsiveness to a number of constrictor agents may be the result of the activation of an intracellular modulator of Ca^{2+}-dependent events associated with excitation–contraction coupling. Receptor stimulation in most blood vessels causes the cleavage of membrane phospholipids to yield diacylglycerol and inositol trisphosphate. The mobilization of intracellular Ca^{2+} is mediated by inositol trisphosphate, whereas diacylglycerol causes the activation of protein kinase C to its Ca^{2+}-sensitive form. Activated protein kinase C phosphorylates a number of intracellular proteins, such that an increased Ca^{2+} sensitivity occurs in both permeabilized as well as intact arteries.[26]

We examined the hypothesis that the nonspecific increase in vascular sensitivity commonly observed in acute vasospasm may be the result of the activation of protein kinase C during the early phase of SAH. In ring segments of rabbit basilar arteries, the sensitivity of the constrictor response to thrombin was increased threefold, whereas the maximal response was augmented by more than 20% by factors released from freshly obtained, collagen-activated human platelets. Pretreatment of basilar arteries with staurosporine, an inhibitor of protein kinase C, blunted this platelet-induced augmentation of the thrombin constrictor response.[20] When similar responses were made in basilar arteries after the endothelium had been disrupted, activated platelets increased the sensitivity to thrombin by 30-fold and the maximal tissue response by 60%, thereby suggesting a protective role for the endothelium in the protein kinase C-mediated increase in vascular tone owing to receptor synergism.[20]

In basilar arteries obtained from a canine model of SAH, inhibition of calmodulin with W-7 causes dilation only of segments in severe spasm, whereas nicardipine, a calcium-entry inhibitor, did not cause dilation of arteries considered to be undergoing either moderate or severe spasm. On the other hand, H-7, an inhibitor of protein kinase C, reduced vessel tone in basilar arteries undergoing either moderate or severe spasm, indicating that acute vasospasm is likely the result of alterations in protein kinase C activity rather than to changes in the calcium–calmodulin pathway.[27] However, it is noteworthy that the extent of dilation owing to H-7 was not related to the degree of vasospasm.

More recently, direct measurements of both protein kinase C activation and diacylglycerol formation support a role for protein kinase C activation during acute vasospasm. The membrane-bound protein kinase C activity was significantly elevated in basilar arteries from dogs with SAH, whereas a corresponding decline in protein kinase C activity was measured in the cytosol of these arteries.[28] Because protein kinase C is translocated to the cell membrane from the cytosol when it is activated, these experiments provide the first direct evidence of a role for protein kinase C in the genesis of acute vasospasm. In a two-hemorrhage model of SAH made in beagles, a significant correlation was found to exist between the diacylglycerol content and reduction in angiographic diameter of basilar arteries.[29] In this study, vasospasm and diacylglycerol content were maximal on d 7 of the experiment, and by d 14, diacylglycerol levels returned to control values as did the caliber of the arteries. The mechanism whereby diacylglycerol levels remain elevated for a prolonged period during acute vasospasm is unclear, since the pool of phosphoinositol is limited, and moreover, protein kinase C activation is known to inhibit receptor-mediated hydrolysis of inositol phospholipids. Of notable interest in the study by Matsui et al.[29] is that diacylglycerol levels return to control levels during the later stages of SAH, suggesting that perhaps protein kinase C activation mediated the early, and not the later, phases of SAH. Such a concept is in keeping with the nonspecific nature of increased vascular sensitivity commonly observed in acute vasospasm.

Conclusion

Cerebral arteries from animal models of subarachnoid hemorrhage demonstrate nonspecific increased sensitivity to constrictor agents during the acute phase of vasospasm. In addition to a decreased dilatory function in such vessels, it is apparent that enhanced sensitivity to Ca^{2+}-dependent mechanisms participating in excitation-contraction coupling may also occur. Evidence to support a causative role for any particular factor present in hemolyzed red cells or activated platelets has not been obtained. Recent studies of acute vasospasm suggest that activated protein kinase C may modulate the nonspecific increased vascular sensitivity observed. Indirect evidence with inhibitors of protein kinase C and direct measurements of diacylglycerol and protein kinase C translocation support such a proposal.

Acknowledgments

This work was supported by USPHS HL 32383 (JAB) and HL 42800 (IL).

References

[1] Toole, J. F. (1990) *Cerebrovascular Disorders* (Toole, J. F., ed.), Raven, New York, pp. 451–469.
[2] Chyatte, D. and Sundt, T. M. (1984) *Mayo Clin. Proc.* **59,** 498–505.
[3] Bevan, J. A. and Bevan, R. D. (1988) *Ann. Rev. Pharmacol.* **28,** 311–329.
[4] Findlay, J. M., Macdonald, R. L., and Weir, B. K. (1991) *Cerebrovasc. Brain Metab.* **3,** 336–361.

5 Cook, D. A. (1984) *Pharmacology* **29**, 1–16.
6 Bevan, J. A., Bevan, R. D., and Frazee, J. G. (1987) *Stroke* **18**, 472–481.
7 Fisher, C. M., Kistler, J. P., and Davis, J. M. (1980) *Neurosurgery* **6**, 1–8.
8 Mayberg, M. R., Okada, T., and Bark, D. H. (1990) *J. Neurosurg.* **72**, 634–640.
9 Peterson, J. W., Roussos, L., Kwun, B. D., Hackett, J. D., Owen, C. J., and Zervas, N. T. (1990) *J. Neurosurg.* **72**, 775–781.
10 Macdonald, R. L., Weir, B. K. A., Runzer, T. D., Grace, M. G. A., Findlay, J. M., Saito, K., Cook, D. A., Mielke, B. W., and Kanamaru, K. (1991) *J. Neurosurg.* **75**, 415–424.
11 Nakagomi, T., Kassel, N. F., Sasaki, T., Fujiwara, S., Lehman, R. M., and Turner, J. C. (1987) *Stroke* **18**, 482–489.
12 Toshima, M., Kassell, N. F., Sasaki, T., Tanaka, Y., and Machi, T. (1992) *J. Neurosurg.* **76**, 670–678.
13 Juvela, S., Kaste, M., and Hillbom, M. (1990) *Stroke* **21**, 566–571.
14 Ross, R. (1986) *N. Engl. J. Med.* **314**, 488–500.
15 Schror, K. and Verheggen, R. (1988) *Trends Pharmacol. Sci.* **9**, 71–74.
16 Conner, H. E., Edwards, L. A., and Feniuk, W. (1989) *Eur. J. Pharmacol.* **174**, 205–213.
17 Chehrazi, B. B., Giri, S., and Joy, R. M. (1989) *Stroke* **20**, 217–224.
18 Saito, A. and Lee, T. J.-F. (1987) *Circ. Res.* **60**, 220–228.
19 White, R. P., Chapleau, C. E., Dugdale, M., and Robertson, J. T. (1980) *Stroke* **11**, 363–368.
20 Germann, P., Laher, I., and Bevan, J. A. (1991) *Stroke* **22**, 1534–1540.
21 Boullin, D. J., Mohan, J., and Grahame-Smith, D. G. (1976) *J. Neurol. Neurosurg. Psychiatry* **39**, 756–766.
22 van Neuten, J. M., De Ridder, W., Van Gorp, L., and De Clerk, F. (1987) *Eur. J. Pharmacol.* **133**, 301–308.
23 Young, H. A., Kolbeck, R. C., Schmidek, H., and Evans, J. (1986) *Neurosurgery* **19**, 346–349.
24 Debdi, M., Seylaz, J., and Sercombe, R. (1992) *Stroke* **23**, 1154–1162.
25 Abel, P. W., Han, C., Noe, B. D., and McDonald, J. K. (1988) *Brain Res.* **463**, 250–258.
26 Laher, I. and van Breemen, C. (1991) *The Resistance Vasculature* (Bevan, J. A., Halpern, W., and Mulvany, M. J., eds.), Humana, Totowa, NJ, pp. 305–317.
27 Matsui, T., Sugawa, M., Johshita, H., Takuwa, Y., and Asano, T. (1991) *Stroke* **22**, 1183–1187.
28 Nishizawa, S., Nezu, N., and Vemura, K. (1992) *J. Neurosurg.* **76**, 635–639.
29 Matsui, T., Takuway, Y., Johsita, H., Yamashita, K., and Asano, T. (1991) *J. Cereb. Blood Flow Metab.* **11**, 143–149.

Chapter 30

Chronic Cerebrovasospasm

Role of Increased Vascular Wall Rigidity

Peter Vorkapic

Chronic cerebrovasospasm (CCV) is the term used to describe the angiographic narrowing of cerebral arteries. CCV is usually a complication of subarachnoid hemorrhage (SAH), which in the majority of instances results from rupture of an intracranial aneurysm. Chronic cerebrovasospasm is closely correlated to the amount of blood in the subarachnoid space,[1] delayed in onset, longlasting,[2] and slowly reversing over several weeks. Its hallmark is refractoriness to pharmacological vasodilator therapy in humans[3] and animals.[4,5] Only few animal models have been developed that reflect the features of CCV seen in the human.[4-6] Structural changes indicative of damage of the vessel wall seem to be responsible for the refractoriness to vasodilator treatment.[7,8] Abnormal active vascular muscle tone resulting from putative spasmogens released from blood, blood clot, and surrounding brain tissue might play a major role in the initiation of events that finally lead to chronic irreversible narrowing of arteries.[9,10] We have developed a model of CCV of the rabbit basilar artery, and studied the longitudinal time-course of angiographic (in vivo) and functional (in vitro) parameters of the vessel wall over a period of 9 d.[5,11] SAH was accomplished by multiple injections of autologous blood (3 mL/kg) through a silastic catheter placed with its tip in the prepontine cistern close to the basilar artery.

From *The Human Brain Circulation*, R. D. Bevan and J. A. Bevan, eds.
©1994 Humana Press

Peak angiographic narrowing occurred after 1 d (54%), and a steady-state constriction of about 70% was observed throughout the rest of the study period. The effect of papaverine (PPV) bolus injection into the vertebral artery during angiography displayed two phases of CCV: The intraarterial bolus injection of PPV completely reversed arterial narrowing within 2 d after SAH. However, beginning on d 3 and increasingly progressing to d 5, the amount of narrowing that was refractory to the vasodilator action of PPV increased. The PPV-insensitive component of arterial narrowing on d 9 was 63.1%. Although an early phase of vasospasm has not been observed in humans,[12] a transient abnormal active vessel contraction owing to putative spasmogens cannot be excluded as an essential and crucial component in the initiation of CCV.[9,10] Papaverine might counteract this active contraction in the early phase of CCV.

During the first 2 d after experimental SAH, we observed transient spontaneous increases in tone (in vitro)—up to 45% of maximum tissue contractility—that were reversed by PPV. When applied topically, PPV relaxes cerebral arteries during operations performed at the acute stage of SAH (personal observation).

A major functional change in the vessel segments examined in vitro was an increase in vessel wall stiffness. This increase was documented by determination of the passive tension–length (T/L) relationship. Expressed as a ratio $T4_{SAH}/T4_C$, vessel wall stiffness increased progressively over the study period, commencing at d 2 and reaching maximum increase at d 9 (270%) (Fig. 1).

Artery wall stiffness was directly related to the PPV-insensitive narrowing of basilar arteries seen on angiography (Fig. 2). It seems likely that the time-course of the PPV-insensitive component of angiographic narrowing reflects changes in vessel wall texture when passive factors dominate the arterial constriction. In a dog model of cerebrovasospasm, compliance and optimum length of basilar arteries for the response to uridine 5'-triphospate were reduced 8 d after SAH.[13]

Endothelium-based acetylcholine-induced vasorelaxation was impaired already on d 1, and progressively diminished to about 50% from d 2 to 9. Loss of endothelial function (release of endothe-

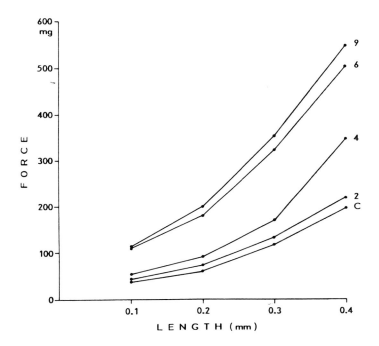

Fig. 1. Longitudinal time-course of in vitro rabbit basilar artery wall stiffness (passive wall force vs length) after experimental subarachnoid hemorrhage (injection of autologous blood). Significant increase in passive wall force occurred 3 d after injection of blood. For clarity only, mean values are shown. C, vessels of sham-operated control rabbits. Numbers to the right of curves are days after subarachnoid hemorrhage.

lium-derived relaxing factor) might enhance the vasoconstrictor influences of substances released from the blood clot (e.g., hemoglobin, serotonin, thrombin). The maximum capacity of the arterial segments to develop active force was markedly reduced at d 3 and progressively declined to d 9 after SAH. The mean reduction in maximum contractility from d 6 to 9 was 52%. Loss of contractility was directly related to PPV-resistant angiographic basilar artery diameter ($r = 0.7949$). Also, we found a positive correlation between vessel wall stiffness and loss of contractility ($r = 0.8493$); the stiffer the artery the greater the loss of contractility. In a monkey model,

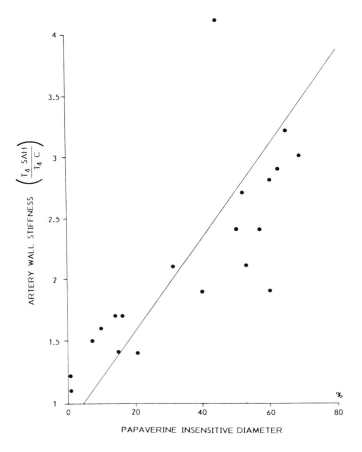

Fig. 2. Graph of relationship between in vivo PPV-insensitive diameter of rabbit basilar artery and artery wall stiffness (ratio of force developed after fourth incremental stretching of vessel segment from experimental and control rabbits) ($r = 0.83316$).

the greatest angiographic narrowing occurred in those vessels that had the least capacity to contract, and the vessels showed degenerative changes of the smooth muscle cell layer.[7] Based on these experimental data, it seems unlikely that active contraction could make an important contribution to chronic cerebrovasospasm.

The mechanisms responsible for the development of chronic cerebrovasospasm are poorly understood. The seeds of CCV are sown early, probably within the first hours after subarachnoid hemorrhage. High concentrations of vasoconstrictor substances released from blood clot are associated with vessel wall damage,[9] followed by nonspecific inflammation and fibrosis.[7,8] Loss of contractility and increased wall stiffness reflect functional damage to the basilar artery wall. Structural changes are consistent with these findings. An increase in the content of Type V collagen in biopsy specimens of arteries taken during surgery 9 and 21 d after SAH has been reported.[8] The results of angioplasty to mechanically dilate narrowed arteries after SAH indicate that structural changes are a dominant feature of cerebrovasospasm.[14]

If chronic cerebrovasospasm follows abnormal smooth muscle contraction resulting from the action of putative spasmogens by causing excessive calcium entry from the extracellular space, it might be expected that CCV would be ameliorated or prevented by calcium channel blockers. In our model, rabbits were treated with clentiazem, a derivative of diltiazem, given 24 h before experimental SAH. Clentiazem prevented the late PPV-insensitive narrowing, the increased artery wall rigidity, the decreased contractility, and the abnormal spontaneous tone excursions. Since the capacity to develop active force and wall compliance was preserved, one can assume that clentiazem interferes with the initial steps in the self-perpetuating cascade of damage and the subsequent vascular wall response. The protective effect of clentiazem is probably the result of the prevention of excessive calcium entry, which prevents calcium overload and subsequent cell damage.[15]

In summary, in our rabbit model of SAH, decreased vessel wall compliance and loss of contractility were the dominant features found to be responsible for the vasodilator-resistant narrowing seen on angiography. CCV is not an active contraction, but is an arterial narrowing owing to structural changes in artery wall texture. Confirmation of these findings needs to be sought in human tissue obtained postmortem.

References

1   Fisher, C. M., Kistler, J. P., and Davis, J. M. (1980) *Neurosurgery* **6**, 1–9.
2   Harders, A. G. and Gilsbach, J. M. (1987) *J. Neurosurg.* **66**, 718–728.
3   Wilkins, R. H. (1986) *Neurosurgery* **18**, 808–825.
4   Varsos, V. G., Liszczak, T. M., Han, D. H., Kistler, J. P., and Vielma, J. (1983) *J. Neurosurg.* **58**, 11–17.
5   Vorkapic, P., Bevan, R. D., and Bevan, J. D. (1991) *J. Neurosug.* **74**, 951–955.
6   Frazee, J. G., Gianotta, S. L., and Stern, W. E. (1981) *J. Neurosurg.* **55**, 865–868.
7   Bevan, J. A., Bevan, R. D., and Frazee, J. G. (1987) *Stroke* **18**, 472–481.
8   Smith, R. R., Clower, B. R., Grotendorst, G. M., Yabuno, N., and Cruise, J. M. (1985) *Neurosurgery* **16**, 171–176.
9   Alksne, J. F. and Greenhot, J. H. (1974) *J. Neurosurg.* **41**, 440–445.
10 Macdonald, R. L., Weir, B. K. A., Runzer, T. D., Grace, M. G. A., Findlay, J. M., Saito, K., Cook, D. A., Mielke, B. W., and Kanamaru, K. (1991) *J. Neurosurg.* **75**, 415–424.
11 Vorkapic, P., Bevan, R. D., and Bevan, J. A. (1990) *Stroke* **21**, 1478–1484.
12 Romner, B., Ljunggren, B., Brandt, L., and Säveland, H. (1989) *J. Neurosurg.* **70**, 732–736.
13 Kim, P., Sundt, T. M., and Vanhoutte, P. M. (1989) *J. Neurosurg.* **71**, 430–436.
14 Zubkov, Y. N., Nikiforof, B. M., and Shustin, V. A. (1984) *Acta Neurochir.* **70**, 65–79.
15 Vorkapic, P., Bevan, J. A., and Bevan, R. D. (1991) *Stroke* **22**, 1409–1413.

Chapter 31

Feeding Artery Rigidity and Hemodynamics of Cerebral Arteriovenous Malformations

Christopher S. Ogilvy, Alynn Klaasen,
Theresa Wellman, Rosemary D. Bevan,
and John A. Bevan

Introduction

Cerebral arteriovenous malformations (AVMs) are vascular abnormalities that result in an excessive shunt of blood from the arterial to the venous system. Although there is brain parenchyma between the vascular channels of an AVM, it is often scarred and abnormal. The purpose of this study is to measure the elasticity of feeding vessels from AVMs obtained at the time of surgical resection. Pressure measurements of feeding arteries and draining veins of AVMs made prior to surgical resection and reported in the literature are reviewed. By combining the results of the in vivo experiments with published observations of pressure in vivo, a theory of how AVM hemodynamics can change over time is proposed.

Materials and Methods

Arterial feeding vessels from human arteriovenous malformations were excised during the resection of the AVM. Great care was taken to manipulate the vessel as little as possible with the surgical

From *The Human Brain Circulation*, R. D. Bevan and J. A. Bevan, eds.
©1994 Humana Press

instruments. Once the vessel was excised, it was placed immediately into a 5°C physiological saline solution containing penicillin, streptomycin, and heparin. The vessels were transported to the laboratory and dissected free from surrounding tissue before experimentation.

Passive Pressure–Diameter Measurements

The passive pressure–diameter relationship of segments of feed arteries to AVMs was measured and compared with prior data obtained from normal human pial artery segments. The apparatus and experimental procedures are described in Chapter 14.[1-4] The vessel was mounted in a pressure–perfusion system arteriograph and, after preliminary procedures, perfused and superfused with a calcium-free physiological saline solution (PSS) containing EGTA (1 mM). Once a plateau was reached indicating that all stretch-induced myogenic tone was lost, a sequential order of pressure steps was carried out up to 200 mmHg in increments of 5 or 10 mmHg, vessel diameter measurements being made at each step. All diameters were normalized to those obtained either at 5–10 or 50–60 mmHg during the initial 30-min setup.

Pressure Measured
from AVMs During Surgical Resection

Several reports describe pressure from the feeding arteries and draining veins of AVMs prior to measurements of surgical resection of the lesion. Typically, a small (25–27-gage) needle is inserted into the vessel to make the pressure measurement. It was possible to identify a total of 57 measurements of feeding artery pressure and 26 measurements of draining vein pressure.[5-10] The systemic blood pressure was reported in 57 of the patients, and central venous pressure was documented in 18. Such pressure measurements must be made safely. If there is any potential for inadvertent venous injury, the pressure in the draining vein cannot be measured.

Results

Elasticity of Feeding Arteries

AVM feeding vessels were relatively noncompliant compared with the normal pial blood vessels (Fig. 1). Under conditions of zero calcium in the surrounding medium when, active smooth

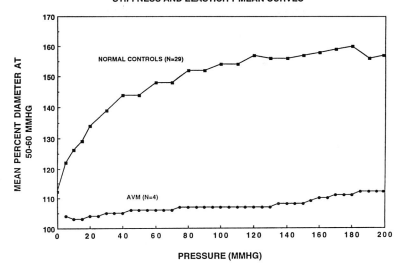

Fig. 1. Elasticity of normal human pial vessels (*n* = 29) and of feeding arteries from arteriovenous malformations (*n* = 4 arms, 24 measurements). Elasticity is expressed as a percent of the amount of vessel diameter increase when the vessel is exposed to incremental increases in transmural pressure from 5 to 199 mmHg. The standard errors for each point are small (1–3%) and are therefore not shown.

muscle tone did not develop, the increase in diameter of 4 AVM feeding arteries was minimal over the pressure range 5–200 mmHg. Vessels ranged in size from 100 to 1200 μm. Normal control vessels were obtained from the cerebral cortical surface of brain overlying central nervous system tumors. By contrast, these showed diameter changes of 30–40% with pressure increments up to 30 or 40 mmHg. The slope of the subsequent increase in diameter with pressure increase was greater than that for the AVM segments. The standard errors of the measurements shown in Fig. 1 were on the order of 1–2%. When points on the AVM curve are compared with points on the control curve for any given pressure value on the X axis using Student's *t*-test, at all pressure levels, the difference is statistically significant.

Pressure Measurements from AVMs

Pressure measurements from AVMs made at the time of surgical excision and presented in the reports noted above were reviewed. Average values were calculated and are shown in Fig. 2. Average mean blood pressure was 78 ± 2 mmHg ($n = 57$). Average feeding artery pressure was 50 ± 2 mmHg ($n = 57$). Pressure in the venous drainage from AVMs was 16 ± 1 mmHg ($n = 26$). Central venous pressure was 7 mmHg ($n = 18$).

Figure 2 also shows an idealized pressure profile for normal brain vasculature. The pressure in medium-sized cerebral vessels (anterior temporal branch of the middle cerebral artery) has been measured in one study during aneurysm surgery.[11] The pressure in this size vessel was approx 90% of the systemic blood pressure. This size of vessel is compatible with the size of feeding arteries to AVMs.

Discussion

Arteriovenous malformations are presumed to be developmental abnormalities, which are formed as direct shunts from the arterial to the venous circulation during gestation. The incidence of hemorrhage of these lesions is greatest in the third, fourth, and fifth decades of life. The fact that AVMs are present for a long time prior to hemorrhage implies that changes occur within the lesions making them more prone to hemorrhage. An analysis of the hemodynamics of these lesions sheds some light on this possibility.

When we measured the elasticity of arteries feeding AVMs, we found them to be extremely stiff-walled conduits (Fig. 1) that show little, if any, response to pharmacologic agents (unpublished data). It is known that these feeding arteries are exposed to high rates of blood flow.[8–10] When arteries are exposed to elevated rates of flow, there is thickening of the vessel wall.[12] The feeding arteries of AVMs are known to have abnormally thickened walls.[13] Indeed, such changes could progress over time to the point where an initially normal vessel could become thickened, noncompliant, and unresponsive to pharmacologic agents. Although the actual pressure in the feeding artery may be lower than normal, the increased flow may be the driving force to induce such changes. Muraszko

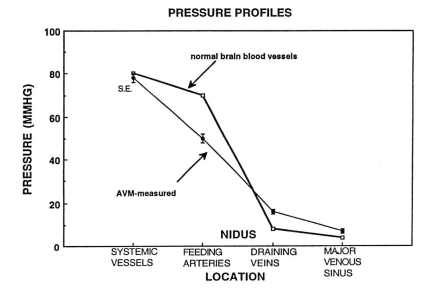

Fig. 2. Pressure profiles measured for AVMs of the brain compared to a hypothetical profile of normal brain blood vessels. SE is standard error of the group mean for values available in the literature *(see text)*.

et al.[14] measured the vascular activity in vitro of feeding vessels from 24 patients with AVMs. They found varying responses to pharmacologic stimuli. Four of the segments were entirely unresponsive to pharmacologic agents.[14]

Figure 2 shows a comparison between pressure measured along the course of AVMs compared with the typical pressure expected in the normal cerebral circulation. The arterial pressure in normal brain medium-sized vessels has been measured to be approx 90% of systemic blood pressure.[11] Feeding arteries to AVMs vary greatly in size. Although some are on the order of 1–3 mm in diameter, others are more comparable to large pial vessels in size. The pressure in pial vessels in experimental animals has been measured to be 50–60% of systemic arterial pressure.[15] Therefore, the idealized "normal brain" blood vessel pressure may overestimate the pressure. The lower pressure in the AVM feeding vessels presumably reflects the lack of distensibility associated with

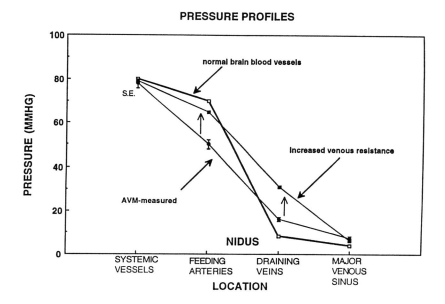

Fig. 3. Pressure profiles are shown as described in Fig. 2. As histopathologic changes occur in the malformation over time, venous resistance may increase. As this occurs, the arterial circuit has little ability to regulate flow into the malformation, and therefore, pressure increases in the nidus of the malformation. This may be why hemorrhage occurs after many years.

their rigid walls. However, such a vessel would not constrict as do normal arteries to an increase in intramural pressure. Thus, increases in systemic arterial pressure would be directly transmitted to the body of the malformation.

The venous system also has a physiologic response to increased blood flow. When vein grafts are placed in the arterial circuit, thickening of the wall occurs over time with intimal proliferation.[16] The pharmacologic response of veins changes as they are exposed to arterial pressure and flow.[17] In AVMs, the venous channels are typically thickened and, at times, can be visibly stenotic on cerebral angiography. Figure 3 demonstrates possible changes that may occur over time if the venous system of the malformation were to develop increased resistance while the arterial side acted as rigid conduits, as we have observed. Venous resistance could increase because of reduction in venous compliance. In addition, venous stenosis and thrombosis are known to occur in AVMs, and are associated with an increased potential for hemorrhage.[18] Seemingly small elevations in venous pressure may be reflected throughout the nidus of the AVM (Fig. 3).

If venous resistance increased over time, the pressure would increase in the nidus of the lesion. It is within this nidus that thin-walled, small-caliber, fragile vessels can be identified. Although the exact location of AVM hemorrhage remains unknown, one could imagine that as these vessels are exposed to higher pressures, hemorrhage may be more likely to occur. Further experiments to evaluate the elasticity of the venous elements of AVMs might shed light on this hypothesis.

References

1 Halpern, W., Osol, G., and Coy, G. S. (1984) *Ann. Biomed. Eng.* **12,** 463–479.
2 Mulvany, M. J. and Halpern, W. (1976) *Nature* **260,** 617–619.
3 Bevan, J. A. and Joyce, E. H. (1988) *Blood Vessels* **25,** 261–264.
4 Bevan, J. A., Garcia-Roldan, J.-L., and Joyce, E. H. (1990) *Blood Vessels* **27,** 202–207.
5 Spetzler, R. F., Hargraves, R. W., McCormick, P. W., Zabramski, J. M., Flom, R. A., and Zimmerman, R. S. (1992) *J. Neurosurg.* **76,** 910–923.
6 Leblanc, R. and Little, J. R. (1990) *Clinical Neurosurgery* (Chapter 20) (Black, P. McL., ed.), Williams and Williams, Baltimore, MD, pp. 299–317.
7 Barnett, G. H., Little, J. R., Ebrahim, Z. Y., Jones, S. C., and Friel, H. T. (1987) *Neurosurgery* **20,** 836–842.
8 Nornes, H. and Grip, A. (1980) *J. Neurosurg.* **53,** 456–464.
9 Nornes, H., Grip, A., and Wikeby, P. (1979) *J. Neurosurg.* **50,** 145–151.
10 Hassler, W. and Steinmetz, H. (1987) *J. Neurosurg.* **67,** 822–831.
11 Little, J. R., Tomsak, R. L., Ebrahim, Z. Y., and Furlan, A. J. (1986) *Neurosurgery* **18,** 716–720.
12 Fry, D. L. (1968) *Circ. Res.* **22,** 165–197.
13 Martin, N. and Vinters, H. (1990) *Intracranial Vascular Malformations* (Barrow, D. L., ed.), AANS, Park Ridge, IL, pp. 1–30.
14 Muraszko, K., Wang, H. H., Pelton, G., and Stein, B. M. (1990) *Neurosurgery* **26,** 190–200.

[15] Baumbach, G. L., Siems, J. E., and Heistad, D. D. (1991) *Circ. Res.* **68,** 338–351.

[16] Lalka, S. G., Unthank, J. L., Lash, J. M., McGue, J. G., Cikrit, D. F., Sawchuk, A. P., and Dalsing, M. C. (1991) *Surgery* **110,** 73–79.

[17] Radic, A. S., O'Donohoe, M. K., Schwartz, L. B., Stein, A. D., Mikat, E. M., McCann, R. L., and Hagen, P.-O. (1991) *J. Vasc. Surg.* **140,** 40–47.

[18] Miyasaka, Y., Yada, K., Ohwada, T., Kitahara, T., Kurata, A., and Irikura, K. (1992) *J. Neurosurg.* **76,** 239–243.

Chapter 32

Effects of Acute Hypertension on Pial Artery Tone

George Osol

Introduction

The arteries that course along the surface of the brain normally operate in a state of partial, sustained constriction (tone) from which either dilation or constriction may occur, as required to maintain normal blood flow. Although its extent varies with arterial size and experimental conditions, basal tone appears to be a widespread vascular phenomenon that has been observed in cerebral arteries from a number of species, in vivo and in vitro (e.g., refs. 1–3). Some degree of arterial constriction is requisite for cerebral blood flow (CBF) autoregulation, which is principally effected by arterial dilation to decreases, and by constriction to increases in transmural pressure.[4]

Whether one accepts the fourth power relationship between flow and the diameter of a tube first described by Hagen and Poiseuille in the nineteenth century, or more recent measurements of blood flow within vascular networks that have the added complexity of geometrical pattern (parallel resistance) and varying arterial diameters (serial resistance) that suggest that a third-order relationship may be more accurate,[5] it is nonetheless clear that lumen diameter is the single most powerful determinant of blood flow under physiological conditions.

From *The Human Brain Circulation*, R. D. Bevan and J. A. Bevan, eds.
©1994 Humana Press

In addition to its contribution to CBF autoregulation, the reflex ability of an artery to constrict with increasing transmural pressure is inherently protective in nature. Large fluctuations in blood pressure normally occur during times of emotional or physical stress, or during certain forms of activity (e.g., weight lifting, sexual intercourse). A failure of the arteries to constrict at a time of acute pressure elevation could lead downstream small arterioles and capillaries to experience abnormally high distending pressures, and thereby produce cellular damage or rupture. This consideration is not purely theoretical, since forced dilatation of the cerebral vasculature during acute hypertension is associated with both hemorrhagic stroke and hypertensive encephalopathy.[6-9]

Case studies in humans suggest that the upper limit of blood pressure that can be tolerated by normotensive individuals is somewhere between 140 and 170 mmHg, although the pressure threshold at which autoregulatory "breakthrough" occurs may actually be fairly discrete. In one person, for example, flow autoregulation was maintained from 110–162 mmHg; when pressure was increased an additional 2 mmHg, to 164 mmHg, CBF suddenly doubled.[8]

In Vivo Studies

Our understanding of the effects of acute hypertension on pial artery tone derives largely from studies on animals in which mean arterial pressure can be increased above the upper limit of CBF autoregulation by the infusion of pressor substances such as angiotensin II or norepinephrine. By such means, arterial pressure can be elevated progressively. These peripherally vasoactive compounds do not cross the blood–brain barrier and are normally metabolized by the cerebral endothelium, so that the responses of the cerebral circulation are considered to be secondary to their effect on intravascular pressure, rather than direct action on the cells within the arterial wall.

Experimental studies of this type have shown that when the systemic pressure is suddenly elevated above the upper limit of CBF regulation, the distending force acting on the vascular wall (wall tension or stress) overcomes the ability of smooth muscle to produce a counterforce sufficient to maintain normal lumen diameter. This results in forced dilatation of the arteries and disruption of the blood–brain barrier,[9–12] an event that occurs initially in postcapillary venules,[13] but has been observed in pial arteries and penetrating arterioles as well.[14]

During an episode of sudden hypertension, cerebral arteries often develop areas of uneven constriction, termed the "sausage-" or "bead–string" phenomenon, which have also been observed in chronically hypertensive animals.[15] Originally thought to represent areas of excessive constriction, or "hypertensive vasospasm,"[16] more recent studies have demonstrated that it is the narrowed portions that possess autoregulatory tone whereas the wider segments have undergone forced dilatation and loss of reactivity to pressure.[17,18]

The potential hemodynamic effects of forced dilatation are threefold. The first, already mentioned above, is that a decrease in flow resistance and subsequent exposure of smaller downstream vessels to excessive transmural pressures may lead to blood–brain damage and edema, or rupture, thereby inducing hypertensive encephalopathy or hemorrhagic stroke. Second, the segmental differences in lumen diameter observed during and after acute hypertension may produce increased flow turbulence and focal changes in shear stress that damage endothelial cells, initiating a positive feedback cycle through which further vascular damage could occur. Third, an increase in flow to one territory of a major artery could produce an intracerebral steal phenomenon, decreasing blood flow to areas that are already marginally perfused, such as the watershed or boundary zones between two major arteries that have a known vulnerability to ischemic lesions.

Regional differences in arterial responses to acute hypertension have also been documented. In one study, acute hypertension was induced in cats by aortic obstruction and intravenous infusion of norepinephrine or angiotensin.[19] Regional cerebral blood flow, measured with microspheres, was increased 159% in the cerebrum, 106% in the cerebellum, and 58% in the brain stem. The authors suggested that regional heterogeneity may be attributed to differences in the fraction of the systemic arterial pressure that is transmitted to smaller arteries. A study in which pressure gradients in the human brain were predicted from measurements of arterial length and radius made from acrylic casts of the cerebral vasculature[20] was cited in support of this hypothesis: Based on differences in the ratio of radius to length, a steeper pressure gradient was predicted in the latter, suggesting that anatomical patterns may contribute to the observed differences. Blood–brain barrier dysfunction during acute hypertension occurred preferentially in the cerebrum of cats[24] but not rats,[12] a finding that serves as a reminder of species differences in the architecture and physiology of the cerebral circulation.

Putative Mechanisms

The cellular mechanisms that underlie forced dilatation in cats have been elucidated by Kontos and his colleagues.[18,21,22] In these studies, discrete episodes of hypertension were induced in anesthetized animals by the intravenous infusion of angiotensin II or norepinephrine. The installation of a cranial window beforehand allowed the investigators to directly observe the pial arteries and arterioles before, during, and after the hypertensive episode. They found arterial responses to be size-dependent, with smaller (<100 μm) arteries dilating initially, whereas larger vessels (>200 μm) remained constricted. Elevating arterial pressure above 200 mmHg produced forced dilatation in the large arteries as well, an event that was frequently irreversible and accompanied by a subsequent loss of reactivity to chemical (hypercapnea) and physical (changes in blood pressure) stimuli, and a significant decrease in oxygen consumption. Scanning and transmission electron microscopy revealed destructive lesions localized primarily in the endothelial cells, although a small percentage of smooth muscle cells (about 5%) were damaged as well.

When animals were pretreated with cyclooxygenase inhibitors, such as indomethacin, or with scavengers of free oxygen radicals (mannitol or superoxide dismutase), both the dilation and the ultrastructural damage associated with acute hypertension were prevented.[18] Additional studies have substantiated these initial observations, leading to the conclusion that acute hypertension may induce the release of an autocoid, possibly bradykinin, that stimulates the release of arachidonate from membrane phospholipids, presumably through the activation of a phospholipase. Increased arachidonate concentrations then initiate cyclooxygenase-mediated prostaglandin synthesis within the vascular wall. The subsequent activation of prostaglandin hydroperoxidase leads to the production and release of a superoxide anion radical that enters the cerebral extracellular space via an anion channel. By dismutation, this gives rise to hydrogen peroxide and the generation of hydroxyl radicals, which damage the endothelium and vascular smooth muscle and render the artery unreactive.[22]

It is unclear whether this mechanism, carefully documented in cats, holds true for other species. In recent years, there has been considerable controversy as to the role of the endothelium in modulating pial artery tone. Using isolated, pressurized vessels in vitro, Harder and colleagues reported that basal tone and reactivity to pressure was abolished in feline cerebral vessels from which the endothelium had been removed.[23] The same researchers, using an apparatus in which two vessels were perfused in series, also demonstrated that intravascular pressure stimulated the release of a transferable endothelial vasoconstrictor substance (as yet unidentified).[24]

Since that time, a number of investigators, working with isolated cerebral, coronary, and skeletal muscle arteries from nonfeline species such as rats or pigs, have demonstrated repeatedly that endothelial removal does not abolish basal tone or arterial responses to pressure.[25-27] This suggests that mechanisms intrinsic to smooth muscle (myogenic) are predominant in most cases (for review, *see* ref. 28). Thus, the cat may be somewhat unique in possessing a mechanism for arterial reactivity to transmural pressure that is largely endothelial in nature.

These rather disparate observations regarding the cellular basis of pial artery tone in cats vs other species raise the question of whether the mechanisms underlying forced dilatation differ as well. If pressure-dependent tone is truly "endogenic" in cats and myogenic in other species, as suggested by the evidence to date, it would not be surprising that forced dilatation, associated with predominantly endothelial lesions in Kontos' studies, led to a complete and irreversible loss of tone in the cat. Endothelial destruction or removal in the rat augments basal tone,[27,29] however, and the pattern of arterial behavior following forced dilatation might be quite different.

In Vitro Studies

With this in mind, we recently applied the in vitro pressurized artery technique[30] to the question of forced dilatation. Pial arteries were obtained from normotensive WKY rats, and pressurized to 75 mmHg. During equilibration, these vessels normally develop a stable tone that reduces lumen diameter by 25–35%, and respond to increases in pressure with additional constriction until the upper limit of the myogenic range (approx 150 mmHg)[31] is attained. Endothelial denudation augments the level of basal tone and does not affect diameter responses to transmural pressure. In one series of experiments ($n = 6$), transmural pressure was increased from 75 mmHg in 25 mmHg increments every 10 min, until forced dilatation (FD) occurred. This event, which occurred at a mean pressure of 161 ± 7 mmHg, was characterized by the appearance of large, transient dilations that were followed by only partial reconstriction. Any further increase in pressure led to a complete and rapid loss of myogenic tone. Following FD, transmural pressure was returned to 75 mmHg, and the arteries allowed to re-equilibrate for 30 min. Endothelial and smooth muscle cell reactivity was tested before and after FD by the application of acetylcholine (ACh, $10 \mu M$) and prostaglandin $F_{2\alpha}$ (PGF$_{2\alpha}$, $5 \mu M$), respectively. The results were as follows:

1. Basal tone, completely abolished during the exposure to high transmural pressure, returned over a period of 10–15 min and, at 30 min, had stabilized to a level that was significantly higher than that measured in the same vessel and at the same pressure prior to FD ($28 \pm 3\%$ before FD vs $36 \pm 5\%$ after FD, $p < 0.05$).
2. Arterial relaxation of ACh was significantly diminished following forced dilatation (dilation, expressed as a percentage of maximal relaxation, was $69 \pm 9\%$ before, and $45 \pm 6\%$ after FD, $p < 0.05$).
3. Constrictions to PGF$_{2\alpha}$ were comparable before vs after FD ($42 \pm 5\%$ vs $46 \pm 9\%$, $p > 0.05$).

Based on these in vitro data, we conclude that, as in the cat, forced dilatation owing to sudden increases in transmural pressure results in selective damage to the endothelium. Smooth muscle cell function appears to be well preserved, however, as manifested by the reappearance of pressure-induced myogenic tone and constriction to $PGF_{2\alpha}$. It is interesting to note that the increase in basal tone following forced dilatation parallels that observed in vessels denuded of the endothelium,[27,29] further suggesting a loss of some tonic inhibitory influence.

Summary

In summary, acute and severe hypertension leads to a loss of intrinsic cerebral artery tone (forced dilatation). Endothelial cells appear to be particularly vulnerable to damage from exposure to high transmural pressures, either acute[23] or chronic,[32,33] and the damage may be related to the generation of oxygen free radicals, particularly of the hydroxyl moiety. Following a return to the normotensive state, the effects of acute pressure elevation on basal tone appear to vary, and may be related to the mechanisms that underlie the expression of pressure-dependent vascular tone.

References

[1] Busija, D. W., Heistad, D. D., and Marcus, M. L. (1981) *Am. J. Physiol.* **241**, H228–H234.

[2] Vinall, P. E. and Simeone, F. A. (1981) *Stroke* **12**, 640–642.

[3] Osol, G. and Halpern, W. (1985) *Am. J. Physiol.* **249**, H914–H921.

[4] Johnson, P. C. (1986) *Circ. Res.* **59**, 483–495.

[5] Mayrovitz, H. N. and Roy, J. (1983) *Am. J. Physiol.* **245**, H1031–H1038.

[6] Heistad, D. D. and Marcus, M. L. (1978) *Circ. Res.* **45**, 331–338.

[7] Tamaki, K. T., Sadoshima, S., Baumbach, G. L., Iadecola, C., Reis, D. J., and Heistad, D. D. (1984) *Hypertension* **6(Suppl. 1)**, I-75–I-81.

[8] Skinhoj, E. and Strandgaard, S. (1973) *Lancet* **1**, 461–462.

[9] MacKenzie, E. T., Strandgaard, S., Graham, D. I., Jones, J. V., Harper, A. M., and Farrar, J. K. (1976) *Circ. Res.* **39**, 33–41.

[10] Strandgaard, S., MacKenzie, E. T., Sengupta, D., Rowan, J. P., Lassen, N. A., and Harper, A. M. (1974) *Circ. Res.* **34**, 435–440.

[11] Johansson, B., Strandgaard, S., and Lassen, N. A. (1974) *Circ. Res.* **34–35**, I-167–I-174.

[12] Johansson, B. B. (1978) *Stroke* **9**, 588–590.

[13] Mayhan, W. G. and Heistad, D. D. (1985) *Am. J. Physiol.* **248**, H712–H718.

[14] Nag, S., Robertson, D. M., and Dinsdale, H. B. (1977) *Lab. Investig.* **36,** 150–161.

[15] Werber, A. H. and Heistad, K. K. (1984) *Circ. Res.* **55,** 286–294.

[16] Byrom, F. B. (1954) *Lancet* **2,** 201–211.

[17] Auer, L. M. (1978) *Acta. Neurochir.* (Wein) **27(Suppl.),** 1–11.

[18] Kontos, H. A., Wei, E. P., Dietrich, W. E., Narari, R. M., Povlishock, J. T., Ghatak, N. R., Ellis, E. F., and Patterson, J. L., Jr. (1981) *Am. J. Physiol.* **240,** H511–H527.

[19] Baumbach, G. L. and Heistad, D. D. (1985) *Am. J. Physiol.* **249,** H629–H637.

[20] Fukasawa, H. (1969) *Tohoku J. Exp. Med.* **99,** 255–268.

[21] Kontos, H. A., Wei, E. P., Navari, R. M., Lavasseur, J. E., Rosenblum, W. I., Patterson, J. L., Jr. (1978) *Am. J. Physiol.* **234,** H371–H383.

[22] Kontos, H. A. (1985) *Cir. Res.* **57,** 508–516.

[23] Harder, D. R. (1987) *Circ. Res.* **60,** 102–107.

[24] Harder, D. R., Sanchez-Ferrer, C., Kauser, K., Stekiel, W. J., and Rubanyi, G. M. (1989) *Circ. Res.* **65,** 193–198.

[25] Kuo, L., Chilian, W. M., and Davis, M. J. (1990) *Circ. Res.* **66,** 860–866.

[26] Falcone, J. C., Davis, M. J., and Meininger, G. A. (1991) *Am. J. Physiol.* **260,** H130–H135.

[27] McCarron, J., Osol, G., and Halpern, W. (1990) *Blood Vessels* **26,** 315–319.

[28] Meininger, G. A. and Davis, M. J. (1992) *Am. J. Physiol.* **263,** H647–H659.

[29] Osol, G., Osol, R., and Halpern, W. (1988) *Proceedings of the Second Symposium on Resistance Arteries,* Perinatology, New York, pp. 162–169.

[30] Halpern, W., Osol, G., and Coy, G. (1984) *Ann. Biomed. Eng.* **12,** 463–479.

[31] Osol, G. and Halpern, W. (1985) *Am. J. Physiol.* **249,** H914–H921.

[32] Mayhan, W. G., Faraci, F. M., and Heistad, D. D. (1987) *Am. J. Physiol.* **253,** H1435–H1440.

[33] Luscher, T. F., Raij, L., and Vanhoutte, P. M. (1987) *Hypertension* **9,** 157–163.

Chapter 33

Changes in the Cerebral Circulation in Chronic Hypertension

Gary L. Baumbach

Introduction

Chronic hypertension profoundly alters the function and structure of cerebral blood vessels. The pressure–flow relationship in the cerebral circulation is altered in chronic hypertension with a shift of the autoregulatory "plateau" to the right.[1] The shift in the autoregulatory plateau is beneficial to the brain, because blood flow is maintained relatively constant during large increases in arterial pressure. At the same time, however, the shift is detrimental because susceptibility to critical reductions in cerebral blood flow during acute hypotension is increased.

Cerebral vascular hypertrophy occurs during chronic hypertension[2] and probably contributes to the shift of the autoregulatory plateau. Another factor that may contribute to this shift is a reduction in external diameter. We have termed this phenomenon "remodeling" to differentiate it from effects of vascular hypertrophy *per se*. In stroke-prone spontaneously hypertensive rats (SHRSP), encroachment on the lumen of cerebral arterioles appears to result in large part from remodeling with a reduction in external diameter, not to hypertrophy *per se*.[3]

Thus, hypertrophy and remodeling would appear to be important adaptive responses of the cerebral circulation to chronic hypertension. One of the aims of this chapter is to consider the

From *The Human Brain Circulation*, R. D. Bevan and J. A. Bevan, eds.
©1994 Humana Press

contributions of hypertrophy and remodeling to altered responses of cerebral blood vessels during chronic hypertension with an emphasis on alterations in cerebral vascular autoregulation. The other aim is to review various factors that may contribute to hypertrophy and remodeling of cerebral blood vessels during chronic hypertension. In relation to hypertrophy, a concept is emphasized that previously has received little attention: Pulse pressure may be an important determinant of hypertrophy in cerebral blood vessels. In relation to remodeling, preliminary evidence is highlighted that suggests that some of the factors that play a prominent role in the development of hypertrophy may not contribute to cerebral vascular remodeling.

Consequences of Structural Change

Hypertrophy vs Remodeling

Two of the major alterations that occur in the cerebral vascular bed during chronic hypertension are increased responsiveness to constrictor stimuli, including acute increases in pressure,[1] and impaired responsiveness to dilator stimuli, such as acute decreases in pressure,[4] seizure,[5] or hypercapnia.[6] The primary mechanism that has been proposed to account for alterations of vascular responsiveness is hypertrophy of the vessel wall with encroachment on the vascular lumen.[7-9] Encroachment results in displacement of vascular smooth muscle toward the lumen. This resets the baseline from which smooth muscle exerts its control of vascular resistance to a higher level. An additional mechanism for encroachment on the vascular lumen is that external diameter of blood vessels decreases during chronic hypertension. A reduction in external diameter would be expected to have the same effect on vascular reactivity and resistance that has been predicted for hypertrophy: encroachment of the vessel wall into the original vascular lumen.

Recently, we examined the effects of chronic hypertension on cerebral arterioles in vivo. We found pronounced hypertrophy of the vessel wall, and also that both external and internal diameter during maximal dilation were reduced in cerebral arterioles of SHRSP.[3] Based on the finding that external, as well as internal, diameter is reduced in SHRSP, we have proposed that cerebral arterioles may undergo structural changes during chronic hypertension that result in remodeling of the arteriolar wall with a reduction in external diameter. Only about 25% of the decrease in internal diameter of cerebral arterioles in SHRSP can be attributed to hypertrophy, whereas about 75% results from reduction in external diameter.[3] Thus, not only does vascular remodeling with reduction in external diameter contribute to encroachment on the lumen of cerebral arterioles in SHRSP, the contribution of remodeling appears to be greater than that of vascular hypertrophy *per se*. Furthermore, we have estimated that remodeling, as well as hypertrophy, contributes to a pronounced shift in the relationship between the degree of smooth muscle shortening and increases in vascular resistance.[10] Vascular remodeling with reduction in external diameter, therefore, contributes importantly to both increased minimal resistance and increased vascular reactivity of cerebral arterioles in SHRSP. In addition, recent findings by Mulvany and his colleagues[11] suggest that remodeling may contribute to altered structure of peripheral resistance vessels in humans with essential hypertension and in spontaneously hypertensive rats (SHR).

Remodeling may have especially important implications in relation to the shift in cerebral vascular autoregulation with chronic hypertension. During chronic hypertension, the pressure–flow relationship in the cerebral circulation is shifted to the right (Fig. 1). Thus, constriction of cerebral blood vessels is enhanced during acute increases in arterial pressure, and vasodilation during hypotension is impaired. Previously, attention has focused on hypertrophy as the primary factor that contributes to the shift in cerebral vascular autoregulation. Recently, we proposed as an additional mechanism that, in the cerebral circulation, vascular remodeling with encroachment on the vascular lumen plays a critical role in the rightward shift of the autoregulatory plateau.[10]

Distensibility and Composition

In addition to encroachment on the vascular lumen by hypertrophy and remodeling, impairment of cerebral vasodilation in chronic hypertension has been attributed to reductions in vascular distensibility. This concept is supported by findings that distensi-

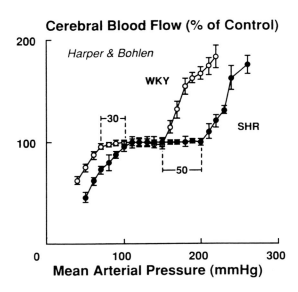

Fig. 1. Effects of chronic hypertension on autoregulation of cerebral blood flow. Autoregulation of cerebral blood flow is shifted to the right in spontaneously hypertensive rats (SHR) relative to normotensive Wistar Kyoto rats (WKY).[15] The magnitude of the shift is greater at the upper than the lower end of the curve, which suggests that enhancement of autoregulatory constriction in SHR is greater than impairment of autoregulatory dilation. The autoregulatory curves were redrawn from Fig. 2 in ref. 15.

bility of large cerebral arteries is reduced in SHR[12] and SHRSP.[13] The concept, however, apparently does not apply to cerebral arterioles. We have found that there is an increase in distensibility of cerebral arterioles during chronic hypertension, despite hypertrophy of the vessel wall.[2] This paradoxical increase in vascular distensibility may be explained by changes in proportional composition of cerebral arterioles that accompany hypertrophy of the vessel wall.[14] The more compliant components in the arteriolar wall, elastin and smooth muscle, are increased. At the same time, the less compliant components, collagen and basement membrane, remain constant. Thus, the more compliant components are disproportionately increased in cerebral arterioles during chronic hypertension.

An implication of the mechanical and structural alterations of cerebral arterioles that accompany chronic hypertension is that increases in arteriolar distensibility may help to preserve dilator capacity of cerebral arterioles. Support for this hypothesis derives from the finding that the autoregulatory range of cerebral blood flow in SHR is extended by 50 mmHg at the upper end of the curve, whereas the lower end of the curve is diminished by only 30 mmHg (Fig. 1).[15] This finding suggests that, during chronic hypertension, the degree of enhancement of autoregulatory constriction may be greater than the degree of impairment of autoregulatory dilation. Thus, not only is the autoregulatory range of cerebral blood flow shifted to a higher level of arterial pressure, but the range may be extended during chronic hypertension.

We speculate that the increase in distensibility of arterioles may tend to counteract encroachment on the lumen by hypertrophy and remodeling of the wall, thus attenuating impairment of vasodilation during acute hypotension and other vasodilator stimuli. Increases in arteriolar distensibility during chronic hypertension, therefore, may contribute to a relative preservation of autoregulatory dilation, which in turn may help to protect the cerebral circulation during severe reductions in arterial pressure. Furthermore, because distensibility of blood vessels is altered by activation of smooth muscle,[16,17] it is likely that the protective effect of encroachment on the lumen during vasoconstriction is preserved despite the increase in arteriolar distensibility.

Determinants of Structural Changes

Intravascular Pressure

Of the various determinants that contribute to vascular hypertrophy, one might assume that arterial pressure *per se* would play an especially important role. Nonetheless, the role of intravascular pressure is far from clear. A common approach is to examine effects of reduction in arterial pressure on vascular hypertrophy. One of the problems with this approach is that many of the methods that have been used to lower arterial pressure also have effects on other potential determinants of vascular hypertrophy. This problem is particularly striking with respect to studies in which pressure is lowered pharmacologically. Several studies have shown convincingly that treatment of hypertension reverses medial hypertrophy in the aorta,[18] arteries in the mesentery,[19] kidney,[20] and cerebrum,[21] and arterioles in muscle.[22] Pharmacological treatment of hypertension, however, influences neurohumoral factors, which may alter the mechanics and structure of blood vessels independently of effects on intravascular pressure. Thus, findings based on treatment or reversal of hypertension do not allow unambiguous separation of the effects of intravascular pressure from neurohumoral effects on vascular structure and mechanics.

An approach that avoids the problems of antihypertensive treatment is to produce local reduction in arterial pressure by ligation of upstream vessels. The advantage of arterial ligation is that neurohumoral factors are the same for blood vessels downstream from the ligation as for vessels of similar size in unligated vascular beds. Using this approach in the hindlimb circulation, Folkow et al.[23] found that reduction of pressure in the hindlimb of SHR attenuated the increase in minimal resistance. This finding suggests that increases in arterial pressure *per se* contribute to development of vascular hypertrophy during chronic hypertension.

Recently, we used arterial ligation to examine the effects of local reduction of arterial pressure in cerebral arterioles.[24] One carotid artery was occluded in 1 mo old, normotensive Wistar Kyoto rats (WKY) and SHRSP. Pial arterioles were examined about 10 mo after placement of the clip. Carotid clipping completely prevented hypertrophy of pial arterioles in SHRSP. We were surprised by this finding because, although clipping reduced pial arteriolar pressure, mean pressure in pial arterioles of SHRSP remained about 30 mmHg higher than in WKY. Furthermore, there was not a significant correlation between cross-sectional area of the arteriolar wall and mean arteriolar pressure, systolic pressure, or circumferential wall tension, which suggests that these factors may not be primary determinants of cerebral vascular growth during normotension or hypertrophy during chronic hypertension. There was, on the other hand, a strong correlation between cross-sectional area and pulse pressure. Based on these findings, we concluded that pulse pressure may play a more important role than mean

Hypertrophy   Remodeling

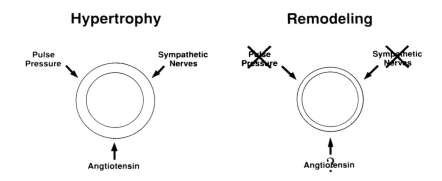

Fig. 2. Possible determinants of vascular hypertrophy and remodeling during chronic hypertension. There is ample evidence to suggest that neural and humoral factors are determinants of vascular hypertrophy. Recent evidence suggests that, of the various parameters of arterial pressure, pulse pressure, rather than mean or systolic pressure, may be an important determinant of hypertrophy. In contrast to hypertrophy, sympathetic nerves and pulse pressure apparently are not determinants of vascular remodeling in cerebral arterioles. On the other hand, there is preliminary evidence to suggest that angiotensin may contribute to cerebral vascular remodeling during chronic hypertension.

pressure, systolic pressure, or wall tension in development of cerebrovascular hypertrophy during chronic hypertension (Fig. 2).

The possibility that pulse pressure may be a determinant of vascular hypertrophy is supported by studies of large arteries and vascular cells in tissue culture. Coarctation of the thoracic aorta in the monkey[25] and dog[26] reduces pulse pressure, but not mean arterial pressure, distal to the coarctation. The reduction in pulse is associated with decreased motion of the aortic wall,[25] and a reduction in DNA and collagen content.[27] In vascular smooth muscle that is grown in culture, DNA synthesis and rate of growth are greater in cells that are subjected to cyclic stretching than in cells that are grown under static conditions.[28] These findings suggest that alterations in cyclic stretching of smooth muscle may influence cellular and extracellular components in the vessel wall and affect vascular growth.

The contribution of increased intravascular pressure to cerebral vascular remodeling during chronic hypertension is unclear. We have found that reduction in external diameter is not prevented in cerebral arterioles of SHRSP during antihypertensive treatment with either hydralazine[29] or carotid clipping,[24] even though cerebral arteriolar pulse pressure is normalized with both treatments. Cerebral arteriolar mean pressure, on the other hand, is not normalized in SHRSP with either treatment.[24,29] These findings indicate that pulse pressure is not a determinant of remodeling in cerebral arterioles of SHRSP (Fig. 2), but do not rule out a role for mean pressure.

Sympathetic Nerves

It is clear that during normotension sympathetic nerves have trophic effects on blood vessels. Chronic sympathetic denervation in rabbits produces a reduction in wall mass of the central ear artery[30] and middle and posterior cerebral arteries.[31] The decrease in wall mass of the ear artery is associated with a reduction in uptake of thymidine by vascular smooth muscle.[32] The latter finding suggests that trophic effects of sympathetic nerves are related, at least in part, to influences on proliferation of smooth muscle.

Sympathetic nerves have trophic effects on arterioles, as well as large cerebral arteries, during normotension. We recently demonstrated that chronic sympathetic denervation reduces cross-sectional area of the vessel wall in pial arterioles of normotensive WKY.[33] Our finding that the decrease in total cross-sectional area of the arteriolar wall results primarily from a reduction in smooth muscle provides support for the concept that trophic effects of sympathetic nerves on blood vessels are directed primarily towards smooth muscle.

Based on findings in normotensive animals, it would not be surprising if sympathetic nerves also contribute to the development of cerebral vascular hypertrophy during chronic hypertension. Hart et al.[34] found that wall-to-lumen ratio was less in denervated than in innervated cerebral arterioles in 1-yr-old SHRSP that had undergone unilateral sympathetic denervation at 3 wk of age. We recently examined cross-sectional area of the vessel wall in first-order pial arterioles of 10–12-mo-old SHRSP that had undergone unilateral sympathetic denervation at 1 mo of age.[33] Cross-sectional area of the arteriolar wall was 44% less in denervated than in innervated arterioles. Although all components in the arteriolar wall (smooth muscle, elastin, collagen, basement membrane, and endothelium) were reduced, the effect of denervation was greatest in smooth muscle. These findings support the concept that sympathetic nerves promote cerebral vascular hypertrophy during chronic hypertension (Fig. 2).

In contrast to their contribution to hypertrophy, it is unlikely that sympathetic nerves contribute to cerebral vascular remodeling during chronic hypertension. In a previous study,[33] we found that unilateral sympathectomy results in a further reduction, rather than an increase, in internal diameter of pial arterioles in SHRSP. This finding indicates that sympathetic nerves do not play a role in remodeling of cerebral arterioles in SHRSP (Fig. 2).

Angiotensin

There are several lines of evidence to suggest that angiotensin may contribute to vascular hypertrophy during chronic hypertension. For example, angiotensin has been shown to stimulate hyperplasia of vascular smooth muscle cells in culture.[35] Furthermore, an ACE inhibitor, captopril, reduces hypertrophy of cremaster arterioles without reducing pressure in one-kidney, one-clip, hypertensive rats.[36] These findings suggest that angiotensin may stimulate vascular hypertrophy independently of its pressor effect (Fig. 2). It should be noted, however, that this concept remains controversial, since there also is evidence that effects of ACE inhibitors on vascular structure may depend primarily on their effects on blood pressure.[37]

In addition to its trophic effects on vascular smooth muscle,[18,35,38] angiotensin may contribute to remodeling of cerebral arterioles. This possibility is supported by our recent finding that treatment with an inhibitor of the angiotensin converting enzyme, but not hydralazine, prevents remodeling of pial arterioles in SHRSP.[29] In contrast to sympathetic nerves and intravascular pulse pressure, therefore, angiotensin may be a determinant of cerebral vascular remodeling during chronic hypertension (Fig. 2).

Acknowledgments

Original studies described in this review were supported by funds from NIH Grants HL-22149 and NS-24621. Gary Baumbach is the recipient of an Established Investigatorship Award from the American Heart Association.

References

[1] Strandgaard, S., Olesen, J., Skinhoj, E., and Lassen, N. A. (1973) *Br. Med. J.* **1**, 507–510.

[2] Baumbach, G. L., Dobrin, P. B., Hart, M. N., and Heistad, D. D. (1988) *Circ. Res.* **62**, 56–64.

[3] Baumbach, G. L. and Heistad, D. D. (1989) *Hypertension* **13**, 968–972.

[4] Jones, J. V., Fitch, W., MacKenzie, E. T., Strandgaard, S., and Harper, A. M. (1976) *Circ. Res.* **39**, 555–557.

[5] Sadoshima, S., Busija, D. W., and Heistad, D. D. (1983) *Am. J. Physiol.* **244**, H406–H412.

[6] Fujishima, M., Sadoshima, S., Ogata, J., Yoshida, F., Shiokawa, O., Ibayashi, S., and Omae, T. (1984) *Gerontology* **30**, 30–36.

[7] Folkow, B. (1978) *Clin. Sci. Mol. Med.* **55**, 3s–22s.

[8] Folkow, B., Hallbäck, M., Lundgren, Y., Sivertsson, R., and Weiss, L. (1973) *Circ. Res.* **32**, I-2–I-16.

[9] Folkow, B., Grimby, G., and Thulesius, O. (1958) *Acta. Physiol. Scand.* **44**, 255–272.

[10] Baumbach, G. L. and Heistad, D. D. (1991) *J. Hypertens.* **9**, 987–991.

[11] Mulvany, M. J. (1991) *Clin. Exp. Pharmacol. Physiol.* **18**, 13–20.

[12] Brayden, J. E., Halpern, W., and Brann, L. R. (1983) *Hypertension* **5**, 17–25.

[13] Toda, N., Okunishi, H., and Miyazaki, M. (1982) *Jpn. Circ. J.* **46**, 1088–1094.

[14] Baumbach, G. L., Walmsley, J. G., and Hart, M. N. (1988) *Am. J. Pathol.* **133**, 464–471.

[15] Harper, S. L. and Bohlen, H. G. (1984) *Hypertension* **6**, 408–419.

[16] Cox, R. H. (1976) *Am. J. Physiol.* **231**, 420–425.

[17] Dobrin, P. B. and Rovick, A. A. (1969) *Am. J. Physiol.* **217**, 1644–1651.

[18] Owens, G. K. (1987) *Hypertension* **9**, 178–187.

[19] Nordborg, C. (1989) *Acta Physiol. Scand.* **135**, 47–56.

[20] Nordborg, C. (1987) *Clin. Exp. Hypertens. A* **A9(10)**, 1567–1584.

[21] Clozel, J.-P., Kuhn, H., and Hefti, F. (1989) *Hypertension* **14**, 645–651.

[22] Stacy, L. D. and Prewitt, R. L. (1989) *Circ. Res.* **65**, 869–879.

[23] Folkow, B., Gurevich, M., Hallbäck, M., Lundgren, Y., and Weiss, L. (1971) *Acta. Physiol. Scand.* **83**, 532–541.

[24] Baumbach, G. L., Siems, J. E., and Heistad, D. D. (1991) *Circ. Res.* **68**, 338–351.

[25] Lyon, R. T., Runyon-Hass, A., Davis, H. R., Glagov, S., and Zarins, C. K. (1987) *J. Vasc. Surg.* **5**, 59–67.

[26] Hollander, W., Kramsch, D. M., Farmelant, M., and Madoff, I. M. (1968) *J. Clin. Invest.* **47**, 1221–1229.

[27] Bomberger, R. A., Zarins, C. K., Taylor, K. E., and Glagov, S. (1980) *J. Surg. Res.* **28**, 402–409.

[28] Leung, D. Y. M., Glagov, S., and Mathews, M. B. (1976) *Science* **191**, 475–477.

[29] Hajdu, M. A., Heistad, D. D., and Baumbach, G. L. (1991) *Hypertension* **17**, 308–316.

[30] Bevan, R. D. and Tsuru, H. (1981) *Circ. Res.* **49**, 478–485.

[31] Bevan, R. D., Tsuru, H., and Bevan, J. A. (1983) *Stroke* **14**, 393–396.

[32] Bevan, R. D. (1975) *Circ. Res.* **37**, 14–19.

[33] Baumbach, G. L., Heistad, D. D., and Siems, J. E. (1989) *J. Physiol. (Lond.)* **416**, 123–140.

[34] Hart, M. N., Heistad, D. D., and Brody, M. J. (1980) *Hypertension* **2**, 419–423.

[35] Geisterfer, A. A. T., Peach, M. J., and Owens, G. K. (1988) *Circ. Res.* **62**, 749–756.

[36] Wang, D.-H. and Prewitt, R. L. (1990) *Hypertension* **15**, 68–77.

[37] Mulvany, M. J. (1991) *Blood Vessels* **28**, 224–230.

[38] Campbell-Boswell, M. A. and Robertson, A. L. (1981) *Exp. Mol. Pathol.* **35**, 265–276.

Chapter 34

Can Vascular Headaches Be Triggered by the Autonomic Nervous System?

Pierre Aubineau and Pierrette Mathiau

Introduction

The pathogenesis of vascular headaches, such as migraines and cluster headaches, remains obscure. The many theories proposed to explain headaches all focus on some particular elements in the cascade of events leading up to the attack.

The prevailing theories, based on the work of Graham and Wolff[1] are that migraine results from a disregulation of undefined origin of intra- and extracranial arteries, producing a painful vasodilation owing to stretching of the intramural C fibers (*see* ref. 2 for review). However, Olesen[3] recently discussed several observations showing that migrainous pain is not always associated with arterial vasodilation. Conversely, dramatic vasodilation experimentally induced in nonmigraineurs is not followed by head pain. Nitrogen derivatives, which were believed to induce headache in migraineurs via their vasodilator action, have recently been shown to primarily activate cerebrovascular sensory nerve fibers.[4] The abnormal vascular behavior associated with certain headaches could thus be an epiphenomenon of the attack, rather than the cause of the pain.

On the other hand, Olesen[3] pointed out that a patient can successively experience various forms of headache, only some of which are associated with abnormal blood flow and the supposed accom-

From *The Human Brain Circulation*, R. D. Bevan and J. A. Bevan, eds.
©1994 Humana Press

panying symptoms, such as aura. This indicates that the different types of headache may form a continuum and, consequently, that they may proceed from a common basal mechanism defined as "a primary vascular nociception." This hypothesis correlates well with the theory recently developed by Moskowitz,[5] who postulated that migraine headache results from sterile inflammation of the meninges and related blood vessels. Briefly, the unknown "primary vascular nociception" activates the trigemino-vascular C fibers whose axon collaterals contain substance P (SP) and calcitonin gene-related peptide (CGRP). This is followed by an axon reflex, which induces release of the neuropeptides, and the inflammatory process, which aggravates the initial pain.

These two complementary theories probably describe several of the mechanisms involved in migraine and other headaches. However, they both leave many questions unanswered. One is the trigger that provokes the "primary vascular nociception." A second is, why are other vascular territories that are also innervated by peptidergic sensory nerves not able to develop a similar disease? In other words, why does the migrainous pain occur only in the head? The sterile inflammation process and the axon reflex are found primarily in peripheral organs, such as the skin, in which they are not associated with migraine-like pain.

The answer to these two basic questions resides probably in some particularity of cephalic blood vessels, in some cellular or structural element that is not present in other vascular beds. Appenzeller[2] recently proposed that this element could be the endothelium. However, although endothelial cells may play a role in this disease, their specificity in the cephalic vascular bed appears to be too limited, spatially and functionally, to explain the particularities of headache pain.

Another possibility that has been repeatedly advanced is that of a specific cerebrovascular innervation, mainly of serotonergic nerve fibers originating in the raphe nucleus (*see* ref. 6 for review). Serotonin (5-HT) appears to play a key role in migraine headache, and 5-HT antagonists and agonists are, to various extents, valuable treatments of headaches.[7-9] Several authors have described abnormal 5-HT metabolism during migraine (*see* ref. 10 for review) and cluster headache.[11-13] As a part of the endogenous pain-control system, the raphe nuclei can play a role in migraine, as in other types of pain, but recent experimental data show the absence of 5-HT-containing or synthesizing nerves in pial blood vessels (vide infra). It is thus very improbable that raphe projections are the specific feature of these vessels that results in the specificity of migraine headache.

Cerebral and facial arteries are innervated by autonomic and sensory nerves and this innervation is usually described as very dense, but "classical." It is rarely pointed out that the classical sympathetic, adrenergic innervation is accompanied by an equally dense parasympathetic, cholinergic innervation that is less classical. In most peripheral vascular beds, cholinergic nerves, when present, share common pathways with adrenergic nerves. On the contrary, the pathways of the two innervations are spatially differentiated in the cephalic vascular bed. The second part of this manuscript summarizes data obtained in animals and humans that show that the duality of these two innervations in cephalic blood vessels can explain how headache is triggered in cases of sympathetic impairment.

Absence of Centrally Originating Innervation in Pial Blood Vessels

Histological and Biochemical Evidence for the Absence of Direct Projections from the Raphe Nuclei

Anterograde Tracing

Only two tracing experiments have been performed to date to verify the existence of a direct link between pial arteries and raphe neurons. Tsai et al.[14] reported that retrograde labeling of the cat middle cerebral artery results in intense labeling of certain dorsal raphe neurons. However, it cannot be excluded with this experimental procedure that the underlying superficial cortical layers, which receive a dense meshwork of dorsal raphe projections, are not reached by the tracer. We recently used anterograde tracing by

Phaseolus vulgaris leucoagglutinin (PHA-L), which allows very precise determination of neuron projections, even at long distances.[15] Eight to 31 d after iontophoretic infusion of PHA-L into the dorsal raphe nucleus, numerous labeled varicose nerve fibers were observed in the cerebral cortex and other brain structures, but no labeled nerve fibers were detected on whole-mounts of large and small cerebral arteries.

Antiserotonin Immunohistochemistry

The earliest studies using anti-5-HT antibodies showed that pial arteries, mainly the largest one, were endowed by a rich plexus of 5-HT-immunopositive nerve fibers.[16–18] However, recent identical experiments performed in animals rapidly fixed by intracardiac perfusion did not confirm this finding. The cerebral blood vessels appeared to be free of 5-HT containing nerve fibers, unless they had been previously incubated in a medium containing 5-HT.[19–21] Sympathectomy,[20] uptake experiments,[21] and electron microscopy[22] have all shown that 5-HT, in fact, accumulates in sympathetic nerve terminals by an active uptake from the extracellular medium. We recently confirmed[15] that 5-HT-immunopositive nerve fibers are not normally present in cerebral vessels, dura mater or femoral arteries of the rat.

Antitryptophan Hydroxylase Immunohistochemistry

Chedotal and Hamel[23] showed that the large and small cerebral arteries of rats and cats contain nerve fibers that are immunopositive to tryptophan-5-hydroxylase (TPH) antibody. TPH is the rate-limiting enzyme catalyzing the transformation of L-tryptophan into 5-hydroxytryptophan (5-HTP). 5-HTP is then decarboxylated into 5-HT by a ubiquitous decarboxylase. Therefore, if TPH is present in a nerve cell, 5-HT must be produced. Chedotal and Hamel concluded that the cerebral artery wall contains a true serotonergic innervation that very likely originates in the raphe.

We have used the same technique to investigate the presence of TPH-immunopositive (TPH-I) nerve fibers not only in cerebral arteries, but also in the femoral artery and the dura mater of the rat.[15] TPH-I nerve fibers were found in all three tissues, but the densest innervation was in the major pial vessels. The presence of TPH-I nerve fibers in the femoral artery strongly suggests that this innervation is of peripheral origin.

Biochemical Determination
of Tryptophan Hydroxylase Activity

The discrepancies between immunohistochemical staining for TPH and 5-HT in cerebral and peripheral blood vessels led us to examine the activity of this enzyme in vitro.[24] Previous neurochemical studies,[16,25] conducted in vivo showed that rat pial vessels may contain significant amounts of 5-HT. The concentration of 5-HT was also found to change by comparable amounts in the brain cortex and in the pial vasculature after lesioning or stimulating the raphe nuclei. When the rat was pretreated with a decarboxylase inhibitor (NSD 1015), pial vessels accumulated 5-HTP.[25] As for 5-HT, accumulation of 5-HTP was markedly decreased, mainly in small pial vessels, by lesioning the dorsal raphe nucleus.[25] These experiments strongly suggested that the TPH-I nerve fibers of pial vessels could synthesize 5-HT and that these fibers represent axonal processes from raphe neurons.

For the reasons developed above (absence of 5-HT-I nerve fibers, presence of similar TPH-I nerves in the femoral artery, and so forth), it appeared possible that some bias could have caused a contamination of the pial vessels by 5-HT or 5-HTP released from extra-vascular nerve terminals, probably those lying in the brain cortex.[20] We therefore measured the TPH activity of intact pial and peripheral blood vessels incubated in vitro with various concentrations of L-tryptophan (or [^{14}C] L-tryptophan) and NSD 1015. The 5-HTP production was measured in the tissue and in the incubation solution by HPLC and by scintillation counting of the [^{14}C] 5-HTP fraction. The 5-HTP production of the pineal gland and of cortex and raphe slices was also estimated under the same experimental conditions. Newly synthesized 5-HTP was found in all brain tissues and incubation solutions, but not in preparations corresponding to pial and peripheral blood vessels. 5-HT synthesized prior to the incubation in NSD 1015 was also present in all brain preparations but not in pial blood vessels. This lack of 5-HT and

5-HT synthesis was not caused by damage to the vascular innervation, since the tyrosine hydroxylase contained in sympathetic
nerve fibers synthesized large amounts of L-dopa from L-tyrosine
under the same experimental conditions.[24]

Thus, if TPH is really present in pial and peripheral blood
vessels, the enzyme is normally inactive. This further differenti-
ates TPH-I cerebrovascular nerves from raphe projections, for
example, those of the cerebral cortex.

Nerve Fibers of Pial Blood Vessels Contain Both 57 kDa (Peripherin) and 68 kDa (NF-L) Intermediate Filaments: Evidence for the Total Absence of Central Projections

Portier et al.[26] demonstrated that the intermediate filament
peripherin is present only in neurons whose axonal processes are
located outside the central nervous system (autonomic and sensory neurons, motoneurons, and so forth). Peripherin is *not* present
in neurons of central structures, such as the raphe nucleus or the
locus ceruleus.[27] On the contrary, the neurofilament NF-L is
present in *all* mature neuronal populations, both central or peripheral. Thus, peripheral neurons contain both filaments, whereas
raphe and locus ceruleus neurons contain only NF-L.

We have used double immunohistochemistry and laser scanning confocal microscopy to show that *all* nerve fibers of the rat
meningeal tissue are immunopositive for both peripherin and
NF-L antibodies.[28] Pial blood vessels and dura mater did not contain axonal processes labeled only by the NF-L antibody that could
belong to raphe or locus ceruleus neurons.

Innervation of Mast Cells of Cephalic Blood Vessels

Morphological Data

Mast cells having various phenotypes are present in most connective tissues, including the tunica adventitia of arteries. In many
species, including man and monkey, pial arteries contain numerous mast cells.[29] In all species, mast cells are also present within the
dura mater. We have shown[30] that the mast cells of rabbit pial

arteries frequently establish close appositions with three types of nerve terminals. One type of nerve terminal is adrenergic (sympathetic) and another is cholinergic (parasympathetic). The third type has the morphological appearance of peptidergic sensory nerve terminals. There are similar contacts between mast cells and autonomic and sensory nerve fibers within the rat dura mater[31–33] and in the human superfical temporal artery[34] (STA). In the latter, these nerve terminals can be morphologically classified as adrenergic, cholinergic, and peptidergic nerves on the basis of their vesicular content.

Action of Neurotransmitters

The cholinergic agonist carbachol induces a marked degranulation of rabbit cerebrovascular and rat dura mast cells.[35] Degranulation results in a massive release of 5-HT into the extracellular fluid. These effects are roughly equivalent to those produced by the mast cell secretagog, compound 48/80. Addition of atropine or verapamil to the incubation solution totally blocks carbachol-induced degranulation and 5-HT release. Preliminary experiments also showed that these actions of carbachol can also be inhibited by noradrenaline, which, alone, has no measurable effects on rabbit mast cells (unpublished observations). Separately, SP and CGRP induce only moderate, but statistically significant, mast cell exocytosis and 5-HT release in the rat dura and rabbit pial arteries (20–60% of the effects induced by 48/80 compound).[36] However, the simultaneous administration of SP and CGRP produces almost complete exocytosis of mast cells and a massive release of granular 5-HT (about 150% of that induced by 48/80 compound).[36]

Observations in Cluster Headache (CH) Sufferers

Morphological Changes in the Superficial Temporal Artery

Biopsies of a branch of STAs on the painful side, obtained from 19 episodic or chronic cluster headache (CH) volunteers (1–5 h after an attack), were compared under the electron microscope to control biopsies obtained from 10 patients undergoing cranial surgery, but free of any kind of headache.[34] In the control group, the mast cells of the STA had intact granules containing electron opaque scroll-shaped matrices and interspersed amorphous material. The mast cells from 17 of the 19 cases of the CH group showed profound alterations that clearly indicated various stages of degranulation, from moderate to total. In the two remaining CH patients, the mast cells were not different from the controls. These two patients had been successfully treated with beta-blockers or methysergide during a period immediately preceding the biopsy. Other CH patients had not been treated for at least 3 d.

Microdialysis in the Vicinity of the Superficial Temporal Artery

We have investigated the possible release of 5-HT and histamine in 11 episodic or chronic CH volunteers who were implanted for 24 h with a sc microdialysis probe. The probe was placed in the immediate vicinity of the STA of the painful side.[13] Four of these patients had one or more CH attacks during this period.

No histamine was detected in any sample from any patient. In the samples collected outside attacks, the concentration of 5-HT was 1.9 ± 0.5 fmol $\cdot$ μL^{-1} (mean $\pm$ SE). The 5-HT concentration was 7.2 ± 1.5 fmol $\cdot$ μL^{-1} during CH attacks, significantly higher than outside attacks. Continuous sampling showed that the 5-HT concentration rose progressively from the onset of the attack to the moment of greatest pain experienced by the patient, and decreased progressively thereafter.

Conclusions

The experimental data summarized above point to three main conclusions.

1. The genesis of migraine pain cannot be attributed to a special innervation of pain-sensitive meningeal blood vessels, i.e., to serotonergic and adrenergic nerve fibers arising directly from the brainstem.
2. Vascular mast cells (intra- and extracranial) are innervated by sympathetic, parasympathetic, and sensory nerve fibers. They are degranulated by acetylcholine, SP, and CGRP, whereas noradrenaline seems to inhibit the exocytosis. A profound degranulation of mast cells of the STA occurs during cluster headache attacks.

3. Cerebrovascular sympathetic nerve fibers may contain TPH and, consequently, may synthesize 5-HT. Large amounts of 5-HT are present in the vicinity of the STA during CH attacks.

We therefore propose that sympathetic dysfunction is at the origin of vascular headaches. Two mechanisms are possible but are not exclusive. The first takes into account the triple innervation of vascular mast cells, together with the distinct neural pathways of the sympathetic and parasympathetic innervations of cephalic blood vessels. A chronic disequilibrium of these innervations owing, for example, to partial sympathetic denervation (pathological or inherited), may favor the cholinergic input to mast cells. In this case, the relative excess acetylcholine may permanently lower the threshold of exocytosis of these cells, so that any supplemental degranulating influence of any kind (sex hormones, parasympathetic hyperactivity, mechanical stimulus, and so forth) may trigger exocytosis. The granular contents are released in the vicinity of sensory nerve terminals. Most of these mast cell products can stimulate and/or durably irritate these nerves and so trigger the "primary vascular nociception" referred to in the introduction. The axon reflex then intervenes, releasing SP and CGRP. SP promotes protein extravasation, and we have shown that both peptides (especially associated) can aggravate mast cell exocytosis. The initial relative excess of parasympathetic input can thus lead, by a positive feedback loop, to a dramatic release of proteolytic, nociceptive, and inflammatory substances from mast cells and sensory nerve terminals.

The second possibility also presupposes damage to the sympathetic nervous system. A TPH-like protein is probably present in sympathetic nerve fibers of cerebral and peripheral blood vessels.[15,37] We have shown that this TPH is inactive under normal physiological conditions. However, a certain plasticity of neurotransmitter synthesis by this innervation raises the possibility of TPH activation under abnormal circumstances. Principal sympathetic ganglionic neurons can synthesize 5-HT when immature[38] or injured.[39] Ex vivo, they also synthesize 5-HT when the culture medium is conditioned by heart cells.[40] Sympathetic TPH activity thus seems to depend on activation–inactivation mechanisms linked to phenotypic changes in principal ganglionic neurons. Such changes toward 5-HT synthesis could explain the presence of 5-HT-containing nerve fibers in temple skin biopsies taken from CH patients in a cluster period, whereas outside this period, the skin does not contain such fibers.[41] The 5-HT locally released during CH attacks[13] could, in this case, come from sympathetic nerve terminals.

There is evidence that 5-HT plays a key role in migraine,[10] as in CH.[11] There is also direct or indirect evidence for the involvement of the sympathetic nervous system in migraine and CH (*see* ref. 2). Sympathetic nerves are also involved in other pains, such as "phantom limb" and neuroma pains.[42] In the latter, it has been stressed that "the damaged [sympathetic] nerves 'sprout' but, trapped in the neuroma, this regenerative effort is abortive."[42] Regeneration generally implies a change in cell phenotype toward dedifferentiation and we have already mentioned (*vide supra*) that immature, injured, or cultured sympathetic neurons can synthesize 5-HT. Therefore, synthesis of 5-HT by lesioned or genetically abnormal sympathetic nerves could well explain their extraordinary role in pain generation.

We thus propose that a hypoactive and/or damaged cephalic sympathetic nervous system can generate cephalalgia. It does this by promoting the degranulating influence of the cholinergic nervous system on vascular mast cells and/or by synthesizing and releasing abnormal painful, vasoactive substances, such as 5-HT. Such mechanisms would also explain how central brain structures, such as the hypothalamus, the raphe nuclei, or the pineal gland are involved in migraine headache, since these structures lead to, or depend on, the balance of the autonomic nervous system.

References

1 Graham, J. R. and Wolff, H. G. (1938) *Arch. Neurol. Psych.* **39,** 731–763.
2 Appenzeller, O. (1991) *Med. Clin. North Am.* **75,** 763–789.
3 Olesen, J. (1991) *Pain* **46,** 125–132.
4 Wei, E. P., Moskowitz, M. A., Boccalini, P., and Kontos, H. A. (1992) *Circ. Res.* **70,** 1313–1319.
5 Moskowitz, M. A. (1990) *Neurology Clinics of North America, Vol. 8, Headache.* (Mathews, N., ed.), Saunders, Philadelphia, pp. 801–815.

6 Bonvento, G., MacKenzie, E. T., and Edvinsson, L. (1991) *Brain Res. Rev.* **16,** 257–263.
7 Solomon, G. D. (1991) *Medical Clinics of North America* **75,** 631–639.
8 Solomon, S. S., Lipton, R. B., and Newman, L. C. (1991) *Clin. Neuropharmacol.* **14,** 116–130.
9 Saxena, P. R. and Ferrari, M. D. (1989) *TIPS* **10,** 200–204.
10 Lance, J. W., Lambert, G. A., Goadsby, P. J., and Zagani, A. S. (1989) *Cephalalgia* **9(Suppl. 9),** 7–13.
11 Waldenlind, E., Ross, S. B., Ekbom, J. S., and Wetterberg, L. (1985) *Cephalalgia* **5,** 45–54.
12 Martelleti, P., Alteri, E., Pesce, A., Rinaldi-Garaci, C., and Giacovazza, M. (1987) *Headache* **27,** 23–26.
13 Aubineau, P., Cunin, G., Brochet, B., Louvet-Giendaj, C., and Henry, P. (1992) *Lancet* **339,** 1294–1295.
14 Tsai, S. H., Lin, S. Z., and Lin, C. J. (1985) *J. Neurosurg.* **16,** 463–467.
15 Mathiau, P., Riche, D., Behzadi, G., Dimitriadou, V., and Aubineau, P. (1993) *Neuroscience* **52,** 645–655.
16 Edvinsson, L., Degueurce, A., Duverger, D., MacKenzie, E. T., and Scatton, B. (1983) *Nature* **306,** 55–57.
17 Griffith, S. G., Lincoln, J., and Burnstock, G. (1982) *Brain Res.* **247,** 388–392.
18 Sano, Y., Takeuchi, H., Yamaha, H., Ueda, S., and Goto, M. (1982) *J. Histochem.* **76,** 277–280.
19 Yu, G. and Lee, T. J. F. (1989) *Blood Vessels* **26,** 33–42.
20 Chang, J. Y., Ekblad, E., Kannisto, P., and Owman, C. H. (1989) *Brain Res.* **492,** 79–88.
21 Chang, J. Y., Hardebo, J. E., and Owman, C. H. (1990) *J. Cereb. Blood Flow Metab.* **10,** 22–31.
22 Jackowski, A., Crockard, A., and Burnstock, G. (1988) *Brain Res.* **443,** 159–165.
23 Chédotal, A. and Hamel, E. (1990) *Neurosci. Lett.* **116,** 269–274.
24 Mathiau, P., Reynier-Rebuffel, A. M., Issertial, O., Callebert, J., Decreme, C., and Aubineau, P. (1993) *Neuroscience* **52,** 657–665.
25 Bonvento, G., Lacombe, P., MacKenzie, E. T., Fage, D., Benavides, J., Rouquier, L., and Scatton, B. (1991) *J. Neurochem.* **56,** 681–689.
26 Portier, M. M., de Nechaud, B., and Gros, F. (1984) *Dev. Neurosci.* **6,** 335–344.
27 Leonard, D. G. B., Gorham, J. D., Cole, P., Green, L. A., and Ziff, E. B. (1988) *J. Cell Biol.* **106,** 181–193.
28 Mathiau, P., Escurat, M., and Aubineau, P. (1993) *Neuroscience* **52,** 667–676.
29 Ibrahim, M. Z. M. (1974) *J. Neurol. Sci.* **21,** 431–478.
30 Dimitriadou, V., Aubineau, P., Taxi, J., and Seylaz, J. (1987) *Neuroscience* **22,** 621–630.

31 Ferrante, F., Ricci, A., Felici, L., Cavallotti, C., and Amenta, F. (1990) *Acta Histochem. Cytochem.* **23,** 637–645.
32 Keller, J. T., Marfurt, C. F., Dimlich, R. V. W., and Tierney, B. E. (1989) *J. Comp. Neurol.* **290,** 310–321.
33 Dimitriadou, V., Buzzi, M. G., Moskowitz, M. A., and Theoharides, T. C. (1991) *Neuroscience* **44,** 97–112.
34 Dimitriadou, V., Henry, P., Brochet, B., and Aubineau, P. (1990) *Cephalalgia* **10,** 221–228.
35 Reynier-Rebuffel, A. M., Callebert, J., Dimitriadou, V., Mathiau, P., Launay, J. M., Seylaz, J., and Aubineau, P. (1992) *Am. J. Physiol.* **262,** R605–R611.
36 Aubineau, P., Henry, F., Reynier-Rebuffel, A. M., Callebert, J., Issertial, O., and Seylaz, J. (1991) *Cephalalgia* **11(Suppl. 11),** 11.
37 Cohen, Z., Bonvento, G., Lacombe, P., Seylaz, J., MacKenzie, E. T., and Hamel, E. (1991) *Society of Neuroscience Abstracts* **17,** 1176.
38 Häppölä, O., Päivärinta, H., Soinila, S., and Steinbuch, H. (1986) *J. Auton. Nerv. Syst.* **15,** 21–31.
39 Häppölä, O. (1988) *Neuroscience* **27,** 301–307.
40 Matsumoto, S. G., Sah, D., Potter, D. D., and Furshpan, E. J. (1987) *J. Neurosci.* **7,** 380–390.
41 Joseph, R., Dhital, K., Adams, J., Burnstock, G., Appenzeller, O., and Clifford Rose, F. (1985) *Migraine Proc 5th Int Migraine Symp London 1984* (Clifford Rose, F., ed.), Basel, Karger, 1985, pp. 162–165.
42 Koltzenburg, M. and McMahon, S. B. (1991) *TIPS* **12,** 399–402.

Chapter 35

Importance
of Cerebrovascular Receptors
in Cluster Headache

Jan Erik Hardebo

Introduction

The intracranial internal carotid artery (ICA) is strongly implicated in the pathogenesis of cluster headache.[1,2] Angiography has demonstrated a dilated ICA with branches from the cavernous sinus level during active periods[3,4] and a narrowed lumen of the proximal (extracavernous) ICA toward the end of an attack.[3] Sympathetic fibers to the human ICA and its branches originate in the superior cervical ganglion and run as the internal carotid nerve along the ICA. Immediately after entering the skull cavity, fibers diverge to form a terminal plexus in the intracranial ICA wall.[5,6] Parasympathetic fibers reach the human intracranial ICA with rami orbitales from the sphenopalatine ganglion, and with the greater deep petrosal nerve from a ganglion along the greater superficial petrosal nerve, and possibly from the otic ganglion.[7,8] Sensory fibers reach the human intracranial ICA within the cavernous sinus through short branches from the ophthalmic trigeminal division,[7–9] with a contribution from the maxillary division at least in the monkey.[9] The question arises whether this innervation exerts a vasomotor action locally. Such action might explain the angiographic findings in cluster headache.

From *The Human Brain Circulation*, R. D. Bevan and J. A. Bevan, eds.
©1994 Humana Press

Transmitters known to be present in these nerves were therefore applied to isolated segments of the human intracranial ICA, and their possible effects on tone were registered. In addition, the reactivity to some other vasoactive agents, of relevance for the acute treatment of attacks of cluster headache (ergotamine, sumatriptan),[10] were tested.[11] It was found that all segments of the intracranial ICA constricted on exposure to a depolarizing potassium solution, noradrenaline, serotonin, sumatriptan, ergotamine, and prostaglandin $F_{2\alpha}$. The maximum contraction (E_{max}) and the concentration at which half maximum contraction occurred (EC_{50}) did not differ significantly between the different segments, and the values were therefore grouped together (Table 1). The vessels started to react to sumatriptan at a concentration of $3 \times 10^{-8}M$. All segments from 3 of the 4 human ICA dilated to a modest and similar extent on exposure to calcitonin gene-related peptide with a mean EC_{50} value for all segments of $8.5 \pm 2.4 \times 10^{-9}M$. Substance P, neurokinin A, acetylcholine, vasoactive intestinal polypeptide, and bradykinin were without effect on tone in all vessel segments.

These findings demonstrate that the whole intracranial segment of ICA in humans is equipped with contractile adrenergic receptors to the sympathetic nerve transmitter noradrenaline, and with dilatory receptors to the sensory nerve transmitter calcitonin gene-related peptide. Thus, this large artery may not simply be a conductance vessel but has the capacity to regulate blood flow downstream on nerve activation or administration of transmitter mimetics. It is known from other cerebral arteries that a continuous activity in the perivascular sympathetic nerves contributes to a constrictory tone at rest.[12]

The present findings offer a rational explanation for the angiographic findings in cluster headache: A sympathetic lesion in the ICA wall is present at the cavernous level during periods of attack, and constriction of the proximal ICA contributes to alleviate the attack. It is well known that administration of agents with vasoconstrictor properties, such as noradrenaline,[13] ergotamine, and sumatriptan,[10] terminate the cluster pain. Also, compression of the ipsilateral common carotid artery alleviates pain.[14] Con-

Table 1

Contractile Response to Noradrenaline, Serotonin, Sumatriptan
(Stimulator of Serotonin$_{1D}$-like Receptors), Ergotamine
(Stimulator of α-Adrenergic and Serotoninergic Receptors),[24]
and Prostaglandin F$_{2α}$ in the Human Intracranial Internal Carotid Artery

	E_{max}, %[a]	EC_{50}, M
Noradrenaline	77 ± 4[b]	2.8 ± 1.4 × 10^{-6}
Serotonin	74 ± 5	6.4 ± 1.2 × 10^{-8}
Sumatriptan	77 ± 5	2.5 ± 1.8 × 10^{-7}
Ergotamine	42 ± 3	6.9 ± 1.6 × 10^{-8}
Prostaglandin F$_{2α}$	84 ± 4	2.1 ± 1.7 × 10^{-6}

[a]E_{max} is expressed in % of contraction induced by a maximally depolarizing potassium solution.
[b]Mean ± SEM of 16 observations in 4 men.

versely, vasodilators such as nitroglycerin, histamine, and alcohol, well-known provocative agents in cluster headache, will initiate an attack.

An obliterating inflammatory process in the cavernous sinus, its outflow sinuses (superior and inferior petrosal sinuses), and to some extent in its inflow vein (superior ophthalmic vein) is found on the painful side in cluster headache sufferers during active periods.[4,15] This process may be responsible for the ipsilateral sympathetic lesion observed in the face as a miosis/ptosis and forehead anhidrosis or by pharmacological tests during active periods.[16–19] A lowered tone in the cavernous ICA and its branch the ophthalmic artery, in combination with a reduced outflow from the cavernous sinus owing to the obliterated sinuses, may cause a venous congestion in the inflamed cavernous sinus, and thus the pain. A further dilation of the ICA and ophthalmic artery will exaggerate the venous congestion and thus provoke an attack, whereas constriction of ICA—by stressful activation of intact sympathetic fibers proximal to the lesion, or by administration of contractile agents—will terminate the attack by alleviating the load on the venous side[2] (Fig. 1).

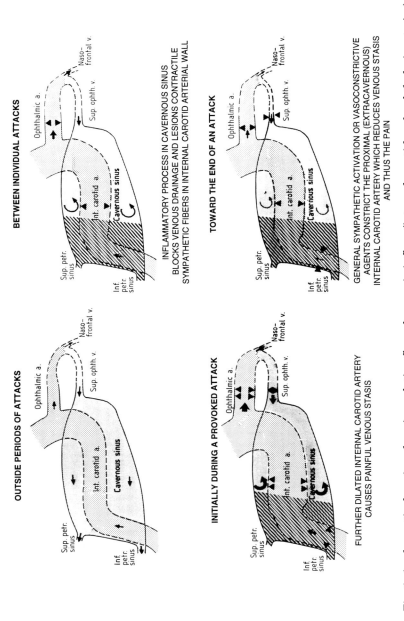

Fig. 1. A schematic drawing showing relative flow changes in inflow (internal carotid and ophthalmic arteries) and outflow vessels (nasofrontal and superior ophthalmic veins, cavernous sinus, and superior and inferior petrosal sinuses) on the painful side in cluster headache. Even when the lumen of the ipsilateral superior ophthalmic vein is narrowed by the inflammatory process, blood will congest in the cavernous sinus after inflow through the contralateral vein, when attacks are induced by vasodilators.

448

That a mere constriction of the ICA may explain why sc sumatriptan alleviates the attack is supported by its very rapid effect (within 15 min)[10,20] as soon as sufficiently high circulating concentrations are reached (after a mean of 10 min).[21] The peak plasma concentration is $1.75 \times 10^{-7}M$ (range $1.33–2.62 \times 10^{-7}M$).[16] The intracranial ICA has vasa vasorum[6] and is located outside the blood–brain barrier. It is therefore reasonable to assume that almost the same concentration can be reached around serotinin$_{1D}$-like receptors in this arterial segment after penetration of the wall of ICA and its vasa vasorum. As presently found, a sumatriptan concentration of this magnitude caused a substantial arterial contraction. Contraction may not be restricted to the ICA but can also involve the external carotid arterial tree and extracranial arteriovenous anastomosis and veins, which also constrict on exposure to sumatriptan and ergotamine.[22,23]

Possibilities exist for dilation of the intracranial ICA if the perivascular pain fibers become activated during cluster headache attacks to release their transmitter calcitonin gene-related peptide. As presently found, the intracranial ICA is equipped at its whole length with vasodilatory receptors for this neuropeptide. The perivascular sympathetic fibers may become further lesioned against bone in the carotid canal if the artery dilates initially during an attack.

References

1 Moskowitz, M. A. (1988) *Headache* **28**, 584–586.
2 Hardebo, J. E. and Moskowitz, M. (1992) *The Headaches* (Olesen, J., Tfelt-Hansen, P., and Welch, K. M. A., eds.), Raven, New York, pp. 569–576.
3 Ekbom, K. and Greitz, T. (1970) *Acta Radiol. Diagnos.* **10**, 177–183.
4 Hannerz, J. (1991) *Headache* **31**, 540–542.
5 Handa, Y., Hayashi, M., Nojyo, Y., Tamamaki, N., and Caner, H. H. (1990) *Exp. Brain Res.* **82**, 493–498.
6 Yasargil, M. G. (1984) *Microneurosurgery*, vol. I, Georg Thieme Verlag, Stuttgart, p. 57.
7 Hardebo, J. E., Arbab, M. A. R., Suzuki, N., and Svendgaard, N. A. (1991) *Stroke* **22**, 331–342.
8 Suzuki, N. and Hardebo, J. E. (1991) *J. Neurol. Sci.* **104**, 19–31.
9 Ruskell, G. L. and Simons, T. (1987) *J. Anat.* **155**, 23–37.
10 (1991) *N. Engl. J. Med.* **325**, 322–326.

[11] Hardebo, J. E. (1992) *Cephalalgia* **12**, 280–283.
[12] Hardebo, J. E. (1989) *Neurotransmission and Cerebrovascular Function*, vol. II (Seylaz, J. and Sercombe, R., eds.), Elsevier, Amsterdam, pp. 193–210.
[13] Ekbom, K. and Lindahl, J. (1970) *Acta Neurol. Scand.* **46**, 585–600.
[14] Ekbom, K. (1975) *Headache* **15**, 219–225.
[15] Hannerz, J., Ericson, K., and Bergstrand, G. (1987) *Cephalalgia* **7**, 207–211.
[16] Drummond, P. D. (1988) *Cephalalgia* **8**, 181–186.
[17] Fanciullacci, M., Pietrini, U., Gatto, G., Boccuni, M., and Sicuteri, F. (1982) *Cephalalgia* **2**, 135–144.
[18] Salvesen, R., Bogucki, A., Wysocka-Bakowska, M. M., Antonaci, F., Fredriksen, T. A., and Sjaastad, O. *Cephalalgia* **7**, 273–284.
[19] Vijayan, N. and Watson, C. (1982) *Headache* **22**, 200–202.
[20] Hardebo, J. E. (1993) *Headache* **33**, 18–21.
[21] Fowler, P. A., Lacey, L. F., Thomas, M., Keene, O. N., Tanner, R. J. N., and Baber, N. S. (1991) *Eur. Neurol.* **31**, 291–294.
[22] Jansen, I., Edvinsson, L., and Olesen, J. (1992) *Acta. Physiol. Scand.* **147**, 141–150.
[23] Den Boer, M. O., Somers, J. A. E., and Saxena, P. R. (1992) *Cephalalgia* **12**, 206–213.
[24] Müller-Schweinitzer, E. (1983) *Gen. Pharmacol.* **14**, 95–102.

Index

A

α-adrenoceptor, 62, 109, 216, 265, 274, 282, 440
α-macroglobulin, 227
α,β-methylene, ATP, 168
21-Aminosteroids, 361
A23187, 168
Acetylcholine, 47, 54, 74, 168
Acetylcholinesterase, 54
Acidosis, 300
Adenosine, 196–200, 300
Adenosine triphosphate, 79
Adrenergic nerve endings, 327
Aging, 33, 271
Alkaline phosphatase, 251
Allotment, 238
Alzheimer's disease, 16, 33, 118
Amplification, 393
Amyloidosis, 32
Anastomosis, 25, 237
Aneurysm, 399
Aneurysmal subarachnoid hemorrhage, 11
Angiotensin, 168, 224, 429
Annihilation coincidence detection, 3
Anti-inflammatory, 368

Arachidonic acid, 168
Artery,
  anterior cerebral, 237, 239, 240
  anterior communicating, 237, 239, 240
  basilar, 168, 240, 243
  human pial, 96, 98, 101, 180
  hypophyseal, 212
  meningeal, 49, 54
  middle cerebral, 54, 237, 239, 242, 374, 367
  pial, 24, 293, 302
  posterior communicating, 237, 239, 240, 243
  resistance, 238, 239, 243, 245, 333
  superficial temporal, 438–440
  vertebral, 237, 238, 240–244
Arterial oxygen content, 10
Arterio-venous malformation, 238, 405, 408
Arteriography, 241
Asphyxia, 259
Aspirin, 168
Atherosclerosis, 23
ATP, 74, 168, 169, 199–201
ATP-sensitive potassium channels (K_{ATP}), 153

451